D1274308

SURGERY, ANESTHESIA, AND EXPERIMENTAL TECHNIQUES IN SWINE

SURGERY, ANESTHESIA, AND EXPERIMENTAL TECHNIQUES IN SWINE

M. Michael Swindle, DVM

Illustrated By

Richard Hughes, LATg

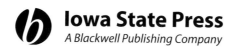

Iowa State Press
A Blackwell Publishing Company

M. MICHAEL SWINDLE received his DVM degree from Texas A&M University, College Station. He is presently Director, Division of Laboratory Animal Resources, and Professor and Chairman, Department of Comparative Medicine, Medical University of South Carolina, Charleston.

Iowa State Press
A Blackwell Publishing Company
2121 State Avenue, Ames, Iowa 50014

Orders: 1-800-862-6657
Office: 1-515-292-0140
Fax: 1-515-292-3348
Web site: www.iowastatepress.com

∞ Printed on acid-free paper in the United States of America

First edition, 1998

Library of Congress Cataloging-in-Publication Data

Swindle, M. Michael
    Surgery, anesthesia, and experimental techniques in swine / M. Michael
Swindle : illustrated by Richard Hughes.—1st ed.
        p.   cm.
    Includes bibliographical references (p.   ) and index.
    ISBN 0-8138-1829-X (alk. paper)
    1. Surgery, Experimental. 2. Swine—Surgery.   3. Swine as labora-
tory animals   4. Veterinary anesthesia.   I. Title.
    RD29.5.S94S944   1998
    617′.007′24—dc21   98-24474

The last digit is the print number: 9 8 7 6 5 4 3 2

To my wife, Paula, and my daughters, Katelyn and Ashley

CONTENTS

PREFACE

This book is meant to be a practical technical guide for the use of swine in biomedical research. The primary intended audience is investigators, veterinarians, and technicians who use swine as experimental animals. Some of the procedures in the book, such as the anesthetic protocols, include information for veterinarians who provide clinical care for pet pigs and for those in agricultural practice.

The surgical sections are written with the assumption that the reader has at least a rudimentary knowledge of surgery rather than as a primer for novices. The sections on anatomy, handling, and anesthesia are written in a more basic format, with the assumption that readers such as physicians and scientists have the ability to perform surgery on swine but do not have sufficient knowledge of the species-specific differences in anatomy and physiology. The descriptions also are intended to be detailed enough to provide an overview for veterinarians and technicians providing collaboration.

The expectation is that this book will provide primary knowledge on the development of porcine biomedical models that involve surgical procedures, especially in laboratories that are unfamiliar with the species. Of course, it is impossible to detail all potential models that can be developed in this species. Consequently, the descriptions of techniques are meant to provide basic principles of performing experiments with an organ or system of interest.

The book is organized by organ systems, and there are substantial differences in the length of the chapters. This is consistent with the primary use of porcine models in cardiovascular and digestive system studies. Many of the uses of swine described in this book are relatively new and reflect the developing interest in using swine to replace other species such as dogs and primates. Examples of this aspect of porcine model development are the musculoskeletal and central nervous system models.

In addition to gross anatomy, images from angiography, endoscopy, and magnetic resonance imaging are included. It is my feeling that these images will be useful to researchers in the rapidly expanding fields of intravascular intervention, endoscopy, and laparoscopy. In the future many of the surgical procedures described in this textbook will be performed using those techniques. However, I describe the surgical techniques as they are performed manually, because the technology for these emerging fields changes daily. More importantly, the manual surgical descriptions are more applicable to most research labs and provide the opportunity to describe the principles of surgery for the various organ systems more accurately.

My original intent was to write this textbook as the sole author, based upon my personal experiences with porcine models. In fact, the majority of the textbook is based upon those experiences and the questions that have been directed to me by investigators from other institutions for two decades. However, it became apparent that, for some aspects of this textbook, I would need the expertise of my colleagues in the Digestive Diseases Center at the Medical University of South Carolina and the Institute of Experimental Clinical Research at the University of Aarhus in Denmark. I am indebted to them for their collaboration. I am deeply grateful to Dr. J.C. Djurhuus for the opportunities and interactions that developed during my visiting professorship with the Institute in Denmark. Much of the previously unpublished information in this book was derived from that opportunity.

I hope that the approach used to complete this textbook will decrease the learning curve for laboratories inexperienced in working with swine. I also hope that it will provide new insights to experienced investigators. The overall goal of the book is to provide guidance for procedures that will lead to the appropriate and humane use of swine in biomedical research.

ACKNOWLEDGMENTS

I acknowledge the great assistance from my faculty and staff at the Medical University of South Carolina. Specifically, I wish to thank Alison C. Smith, DVM, and Kathy Laber-Laird, DVM, MS, for their editorial and scientific input. Beth Greene was extremely helpful with the formatting of the illustrations and, of course, Richard Hughes who provided the original illustrations. I also thank Debra Allston for typing the manuscript and Mary Strobel for her help with the references. Terry Fisher, manager of the swine program at Charles River Laboratories, was also helpful as a reviewer of the husbandry and management sections.

CONTRIBUTING AUTHORS

ROBERT H. HAWES, MD
Professor of Medicine
Chief of Endoscopy
Digestive Disease Center
421 North Tower
Medical University of South Carolina
171 Ashley Avenue
Charleston, S.C. 29425-5121

RICHARD HUGHES, LATG
Department of Comparative Medicine
Medical University of South Carolina
770 MUSC Complex
Suite 135, Room 648
Charleston, S.C. 29425-5121

WHITFIELD KNAPPLE, MD
Instructor of Medicine
Digestive Disease Center
421 North Tower
Medical University of South Carolina
171 Ashley Avenue
Charleston, S.C. 29425-5121

M. MICHAEL SWINDLE, DVM
Diplomate, American College of
    Laboratory Animal Medicine
Professor and Chairman, Department of
    Comparative Medicine
Professor, Department of Surgery
Medical University of South Carolina
770 MUSC Complex

Suite 135, Room 648
Charleston, S.C. 29425-5121

JENS C. DJURHUUS, MD, DMSc
Professor
The Institute of Experimental Clinical
    Research
Aarhus University
Aarhus, Denmark

STEEN B. KRISTIANSEN, MS
The Institute of Experimental Clinical
    Research
Aarhus University
Aarhus, Denmark

ERIK LUNDORF, MD
The MR Center
Aarhus University Hospital
Section SKS
Aarhus, Denmark

MICHAEL RAHBEK SCHMIDT, MS
The Institute of Experimental Clinical
    Research
Aarhus University
Aarhus, Denmark

ELISABETH V. STENBØG, MD
The Institute of Experimental Clinical
    Research
Aarhus University
Aarhus, Denmark

SURGERY, ANESTHESIA, AND EXPERIMENTAL TECHNIQUES IN SWINE

1 BIOLOGY, HUSBANDRY, HANDLING, AND ANATOMY

Introduction

Swine are being used extensively in biomedical research with a significant increase occurring in recent years. They are replacing other mammalian species such as the dog as animal models, as well as being developed as a model on their own merit. This increased use of swine in the laboratory would not be occurring if technical procedures for handling, husbandry, and anesthetizing the species were not being refined during the same time period.

Major symposia on the use of swine in biomedical research have been organized in the last decade and have resulted in proceedings books, which provide a vast amount of baseline information on the species (Swindle, 1992; Tumbleson, 1986; Tumbleson and Schook, 1996). Much of the information in these books is based upon the description of a particular laboratory's model and may not provide enough detailed information overall for persons not familiar with the species.

Other reference books on swine provide information on specific experimental fields (Stanton and Mersmann, 1986; Swindle, 1983) in addition to the general references on anatomy and biology referenced in this chapter.

The purpose of this textbook and this chapter is to provide concise technical data on the use of swine in the laboratory, with an emphasis on surgically produced models. This chapter includes an overview of the breeds of swine that appear most commonly in the recent literature not of all the breeds of swine that are available.

Breed Selection

All domestic and miniature swine are *Sus scrofa domestica,* as are many of the feral strains of swine found throughout the world. However, they differ substantially from each other in appearance, behavior, and size. Within this textbook, all commercially available breeds of swine raised mainly for meat production are referred to as domestic farm breeds, unless the breed is of particular importance to the model being described. When the breed is mentioned, the most common breeds of domestic swine found in the literature are Yorkshire, Landrace, Duroc, and crossbred animals. Breeds of miniature swine are both naturally occurring and commercially bred for research or for pets. Miniature swine are referred to by their particular breed if it is mentioned in the references. The most commonly used breeds of miniature swine that are commercially available and that appear in the recent biomedical literature are the Yucatan miniature (Fig. 1.1) and the micro varieties: the Hanford (Fig. 1.2); the Göttingen (Fig. 1.3); the NIH; and the Sinclair S-1 (Hormel) (Fig. 1.4) . Other breeds of miniature pigs are available in limited markets and are not currently widely cited in the literature. These include the Ohmini, Pitman-Moore, Chinese Dwarf, Vietnamese Potbellied (Fig. 1.5), and the recently developed Panepinto (Fig. 1.6), to name a few. Some of these breeds were the foundation stock for miniature breeds currently in use such as the Hanford, Sinclair, and Göttingen. Panepinto (1986) has written a summary of the derivation of the various breeds of miniature swine. Of the breeds currently important to biomedical research, as listed above, only the Yucatan is a naturally occurring miniature breed.

The main difference between commercial breeds and miniature breeds is size at sexual maturity. Miniature breeds were purposely developed to provide a slower-growing porcine model that would be manageable at sexual maturity. Domestic swine exceed 100 kg body weight at sexual maturity and will continue to grow at an accelerated rate that is breed and diet related. It is not unusual to have a domestic pig at 12 months of age exceed 200 kg. In contrast, most breeds of miniature pigs weigh 12–45 kg at sexual maturity (Fisher, 1993; Swindle et al., 1994).

It is neither cost effective nor user friendly to attempt to use domestic breeds for chronic models merely to save money on the purchase price. The increased cost of feed, husbandry considerations, and personnel safety issues quickly negate any perceived savings. Also, the rate of growth of domestic swine on long-term projects scientifically skews the results unless growth is part of the hypothesis. Rather, the breed of animal should be selected on the basis of biological characteristics necessary to conduct the experimental study.

All investigators should describe accurately the swine used in their particular research in the materials and methods section of manuscripts. Essential information for meaningful comparison to other studies includes the anesthetic methods, breed, weight, age, and gender. Information that may be important in particular research protocols or for some journals includes the source of the

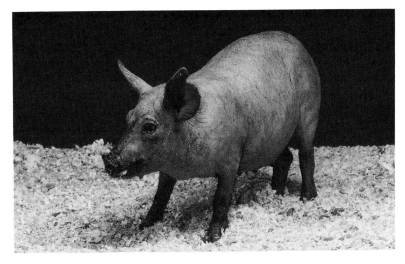

FIGURE 1.1   Yucatan miniature pig. *Courtesy of Charles River Laboratories, Inc.*

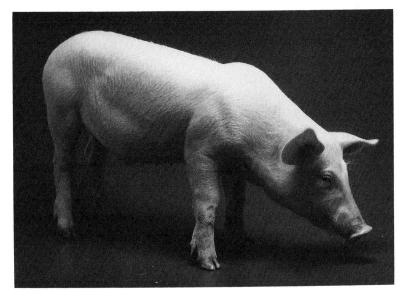

FIGURE 1.2   Hanford miniature pig. *Courtesy of Charles River Laboratories, Inc.*

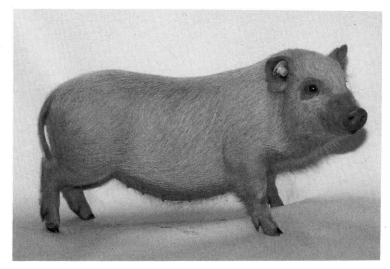

FIGURE 1.3   Göttingen miniature pig. *Courtesy of Ellegaard Göttingen Minipigs.*

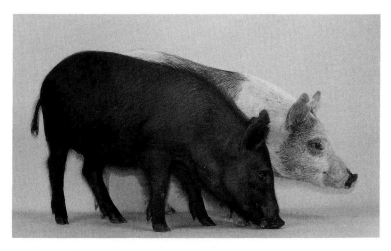

FIGURE 1.4   Sinclair S-1 (Hormel) miniature pigs. *Courtesy of Sinclair Research Center, Inc.*

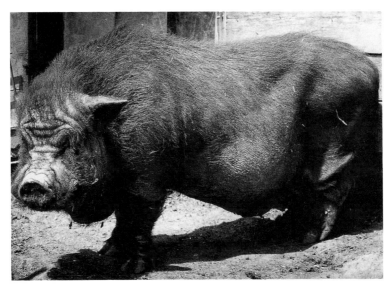

FIGURE 1.5   Vietnamese potbellied miniature pig. *Courtesy of Linda Panepinto and Associates.*

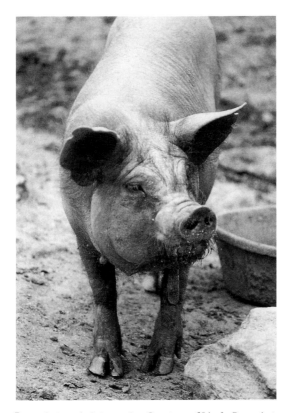

FIGURE 1.6   Panepinto miniature pig. *Courtesy of Linda Panepinto and Associates.*

animal, its health status, and a description of the housing environment, diet, and pertinent genetic information. A recent attempt has been made to standardize the description of animal studies in cardiopulmonary resuscitation research because of the problems associated with making meaningful comparisons of results between laboratories (Idris et al., 1996). This document may be helpful as a blueprint for other areas of research that require comparisons between laboratories.

Biology

In the appendix, Tables A1, A2, A15, A20, A23, and A24 provide biological values for growth, development, and body weights of miniature swine used in research. If a particular breed of pig is not listed in the tables, then the comparison to the normals should be based on age. Within this chapter, only the general biological characteristics of swine that should be of practical importance to biomedical researchers and laboratory animal personnel is discussed. A complete reference book on the biology of domestic swine has been published (Pond and Houpt, 1978), and information on the biology and diseases of domestic swine with an emphasis on data important to commercial production of food animals is also available (Leman et al., 1992). Recent reference books have been written on the Vietnamese potbellied pig for pet owners and veterinary practitioners (Boldrick, 1993; Reeves, 1993). However, a concise reference book on the breeds of miniature swine important to biomedical research is not available, and this textbook emphasizes that aspect of the biology and husbandry. Additional information is found in the system chapters and the appendices of this book.

Taxonomy and Nomenclature

Swine are ungulate (hoofed) mammals. The taxonomic classification of the species used in research is Phylum Chordata, Class Mammalia, Order Artiodactyla, Family Suidae, Genus *Sus*, Species *scrofa*, Subspecies *domestica*. Agricultural terminology is typically used in the literature and may cause some confusion to investigators not familiar with the terms. Some common definitions are listed below:

Swine	Refers to the whole species or multiple animals
Pig	Newborn animal. Sometimes this term is used interchangeably with swine or to denote a single animal.
Shoat	Weaned animal
Gilt	Immature female
Sow	Sexually mature female
Barrow	Castrated male
Boar	Sexually mature male
Porcine	Adjective used to describe anything pertaining to swine

Reproduction

The sow has a bicornuate uterus and is polytocous. The gestation period is typically 114 days (range, 110–116 days) for the larger breeds, with the miniature breeds usually having a shorter gestation by a few days. Swine are weaned around 4–6 weeks of age (range, 3–8 weeks) and may start to eat solid food (creep feed) as early as 2–3 weeks of age.

The average estrous cycle is 21 days (range, 18–24 days), with estrus being typically 2 days (range, 1–5 days). In commercial operations, sows are usually mated twice when they are showing vulvar swelling and willingly accept the boar. Ovulation occurs 30–36 hours after the onset of estrus.

Sexual maturity ranges from 3–7 months with most miniature breeds being sexually mature at 4–6 months of age. Sows will rebreed as soon as 3–9 days after parturition and may have approximately two litters per year for 5–6 years (Frandsson, 1981). The litter size varies greatly between breeds and may range from 4 to 20, however, attrition of the newborn may substantially reduce the number of animals weaned. In general, litter size is reduced with miniature swine.

In the appendix, Tables A2, A7–A14, A16, and A17 provide reproductive values for miniature swine.

Growth and Development

Birth weights of pigs depend upon the breed, the nutritional status of the sow, and the size of the litter, and range from 0.5 kg in the smaller miniature pigs to 1–2 kg in domestic swine (Fisher, 1993; Swindle et al., 1994).

Newborn pigs require an external heat source such as a heat lamp to provide an ambient temperature that is close to normal body temperature to prevent cold stress. They do not have brown fat, nor do they mobilize glycogen and lipid stores for thermal control. This ability to regulate temperature gradually improves with physiological maturity over the first few days of life (Consortium for Developing a Guide for the Care and Use of Agricultural Animals, 1988).

Pigs are mobile shortly after birth. They nurse almost hourly in the first few days of life. In large litters, they may have to compete with littermates for adequate nutrition, depending upon the number of nipples on the sow.

The growth rate of domestic swine is significantly different from that of miniature breeds. Domestic swine are bred and managed to grow to 100–110 kg of body weight within 150–200 days of age. Their daily weight gain can be between 0.2 and 1.0 kg depending upon husbandry and nutritional circumstances within a particular age group. The weight range of 12–45 kg for miniature breeds at the same age provides a vivid contrast of the differences in growth rate (Fisher, 1993; Swindle et al., 1994).

The epiphyses of the long bones are not completely closed in domestic swine until approximately 3.5 years. Miniature swine vary depending upon the stature of the animal. For example, Yucatan microswine have epiphyseal closure at 1.5–2.0 years, whereas standard Yucatans have closure at 3.0–3.5 years.

Even though the commercial life span of domestic swine is less than 6 months for meat production and less than 5 years for breeding stock, their general life spans may be 15–25 years depending upon the breed and environmental circumstances.

Nutrition

Swine are true omnivores and will consume a wide variety of diets and test substances. Specific test diets, such as those for inducing atherosclerosis, are discussed with the model descriptions within this book when appropriate.

Commercial pig food is designed to enhance the growth rate of domestic swine and may contain food additives such as antibiotics or growth stimulants. The feeding of the various rations to swine within particular weight groups is a science based upon optimum muscle growth. Ad libitum feeding of swine for long-term projects may produce obesity without any particular gain in nutritional value. Because this rapid weight gain is undesirable in miniature swine, commercial feed manufacturers have developed diets specifically for these breeds. The diets are designed to limit weight gain without causing nutritional deficiencies, which may occur if regular commercial diets are restricted only on a weight or volume feeding basis. Experience has shown that the feeding of miniature swine diets to domestic swine does not cause nutritional disorders, however, chronically housed animals should have their body weight and general condition monitored (Fisher, 1993; Swindle et al., 1994).

Generally, the miniature pig diets are lower in protein and higher in fiber than commercial diets. Usually, the diets are made in three formulations: starter diet, grower diet, and breeder and lactation diet. Starter feeds (creep feed) are usually fed free choice within the first few weeks of life. The other diets are then usually fed at a rate of 2%–3% of the body weight per day of rations containing 3–3.2 kcal/g of metabolizable energy. For most feeds this calculates to approximately 0.2–2.5 kg of feed per day depending upon the weight of the pig. The manufacturer's recommendations should be followed. Swine can be fed either the entire day's ration in a single feeding or the calculated ration can be split into two feedings a day (National Research Council, 1988).

Presurgical fasting of 8–12 hours will empty the stomach and small intestine; the colon usually requires 48–72 hours. If a prolonged fast is required for some procedures, nutrition may be maintained by providing oral, flavored electrolyte and glucose solutions that are commercially available from grocery stores (i.e., Gatorade). These liquids do not interfere with endoscopic or laparoscopic procedures because they do not leave residue. Bedding and chewable objects should be removed from the cage of an animal being fasted for surgery (Swindle, 1983; Swindle et al., 1994).

In the appendix, Table A3 provides guidelines for feeding and nutrition of miniature swine.

Hematology

Hematologic and plasma biochemical values for swine vary to some degree with environmental conditions, health status, breed, age, and gender. However, normal values are generally comparable and tables of values from various breeds of swine are included in the appendix.

Several general statements may be made concerning these values in swine. The hematocrit is physiologically low in neonatal swine, which requires the administration of iron dextran injections (100 mg im) during the nursing period. Swine generally have a higher percentage of neutrophils than lymphocytes, but this can be variable (Pond and Houpt, 1978). The blood volume of adult swine is 61–68 ml/kg. The 2N chromosome number is 38.

In the appendix, Tables A4–A14, A18, A19, A21, and A22 provide hematology and serum chemistry values for miniature swine.

Behavior

Swine are social animals and prefer to be in contact with other members of their own species. To avoid stress and potential disease transmission in the laboratory setting, they should not be mixed with other species. They can be housed in socialized groups, however, dominance fighting will occur when new animals are mixed into the group. Single housed animals should be able to see animals in other pens; this can be accommodated by using vertically slatted cage sides to allow them to see and touch each other. Dominant animals will bite the tails and ears of submissive animals, especially at feeding time. This can be minimized by housing problem animals separately and by providing longer or separate feeding troughs (Consortium for Developing a Guide for the Care and Use of Agricultural Animals, 1988; Fisher, 1993; Panepinto, 1986; Swindle et al., 1994).

Swine cannot bend to groom themselves and will scratch against the side of the cage. They tend to be cannibalistic if a sick or injured animal is housed with them. For this reason, it is best for animals that have had surgery to be housed singly.

Swine develop a dunging pattern and will defecate at the opposite end of the cage from where they are fed. The cage should, therefore, be designed to have their food and water separate from the area where they are supposed to defecate.

Swine primarily are sedentary animals and will seldom exercise on their own. Generally, they will only move when aroused by activity such as feeding or the introduction of personnel or new swine. They tend to move around the perimeter of their area of confinement rather than in the center.

Swine have a rooting behavior and like to use their snouts to dig through bedding or pastures. In artificial environments, such as those that are likely to be found in research institutions, it is best to provide them with toys. Large Teflon balls can be used to provide an object that can be rooted and thrown, and they are easily sanitized. Swine also like to pull on objects such as chains hung from the ceiling or roof of the cage. However, these objects for psychological well-being must be carefully selected to minimize damage to the cage or animal (Panepinto, 1986; Swindle et al., 1994).

Husbandry

In the United States, two sets of regulatory guidelines exist for laboratory swine: one for biomedical research (Public Health Service, 1996) and one for agricultural research (Consortium for Developing a Guide for the Care and Use of Agricultural Animals, 1988). These guidelines are contradictory for specified cage size. The cage sizes recommended are listed in Tables 1.1 and 1.2.

No consensus exists on the best type of caging to use for swine in the laboratory setting. Most research facilities are not dedicated to swine housing and require flexibility in housing other types of large animals in the same facility. Some general standards related to research housing are discussed later in this chapter.

Swine require flooring that provides for secure footing and a surface for wearing down their hooves. The flooring also needs to be easily sanitized. Swine can become stressed with slippery flooring and develop such symptoms

Table 1.1. National Institutes of Health Guide, 1996: Recommended space for commonly used farm animals

Swine/enclosure	Weight (kg)	Floor area animal (ft²)
1	< 15	8
	Up to 25	12
	Up to 50	15
	Up to 100	24
	Up to 200	48
	> 200	> 60
2–5	< 25	6
	Up to 50	10
	Up to 100	20
	Up to 200	40
	> 200	> 52
>5	< 25	6
	Up to 50	9
	Up to 100	18
	Up to 200	36
	> 200	> 48

SOURCE: Adapted with permission from the Guide for Care and Use of Laboratory Animals. Copyright (1996) by the National Academy of Sciences. Courtesy of the National Academy Press, Washington, DC.

Table 1.2. Agricultural Guide, 1988: Minimum floor area recommendations for swine used in agricultural research and teaching

	Individual (per pig)		Groups (per pig)	
Stage of production	m²	ft²	m²	ft²
Litter and lactating sow, pen	3.15	35	...	...
Litter and lactating sow, sow portion of crate	1.26	14	...	...
Nursery, 5–27 kg (12–60 lb) body weight	0.54	6	0.16–0.37	1.7–4.0
Growing, 27–57 kg (60–125 lb) body weight	0.90	10	0.37–0.56	4.0–6.0
Finishing, 57–104 kg (125–230 lb) body weight	1.26	14	1.49	16.0

SOURCE: Adapted with permission from the Guide for the Care and Use of Agricultural Animals in Agricultural Research and Teaching. Copyright (1988) by the Consortium for Developing a Guide for the Care and Use of Agricultural Animals in Agricultural Research and Teaching. Champaign, IL.

as stress ulcers. Several types of flooring have been used with different degrees of success. Concrete or seamless epoxy floors should have grit added to provide for secure footing. These types of floors are best utilized with deep bedding of wood shavings or straw. These floors, plus the bedding, provide an outlet for the rooting behavior of the species. Plastic-coated metal grid floors provide good sanitation, especially if they are raised above the floor level. However, swine will pull the plastic off the metal with the first sign of a tear. In the authors experience, diamond-shaped grids of approximately five-eighths inch openings provide the best all-around characteristics for housing swine of multiple sizes (Fig. 1.7). Newer fiberglass slatted-rail types of flooring can be used in the same manner as the expanded metal floors (Fig. 1.8). They provide good sanitization and are not easily damaged. They are also lighter and can be removed easily for sanitization. The spacing between the grids should be approximately one-half inch, to keep the animals from catching their hooves in the floor. These grids can also be manufactured to provide a gritty surface to provide for hoof wear. Rails and grids can be manufactured from aluminum and wood, however, care must be taken to make sure that the floors will support the weight of large animals and that they can be easily sanitized. Wood is, actually, inappropriate except for some agricultural settings. If the flooring does not maintain wear on the hooves of chronically housed animals, then they will have to be trimmed with hoof nippers approximately every 3-6 months.

Swine do not climb, but they may stand on their rear legs and lean against the cage to see other animals in some circumstances. They also use the sides of the cage to scratch themselves. If they cannot see other animals, they will use their snouts to try to open the cage. Also, if there is any loose-fitting area of the cage, swine will manipulate it with their snouts; consequently, the cage should

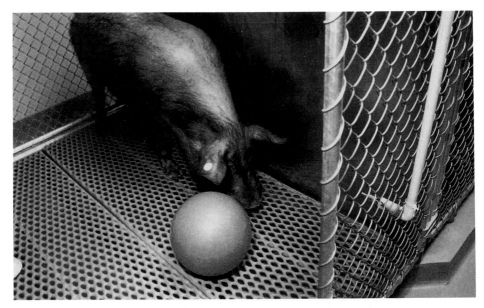

FIGURE 1.7   Yucatan miniature pig housed in a chain-link pen with a plastic-coated expandable metal floor.

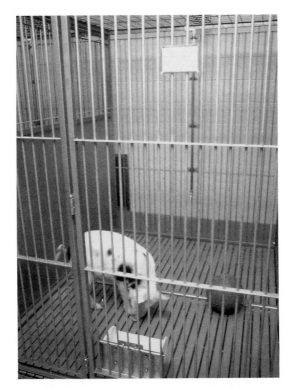

FIGURE 1.8   Hanford miniature pig housed in a stainless steel pen with fiberglass slatted floors.

be sturdy and free of any surface that can be manipulated or torn by the animals. Chain-link fencing can be used for small swine, but care should be taken to ensure that the sides of the cage meet the flooring securely to prevent animals from catching their hooves. If aluminum or stainless steel sides are used, the edges should be rounded and the bars sturdy. Vertical bars are preferred for swine and ruminants, however, these will not be as satisfactory for dogs. Cages can be manufactured to provide solid side panels that can be used to replace slotted panels when required.

Food bowls should be secured to either the side of the cage or to the floor. Easily sanitized stainless steel or Teflon feeders are preferable to the rubber feeders frequently used in agricultural settings. When the feeders are attached to the sides of the cage, guillotine-type closures should be avoided. In its anxiety to eat, the pig may slam it shut and injure the caretaker when food is being delivered.

Swine readily utilize automated watering systems, which are preferred to the use of water bowls because they provide a constant source of water without contamination and cannot be spilled like bowls. If bowls are utilized, they should be secured to the side of the cage. Water deprivation can result in dehydration and a syndrome known as "salt poisoning." This results in an encephalitic clinical presentation in affected animals and may be fatal (Leman et al., 1992). For this reason, water is not withheld presurgically in swine except in cases in which it is absolutely essential for gastric procedures. Placement of the food and water sources should be selected with the dunging pattern of the swine using the cage in mind.

Cages without bedding are best washed with a hose once or twice daily to eliminate odor. The animals should be removed from the cage during the hosing procedure to avoid being wetted and chilled. However, they readily accept baths and can be periodically washed with mild soap and warm water. They also develop dry skin in some housing conditions and can be rubbed with moisturizing oils or ointments to prevent scaling and flaking of the skin. If deep bedding is used, the cage can be spot cleaned daily because of the dunging pattern and the bedding changed once or twice weekly. Swine tend to keep cleaner in bedding than in cages that are hosed. Drains should be large and easily flushed. If bedding is used, then the drains should be covered with solid caps to avoid blockage. The main disadvantage of using bedding in surgical protocols is that swine will eat it when fasted (Fisher, 1993; Panepinto, 1986; Swindle et al., 1994).

If modular units are utilized, they may be taken apart and cleaned in a cage washer to sanitize the cage between uses by different animals or every 1–2 weeks with chronically housed animals. Pressure washers may be used to clean caging units in place.

The recommended temperature range for housing laboratory swine is 16°–27°C (61°–81°F) in the Public Health Service (1996) guide. The Consortium for Developing a Guide for the Care and Use of Agricultural Animals (1988) provides preferred ranges of temperatures depending upon the age of the animal. Generally, their standards recommend 26°–32°C (79°–90°F) for animals less than 15 kg, 18°–26°C (64°–79°F) for swine 15–35 kg, and 10°–25°C (50°–77°F) for larger swine. Increased environmental temperatures are appropriate for postsurgical care and other stressful situations and may be provided by suspended heat lamps. Normal swine are capable of surviving temperatures outside this range, especially at the lower end of the scale; however, environmental control is an essential part of the research environment and should be provided.

Standard laboratory animal practice is to provide 10–15 air changes per hour with 100% fresh outside air. Relative humidity ranges of 30%–70% are also standard. This type of ventilation greatly aids reducing odor and minimizing ammonia levels, which can contribute to respiratory disease. Location of the air ducts will depend upon the design of the facility, however, care should be taken to ensure that the temperature is controlled at the floor level to prevent the pigs from becoming chilled (Public Health Service, 1996).

The photoperiod for swine is not as critical as for other species and they may be provided with up to 16 hours of light in the laboratory setting (Consortium for Developing a Guide for the Care and Use of Agricultural Animals, 1988).

Disease Prevention

Vaccination of swine depends upon the source of the animals, the length of time they are housed, and the protocol. Most of the vaccinations are given to neonatal and weanling animals, except those in breeding programs. The attending veterinarian should use professional judgment to establish the vaccination protocol. Vaccination injections are conventionally given in the neck (Leman et al., 1992). The agents against which prophylaxis may be provided includes *Erysipelothrix, Pasteurella, Bordetella, Escherichia, Clostridium,* Parvovirus, and Rotavirus.

Swine require the trimming of needle teeth during the first day of life to prevent damage to the nipples of the sow and to their siblings. Newborn animals also should have the umbilicus cleaned with iodine solution. An iron dextran injection is given to 3-day-old animals to protect against the physiologic anemia that occurs in animals not housed on soil. Swine are susceptible to vitamin E/selenium deficiencies, and care must be taken to ensure that an adequate level is provided in the feed (Fisher, 1993).

In agricultural settings, castration and hernia repair are performed on neonates. However, it is not usually routine for miniature swine from commercial producers. If these surgeries are performed in an agricultural setting, it is not unusual to see incisional infections. Observation of animals upon receipt from the supplier should include an inspection for problems related to these surgeries.

All animals should be examined for health problems by the attending veterinarian upon receipt. It is good practice to isolate and quarantine animals upon arrival away from animals already on the premises. It is also good practice to house animals from different suppliers in separate rooms. Animals purchased from auctions are probably from mixed sources and should be considered to have an increased health risk, similar to that when receiving dogs from municipal pounds. When purchasing animals, it is best to limit suppliers to those who have been determined to have high standards of husbandry and disease control. Specific pathogen–free (SPF) is a specific proprietary term in swine (National SPF, 1994; Saffron and Gonder, 1997). This means that the herd of animals has been certified by veterinary and gross necropsy examinations to be free of the specific diseases of atrophic rhinitis, pneumonia, swine dysentery, lice, mange, pseudorabies, and brucellosis. Although this certification does not guarantee that swine will be free of all diseases, it is a gold standard among swine producers and provides the best assurance that swine will be of a suitable condition for surgical protocols. Higher standards are required for animals used in xenografic procedures (Swindle, 1996). Zoonotic diseases are discussed in Chapter 14.

Dosages of antimicrobial agents that have been utilized in laboratory swine are included in the appendix (Table A25).

Restraint and Handling

Agricultural methods of restraining swine are inappropriate for laboratory settings. These methods include snout tying, hog tying, and suspending animals by their rear legs. Such methodologies are stressful and make chronically housed animals timid and potentially aggressive toward their handlers. These animals are easily trained and can be restrained in sling apparatuses, such as the Panepinto sling (Panepinto et al., 1983) (Fig. 1.9). With small animals, their weight can be supported in the handler's arms, like other species such as the dog. Larger animals may be herded and restrained against the side of the cage with hand-held panels. Squeeze chutes may be appropriate in some circumstances for very large animals if care is taken to avoid trauma to the animal. Swine can also be trained to walk with a leash and harness (Houpt, 1986; Panepinto, 1986; Swindle et al., 1994).

Swine respond well to food treats for training, and food may be used to calm them during long-term restraint in slings. Foods that have been used successfully include dog biscuits, carrots, candy, donuts, and cookies.

If complete restraint is required, it is best to utilize short-term anesthetics and chemical restraint agents (Chapter 2).

Administration of Medications and Injections

Oral medications can be administered by multiple methods. The easiest method is to mix the medication with food. In the case of substances with a

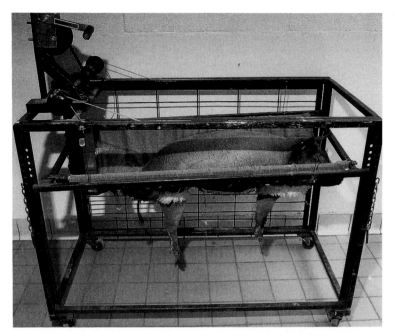

FIGURE 1.9   Yucatan pig restrained in a humane restraint sling (Panepinto sling).

foul taste, they may be placed inside gelatin capsules. Medications can be mixed with chocolate syrup or canned cat food or dog food. Swine will consume these substances quickly and without substantial chewing, thus, breaking capsules and tablets is seldom necessary. Balling guns have been utilized in agricultural settings (Fig. 1.10). If these devices are required, then it is best to restrain the animals in a sling and utilize equipment with flexible necks to avoid trauma to the pharynx and larynx. Swine can also be readily medicated using stomach tubes if the animal is restrained in a sling. Stomach tubes should be approximately the size of the trachea and have rounded tips. The tube should be lubricated and passed slowly through the side of the mouth. Medication should be administered quickly and the tube removed. If precautions are not taken, swine may sever the tube with their incisors. Mouth gags may be utilized in smaller swine, however, larger swine are too powerful for the handler to hold the mandible closed around it (Swindle et al., 1994).

Intramuscular (im) and subcutaneous (sc) injections may be given in the rear legs or neck. In the rear leg, the gluteal, semimembranosus, and semitendinosus muscles may be used (Fig. 1.11). Care should be taken to avoid the sciatic nerve. The flank may be utilized for im injections, however, sc injections require that the pigs be larger and have a layer of fat to separate the skin from the underlying muscles. Muscles on the sides of the neck or behind the ears may be utilized in small swine; however, injections given in this area in larger swine will be sc rather than im because of the layers of fat that develop. Expe-

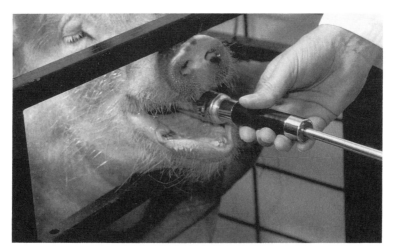

FIGURE 1.10   Balling gun with a flexible neck being used to administer a capsule.

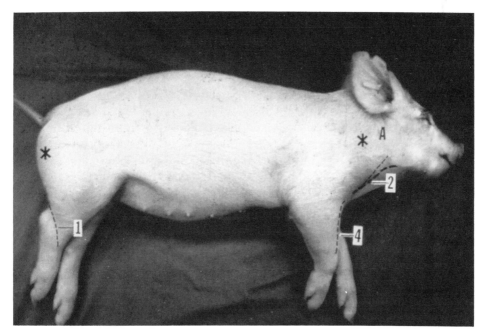

FIGURE 1.11   Injection sites on a pig. *—Sites for im injection, *A*—Mandibular arterial
pulse, *1*—Lateral saphenous vein, 2—External jugular vein, *4*—Cephalic
vein. *Reprinted with permission from Bobbie and Swindle, 1986, in M.E.
Tumbleson (ed), Swine in Biomedical Research, Vol. 1, New York: Plenum
Press.*

rience has shown that this does not present a problem for injectable anesthetics, and this area is preferred because larger-volume injections can be given with less pain to the animal than im injections in the rear legs. Animals should be restrained in a sling or with panels when given injections with a hypodermic needle. It is seldom necessary to use a needle larger than 20 gauge. A method that does not require restraint is to use a slapping motion to instill a butterfly catheter into the side of the neck and allow the animal to recover from the insertion. The medication can then be administered through the butterfly catheter while the animal is walking around the cage (Swindle et al., 1994; Swindle, 1983).

Intraperitoneal (ip) injections may be given in the lower quadrants of the abdomen off the midline. Intrathoracic injections should be given in the dorsocaudal intercostal spaces if they are required by research protocol. Methodologies for giving injections and taking samples in the subarachnoid space and cisterna magna are discussed in Chapter 11.

Intravenous (iv) injections and venipuncture for sampling or implanting catheters can be performed in a variety of locations (Figs. 1.11–1.15). Procedures for chronic catheterization and percutaneous catheterization for cardiovascular procedures are discussed in Chapters 4, 9, and 12. The standard methodology for withdrawing blood samples in agricultural settings utilizes the precava. The use of large-gauge (14-16 ga) 3- to 5-inch "hog needles" is unnecessary except in large breeding stock. For swine less than 50 kg, the largest needle size that is required is 20 gauge 1.5 inches. Animals may be restrained in a sling or on their backs with the forelegs retracted caudally. In order to avoid injury to the vagus nerve, the needle is inserted into the right side of the neck, lateral to the manubrium sterni, and directed at a 30- to 45-degree angle toward the left shoulder. A popping sensation will be felt when the needle enters the vein, and then blood can be readily withdrawn. This method can also be utilized for sequential venipuncture, but hematomas form in the area after the needle is withdrawn; therefore, it is best reserved for procedures that do not require withdrawal more often than weekly (Panepinto et al., 1983; Swindle, 1983; Swindle et al., 1994).

General Anatomy

Several textbooks describing the detailed anatomy of swine are available (Getty, 1975; Gilbert, 1966; Popesko, 1977; Sack, 1982). A recent review article compares the anatomy and physiology of swine as it applies to their use as research animals (Swindle and Smith, 1998). Specific aspects of anatomy important to surgical procedures are included in the introduction to the various system chapters. This section provides an illustrated introductory overview of the gross anatomy of swine.

The vertebral formula is C7, T14–15, L6–7, S4, Cy20–23. There are seven sternal and seven asternal ribs. If a 15th rib is present, it is usually floating rather than being attached to the cartilage of the costal arch. The clavicle is absent. In the forelimb, there are eight carpal bones, four metacarpal bones (2–5), and three phalanges; proximal and distal sesamoid bones are present. In the hind limb, there are eight tarsal bones, four metatarsal bones, and phalanges with sesamoid bones present (Fig. 1.16).

The musculature of the pig is massive, as would be expected of an animal that has been bred predominantly for meat production (Fig. 1.17).

The unique features of the gastrointestinal tract include the torus pyloricus in the pyloric region of the stomach, the mesenteric vascular arcades, and the spiral colon. The torus pyloricus is a muscular and mucoid glandular structure adjacent to the pylorus, which is involved in the functional closure of the ori-

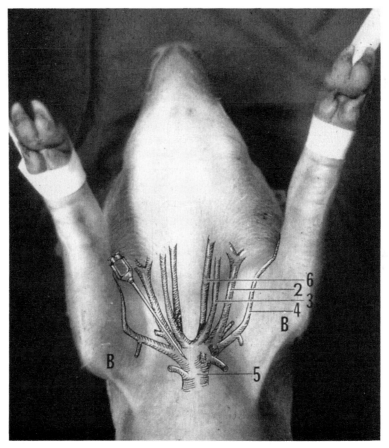

FIGURE 1.12   Blood vessels of the neck. *B*—Site of radial arterial pulse, *2*—External jugular vein, *3*—Internal jugular vein, *4*—Cephalic vein, *5*—Precava, *6*—Carotid artery. *Reprinted with permission from Bobbie and Swindle, 1986, in M.E. Tumbleson (ed), Swine in Biomedical Research, Vol. 1, New York: Plenum Press.*

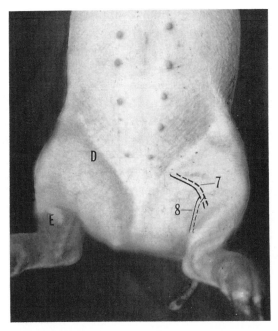

FIGURE 1.13   Blood vessels of the medial thigh. *D*—Site of femoral arterial pulse, *E*—Site of saphenous arterial pulse, *7*—Femoral artery and vein, *8*—Medial saphenous artery and vein. *Reprinted with permission from Bobbie and Swindle, 1986, in M.E. Tumbleson (ed), Swine in Biomedical Research, Vol. 1, New York: Plenum Press.*

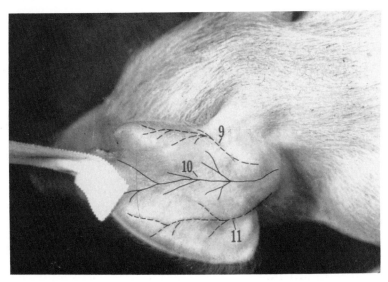

FIGURE 1.14   Blood vessels of the ear. *9*—Medial auricular vein, *10*—Auricular artery, *11*—Lateral auricular vein. *Reprinted with permission from Bobbie and Swindle, 1986, in M.E. Tumbleson (ed), Swine in Biomedical Research, Vol. 1, New York: Plenum Press.*

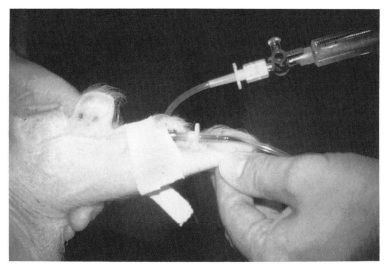

FIGURE 1.15   Intravenous catheter with a three-way valve in the auricular vein.

fice. The small intestine is arranged in a series of coils from the stomach to the pelvis, dorsal and lateral to the spiral colon. The bile duct and pancreatic ducts enter the duodenum separately in the proximal portion in the right upper quadrant. The mesenteric vascular arcades form in the subserosa of the intestine rather than the mesentery, giving a fanlike appearance. The spiral colon contains the cecum, the ascending, transverse, and main portion of the descending colon arranged in a series of centrifugal and centripetal coils in the left upper quadrant of the abdomen, caudal to the stomach. The descending colon continues caudally on the left side to become the rectum (Figs. 1.18–1.21).

The kidneys are usually ventral to the transverse processes of the first four lumbar vertebrae with the left kidney usually more cranial than the right one. The adrenal glands are craniomedial to the hilus of the kidneys. The right gland is attached to the vena cava (Fig. 1.22).

The male urogenital system contains large vesicular glands, a prostate and bulbourethral glands, as accessory genital glands. The scrotum and testicles are ventral to the anus and more caudal than ventral on the perineum. The fibromuscular penis has a sigmoid flexure and terminates in a corkscrew-shaped tip in the preputial diverticulum, caudal to the umbilicus (Fig. 1.23). The female urogenital tract has long, flexuous fallopian tubes and a bicornuate uterus with a small body. The urethra enters the vagina on the ventral floor within the pelvic cavity, cranial to the vestibule (Fig. 1.24). There are 10–12 paired mammary glands on the ventral abdomen.

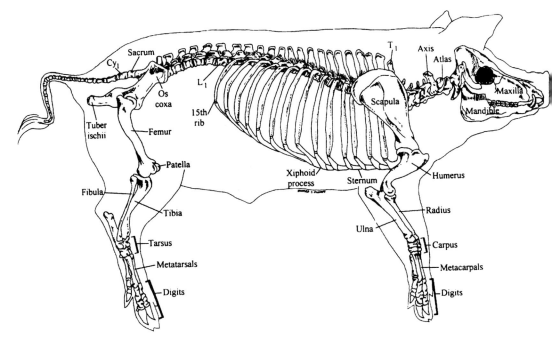

FIGURE 1.16   Skeleton of the pig.

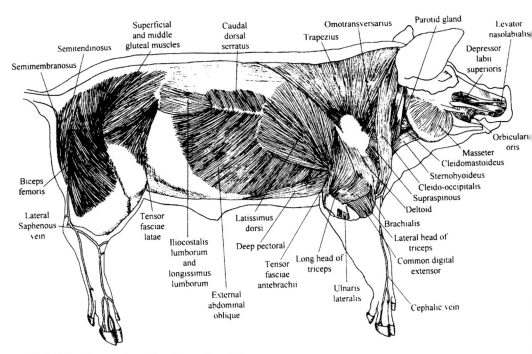

FIGURE 1.17   Superficial muscles of the pig.

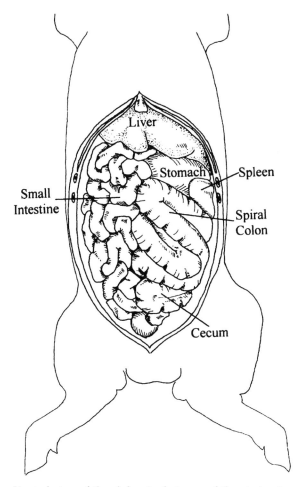

FIGURE 1.18   Ventral view of the abdominal viscera of the pig in situ.

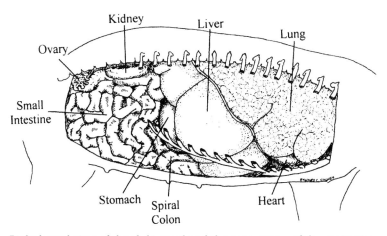

FIGURE 1.19   Right lateral view of the abdominal and thoracic viscera of the pig in situ.

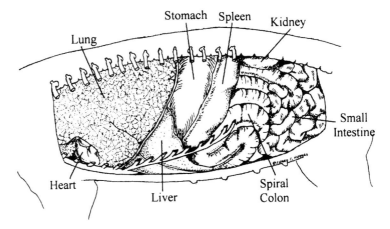

FIGURE 1.20   Left lateral view of the abdominal and thoracic viscera of the pig in situ.

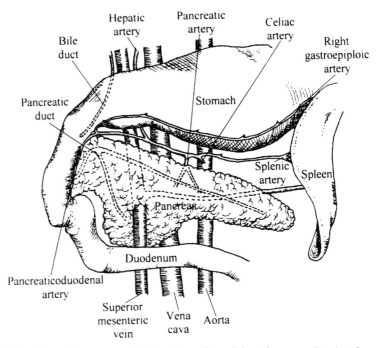

FIGURE 1.21   Ilustration of the pancreatic blood supply and ductal system. *Reprinted with permission from Stump et al., 1988, Pancreatectomized swine as a model of diabetes mellitus, Lab. Anim. Sci. 38(4): 439–443.*

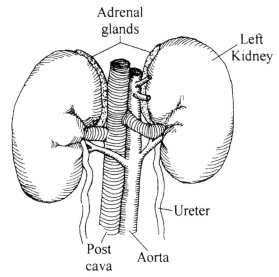

FIGURE 1.22   Ventral view of the kidneys and adrenal glands.

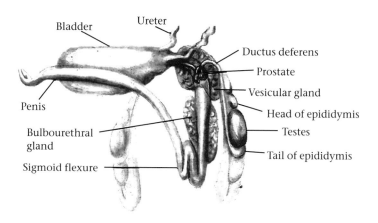

FIGURE 1.23

Left lateral view of the male urogenital system. *Reprinted with permission from Swindle, 1983, Comparative Anatomy of the Pig, Charles River Technical Bulletin, Charles River Laboratories, Inc.*

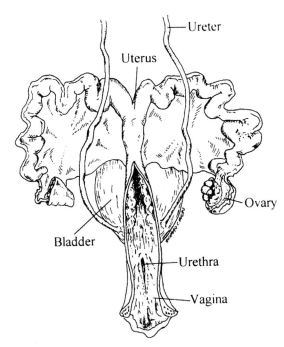

FIGURE 1.24   Dorsal view of the female reproductive tract.

The larynx is prominent with a large vestibule that narrows caudally because of internal compression of the cricoid cartilage. There are middle and lateral ventricles that have to be avoided during intubation (Chapter 2).

The thyroid gland is located on the ventral midline of the trachea at the level of the thoracic inlet. A pair of parathyroid glands can be found associated with the craniomedial portion of the thymus in the neck (Fig. 1.25). The lymph nodes have an inversion of the cortex and medulla. Histologically, this presents a unique appearance with the more central location of the germinal centers (Fig. 1.26).

The trachea extends from C4–5 to T5 where it bifurcates into the bronchi. At T3, it provides a bronchus to the apical lobe of the right lung. The lungs are composed of apical, middle, and diaphragmatic lobes, with an accessory lobe to the right lung. The intralobular fissure is incomplete between the left apical and middle lobes.

The heart extends from T2 to T7 and has sternal contact the majority of the caudal distance. The left azygous vein is the most unique feature of the external anatomy. It curves caudoventrally from the dorsal thorax across the dorsal surface of the heart to enter the right atrium in the coronary sinus.

Unique aspects of the vasculature and the other visceral organs are discussed in the various system chapters.

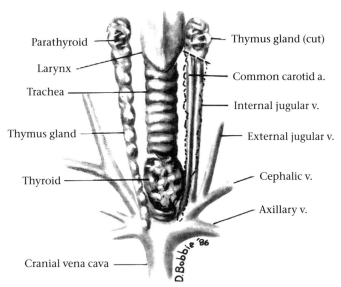

FIGURE 1.25   Diagram of the ventral aspect of the trachea and glandular structures of the neck. *Reprinted with permission from Swindle, 1983, Comparative Anatomy of the Pig, Charles River Technical Bulletin, Charles River Laboratories, Inc.*

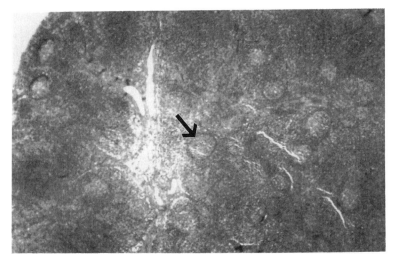

FIGURE 1.26   Cross section of a lymph node demonstrating the inversion of the cortex and medulla. A germinal center is illustrated with an arrow (×100, Hematoxylin and Eosin stain).

Model Selection

The principles for selecting swine as a model are similar to those of other species, and the proceedings books referenced in the introduction to this chapter contain the descriptions of many diverse biomedical models that have been developed in this species. This textbook details many of the surgical procedures utilized in the development of induced porcine models.

One of the principal concerns when considering the use of swine is the age of the animal. Because swine grow rapidly, and if small domestic pigs are used as biological models, the physiologic process being studied may be defined as that of a pediatric rather than an adult model. This may require that the animal selected be either a miniature pig or a larger domestic animal if maturity is a factor to be considered in the experiment.

Likewise, if a chronic experiment is planned, then the growth of the animal is a consideration, especially if biomaterials are implanted. As a general rule, the growth of sexually immature domestic swine over a 3-week period will be significant enough to have an impact on the physiologic parameters of the study. Consequently, the use of miniature breeds should be considered for experiments in which growth could be a factor.

Also as a general rule, miniature pigs are more mature at a given body weight than are domestic swine, and this should be considered if maturity of the system or wound healing characteristics are a factor in the experiment.

When comparing experiments between laboratories, animals should be matched for age, weight, gender, and breed. Because of the line-breeding that occurs in herds of commercial animals raised for food, there may even be differences between animals of the same breed from different herds. Animals bought from the same supplier may be siblings or otherwise closely related; therefore, the relatedness of the animals should be considered if it is a potential factor in the experiment. Consequently, if differences are noted in experiments between laboratories, the genetic factors should be considered.

Most of the porcine models are selected because of the close comparisons of the physiology of the various systems. In the literature, most of the models involve either the cardiovascular or the digestive systems. This textbook reflects that fact by the disparity of the sizes of the various system chapters. The reasons for selection of the models of the different body systems is discussed within those chapters.

A list of general references, which may be useful in providing information on the use of swine as animal models in biomedical research, is provided.

References

Boldrick, L. 1993. Veterinary Care of Pot-Bellied Pet Pigs. Orange, CA: All Publishing Co.
Consortium for Developing a Guide for the Care and Use of Agricultural Animals. 1988.

Guide for the care and use of agricultural animals in agricultural research and teaching. In Agricultural Animal Care Guide.Washington, DC: Consortium for Developing a Guide for the Care and Use of Agricultural Animals.

Fisher, T.F. 1993. Miniature swine in biomedical research: Applications and husbandry considerations. Lab. Anim. 22(5): 47–50.

Frandsson, R.D. 1981. Anatomy and Physiology of Farm Animals, 3rd ed. Philadelphia: Lea and Febiger.

Getty, R. (ed). 1975. Sisson and Grossman's the Anatomy of the Domestic Animals— Porcine, Vol. 2. Philadelphia: W.B. Saunders, pp. 1215–1422.

Gilbert, S.G. 1966. Pictoral Anatomy of the Fetal Pig, 2nd ed. Seattle: University of Washington Press.

Houpt, T.R. 1986. The handling of swine in research. In Stanton, H.C., and Mersmann, H.J. (eds), Swine in Cardiovascular Research, Vol. 1. Boca Raton, FL: CRC Press, pp. 25–38.

Idris, A.H., L.B. Becker, J.P. Omato, J. Hedges, N. Chandra, R.O. Cummins, U. Ebmeyer, H. Halperin, R. Kerber, K. Kern, P. Safar, P. Steen, M.M. Swindle, J. Tsitlik, I. von Planta, M. von Planta, R. Wears, and M.H. Weil. 1996. Utstein-Style guidelines for uniform reporting of laboratory CPR research. Circulation 94(9): 2324–2336. Simultaneous publication in Ann. Emerg. Med. Resuscitation 33(1): 69–84.

Leman, A.D., B.E. Straw, W.L. Mengeling, S. D'Allaire, and D.J. Taylor (eds). 1992. Diseases of Swine, 7th ed. Ames: Iowa State University Press.

National Research Council. 1988. The Nutrient Requirements of Swine, 9th ed. Washington, DC: National Academy Press.

National SPF Swine Accrediting Agency. 1994. Rules and regulations. Conrad, IA: National SPF Swine Accrediting Agency.

Panepinto, L.M. 1986. Character and management of miniature swine. In Stanton, H.C., and Mersmann, J.H. (eds), Swine in Cardiovascular Research, Vol. 1. Boca Raton, FL: CRC Press, pp. 11–24.

Panepinto, L.M., R.W. Phillips, S.W. Norden, P.C. Pryor, and R. Cox. 1983. A comfortable minimum stress method of restraint for Yucatan miniature swine. Lab. Anim. Sci. 33(1): 95–97.

Pond, W.G., and K. Houpt. 1978. Biology of the Pig. Ithaca, NY: Comstock Publishing Associates.

Popesko, P. 1977. Atlas of Topographical Anatomy of the Domestic Animals, 2nd ed., Vol. 1. Philadelphia: W.B. Saunders Company.

Public Health Service. 1996. Guide for the Care and Use of Laboratory Animals. Washington, DC: National Academy Press.

Reeves, D.E. 1993. Care and Management of Miniature Pet Pigs. Santa Barbara, CA: Veterinary Practice Publishing Co.

Sack, W.O. 1982. Essentials of Pig Anatomy and Harowitz/Kramer Atlas of Musculoskeletal Anatomy of the Pig. Ithaca, NY: Veterinary Textbooks.

Saffron, J., and J.C. Gonder. 1997. The SPF pig in research. ILAR J. 38(1): 28–31.

Stanton, H.C., and H.J. Mersmann. 1986. Swine in Cardiovascular Research, Vol. 1 and 2. Boca Raton, FL: CRC Press, Inc.

Swindle, M.M. 1983. Basic Surgical Exercises Using Swine. Philadelphia: Praeger Press.

Swindle, M.M. 1992. Swine as Models in Biomedical Research. Ames: Iowa State University Press.

Swindle, M.M. 1996. Considerations of specific pathogen free swine (SPF) in xeno— transplantation. J. Invest. Surg. 9(3): 267–271.

Swindle, M.M., and A.C. Smith. 1998. Comparative anatomy and physiology of the pig. Scand. J. Lab. Anim. Sci. 25(Suppl 1): 1-10.

Swindle, M.M., A.C. Smith, K. Laber-Laird, and L. Dungan. 1994. Swine in biomedical research: Management and models. ILAR News 36(1): 1–5.

Tumbleson, M.E. 1986. Swine in Biomedical Research, Vol. 1–3. New York: Plenum Press.

Tumbleson, M.E., and L.B. Schook. 1996. Advances in Swine in Biomedical Research, Vol. 1 and 2. New York: Plenum Press.

2 ANESTHESIA AND ANALGESIA

Introduction

The purpose of this chapter is to provide practical advice on anesthetic procedures in swine. A recent publication (Smith et al., 1997) provides an exhaustive review of most of the potential agents that may be used in anesthesia in laboratory swine. An emphasis on the physiologic effects of injectable anesthetics and cardiopulmonary bypass procedures is included in that publication. Recent veterinary publications (Riebold et al., 1995; Thurmon and Benson, 1996) provide an overview of anesthesia in swine with an emphasis on agricultural and pet pig procedures. Reviews of agents used in cardiovascular research (Thurmon and Tranquilli, 1986) and laboratory animal medicine (Flecknell, 1987; Hawk and Leary, 1995; Kohn et al., 1997) are also available.

Anesthetic protocols for experimental procedures should be selected with consideration of the potential physiologic complications on the experiment. For example, no anesthetic protocol has been developed that is without effects on cardiovascular hemodynamics; however, the effects may be minimized by judicious selection of the agents. This chapter discusses the most commonly used protocols in research and makes specific recommendations for their selection.

Endotracheal Intubation

Endotracheal intubation should be performed on all swine when they undergo general anesthesia. The procedure is easily performed when the species-specific anatomic considerations are understood. The laryngeal passage is narrow, and the vocal cords and blind folds are easily traumatized if too large a tube or too much force is used during intubation. The lateral folds of the larynx can be easily ruptured and the tube passed into the subcutaneous tissues.

Swine may be intubated from any position. The most common positions are dorsal and sternal recumbency. The dorsal recumbency position tends to be easier for swine less than 50 kg when personnel are used to human intubation. Straight laryngoscope blades with a curved tip are the best for swine. Standard laryngoscope blades, 195 mm or longer, are sufficient for swine less than 50 kg. For larger animals, modified blades with 3- to 5-cm extensions are optimal.

When intubating swine in dorsal recumbency, assistance with holding the jaws open is not necessary and a simplified atraumatic method of intubation has been published (Swindle, 1991). When the pig is placed in sternal recumbency, an assistant must hold the jaws open with gauze strips, or a mouth gag should be used. The method of unassisted intubation in dorsal recumbency is pictured (Fig. 2.1) and illustrated (Fig. 2.2).

After the laryngoscope is passed into the pharyngeal cavity, the tip is used to displace the epiglottis from the soft palate. After this procedure, the epiglottis and laryngeal aperture are easily seen, and the larynx is sprayed with a topical anesthetic, such as lidocaine, to prevent laryngospasm. The tip of the epiglottis is caught with the tip of the curved laryngoscope blade and displaced ventrally against the tongue. At this point, the vocal cords can be observed moving with each breath. The handle of the laryngoscope is tilted toward the operator at approximately a 45-degree angle. This will result in the larynx being flattened against the ventral surface of the neck; this can be seen readily from the outside. This maneuver will result in the laryngeal passage being straightened. The tip of the endotracheal tube is placed into the laryngeal cavity from the side of the oral cavity while watching the positioning of the tube along the laryngoscope blade. After the tip of the tube is in place, it is passed into the trachea while simultaneously rotating it in a screw-like fashion to facilitate passage through the aperture. Resistance should not be felt if the angle of the laryngoscope blade is correct and the size of the endotracheal tube is not too large.

When using this method, the use of stylets or other assist devices is unnecessary. A range of endotracheal tubes from 4.5 to 8.0 mm outside dimension is sufficient for most swine used in biomedical research. The size of the tube required can be estimated by palpation of the trachea prior to intubation. As a general rule, most 20- to 30-kg swine can be intubated with 6.5- to 7.5-mm tubes.

With practice, small swine can be intubated without a laryngoscope. The technique involves placing the pig in dorsal recumbency and pinching the dorsum of the larynx between the thumb and forefinger of one hand. This pinching movement should elevate the larynx and close the esophageal passage. A popping will be felt when the epiglottis is displaced ventrally from the soft palate. The endotracheal tube is then passed blindly through the oral cav-

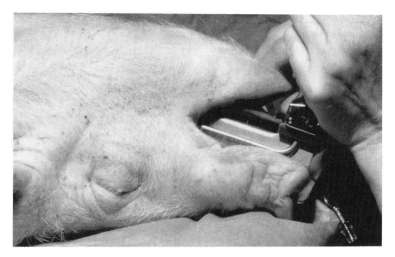

FIGURE 2.1   Proper angle for holding the laryngoscope blade when intubating a pig
                    in dorsal recumbency.

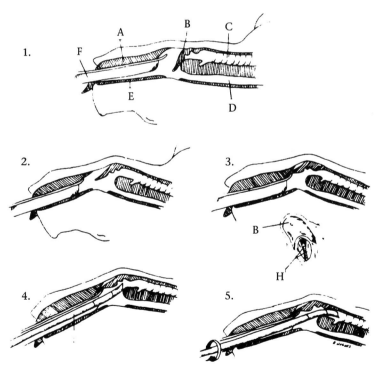

FIGURE 2.2   Stepwise illustration of the process of endotracheal intubation.
                    A-Tongue, *B*-Epiglottis, *C*-Trachea, *D*-Esophagus, *E*-Hard palate,
                    F-Laryngoscope blade, *G*-Endotracheal tube, *H*-Vocal cords. *Reprinted
                    with permission from Swindle, 1994, Anesthetic and Perioperative Techniques
                    in Swine, Charles River Technical Bulletin, Charles River Laboratories, Inc.*

ity with the other hand. This methodology can best be utilized in small swine in which the larynx can be easily manipulated from the outside.

Regardless of the methodology utilized, a free passage of air should be felt and heard when the pig is properly intubated. The two most common problems are inadvertent closure of the laryngeal opening with the laryngoscope and placement of the tube in the esophagus. With traumatic methodologies, the larynx may also either be ruptured through one of its membranes or traumatized sufficiently to produce laryngeal edema. Any gasping or cyanosis is a sign of improper tube or laryngoscope placement. Cyanosis can easily be observed in the snout or nipples of pigs with light-colored skin. The technique of tracheostomy is described in Chapter 9, should it be indicated.

Special Perioperative Considerations

Consideration should be given to several issues concerning perioperative care and monitoring of swine while under anesthesia. These issues include methodologies to provide homeostasis and prevent other potentially fatal complications. The general principles of proper anesthesia and monitoring are applicable to swine, but some issues are species specific (Smith et al., 1997; Smith and Swindle, 1994).

Preoperative Fasting

Swine have rapid intestinal transport times in the upper gastrointestinal tract (GI) and require only a few hours to empty the stomach. Consequently, a fast of solid food for 6–8 hours preoperatively is sufficient for most surgical procedures. Water may be provided up until the time of surgery. Swine will readily consume most liquid diets and flavored drinks if they are required, to prevent hypoglycemia for prolonged fasts, such as for colonic procedures. Bedding should be removed from the cages of swine being fasted, because they will readily consume it if not provided food. Issues of fasting specifically applicable to GI procedures are discussed in Chapter 4.

Intravenous Fluid Administration

The sites for administration of intravenous (iv) fluids are discussed in Chapter 1. Once iv access is obtained, maintenance fluids should be administered for all anesthetic procedures requiring more than short-term chemical restraint. The rate of administration should be 5–10 ml/kg/h with isotonic solutions, unless a problem or specific indication for a different rate of administration is observed. A flow rate of approximately 3–5 ml/h is required to maintain patency of iv catheters.

Thermal Support

The relatively hairless skin, the common use of alcohol in skin preparation for surgery, and administration of chemical restraint agents that induce peripheral vasodilation make swine more susceptible to hypothermia than most other animal species. Rectal temperature should be continuously monitored and not allowed to decrease below 36°C (normal, 38°–39.5°C). The use of circulating hot water blankets and complete draping of the anesthetized animal are usually sufficient to prevent hypothermia. More intense methods, such as administration of warmed iv fluids and increasing the room temperature, may be necessary for some highly invasive procedures or if hypothermia occurs.

Cardiac Monitoring and Arrhythmias

Swine are susceptible to anesthetic-induced cardiac arrhythmias and, as a minimum, should be monitored by electrocardiogram (ECG) during anesthesia. For prolonged and invasive procedures, especially those involving the cardiothoracic system, blood pressure and blood gases should also be monitored. Pulse oximetry is useful, and finger cuffs can be placed either on the ears, tail, or the dew claws. Peripheral blood pressure cuffs are most reliable for the coccygeal and median saphenous arteries. Peripheral arterial access in the median saphenous artery or using the methodologies described for arterial access in Chapters 9 and 12 can be utilized to measure blood gases.

Cardiac arrhythmias are more likely to be a problem during manipulation of the heart or central vessels or when using anesthetics such as xylazine and halothane, which have a proarrhythmic effect on the myocardium. Farm animals appear to be more susceptible than miniature breeds. Most of the fatal cardiac arrhythmias can be prevented by the administration of bretylium 3–5 mg/kg iv given by slow injection every 30 minutes during cardiac manipulation (Horneffer et al., 1986; Schumann et al., 1993). Lidocaine (2–4 mg/kg iv) can be administered as a continuous iv infusion 0.3 mg/kg/h as an antiectopic and antivasospasmotic agent. Other cardiovascular support agents can be administered as indicated and the dosages are included in the appendix.

If ventricular fibrillation occurs, then defibrillation should be attempted with 10-joule countershock for internal paddles or 200 joules for external paddles. The principles of treatment of this potentially fatal condition are the same as for other species.

Malignant Hyperthermia

Malignant hyperthermia is a genetic condition in certain breeds of domestic swine, such as the Landrace, Yorkshire, and Pietrain. The condition is transmitted as an autosomal dominant gene (Hal genotype). The ryanodine receptor gene (ryr-1 locus) is the probable site (Geers et al., 1992; Houde et al., 1993). The condition has not been reported in miniature swine.

The condition is induced by stress (porcine stress syndrome) or by many anesthetic and paralytic agents. Susceptible animals can be screened genetically or by testing for abnormal creatine phosphokinase serum levels. The condition may also be prevented by the prophylactic intramuscular (im) or iv administration of dantrolene 5 mg/kg (Anderson, 1976; Ehler et al., 1985; Smith et al., 1997).

If malignant hyperthermia is encountered, it is associated with elevated rectal temperatures and skeletal muscle rigidity. Elevated CO_2 levels and associated cardiovascular responses such as tachycardia occur rapidly at the onset. The condition is rapidly fatal in susceptible animals. If encountered, it may be treated by discontinuing the triggering agent, cooling of the animal, and administration of dantrolene; however, it is best to avoid sources of animals that have the condition, rather than using screening methods or pharmaceutical interventions to prevent the disease.

Paralytic Agents

Paralytic agents may be indicated for some procedures either to paralyze the diaphragm during cardiac surgery or to provide increased muscle relaxation. Paralytic agents should not be administered during surgery until it is established that surgical analgesia has been obtained. For example, the use of paralytic agents is helpful to paralyze the diaphragm during cardiac surgical manipulations. The thoracotomy can be performed without the administration of paralytic agents to ensure that analgesia levels are sufficient. It is unnecessary to administer these agents throughout the surgical procedure in most cases.

Paralyzed animals should be monitored for an increase in heart rate or blood pressure as an indication of inadequate analgesia. The initial administration of pancuronium (0.02–0.15 mg/kg, 0.003–0.030 mg/kg/h iv infusion) is associated with a physiologic increase in heart rate. Vercuronium (1 mg/kg) does not affect the heart rate (Smith et al., 1997).

Anesthetic Monitoring

Anesthetic monitoring can be performed by monitoring heart rate and blood pressure as described above. This methodology is more sensitive than the muscular or ocular reflexes that are commonly used in veterinary medicine. Ocular reflexes are difficult to observe in swine because of the depth of the orbit and the frequently used combinations of drugs in porcine anesthesia that can make meaningful observations obscure. Muscular reflexes can be induced by pinching at the coronary band of the hoof, the tip of the ear, or the tail or by observing mandibular jaw tone. Jaw tone seems to be the most reliable and is the preferred method of observing muscular reflexes. Rigidity of the mandibular muscles should be taken as an indication that the anesthetic level is light (Swindle, 1983).

Ventilation Rates

The pulmonary tissue of swine is sensitive to overventilation and may rupture and cause emphysematous bullae, pneumothorax and pneumoperitoneum. Pneumatosis intestinalis may occur in severe cases. The ventilatory pressure for swine should be 18–22 cm H_2O. The tidal volume for swine is 5–10 ml/kg. The respiratory rate varies depending upon the anesthetic and individual animal characteristics. For swine 20-40 kg on inhalational anesthesia, a rate of 12–15 breaths per minute is usually sufficient, however, monitoring with pulse oximetry, arterial blood gases or end tidal CO_2 should be performed to ensure proper ventilation (Smith et al., 1997; Swindle, 1983).

Preanesthetic Agents

Preanesthetic agents are useful to relieve anxiety, abolish the vagal reflex, decrease the amount of general anesthetic required, and facilitate handling. These agents fall into the categories of anticholinergics, sedatives, and tranquilizers. The use of preoperative and intraoperative analgesics is discussed under analgesics.

Anticholinergics

Atropine (0.05 mg/kg im or 0.02 mg/kg iv) and glycopyrrolate (0.004–0.01 mg/kg im) are used preoperatively to dry bronchiole secretions and abolish the vagal reflex during endotracheal intubation or suctioning. It is also useful to counter the bradycardia that is associated with the use of some anesthetic agents. Routine use of these agents is not required, and the physiologic effects of tachycardia and vagal blockade should be considered when designing the protocol (Smith et al., 1997; Swindle, 1983).

Tranquilizers and Sedatives

The phenothiazine, benzodiazepine, and butyrophenone tranquilizers are the most commonly used agents for preanesthesia. All of these agents have been combined with dissociative agents to induce anesthesia and are discussed in that context below. Of the phenothiazines, acepromazine [1.1–2.2 mg/kg im, iv, or subcutaneously (sc)] is the most commonly used agent. It is associated with peripheral vasodilation and α-adrenergic blockade in higher dosages. Its effects as a sole agent last for 8–12 hours (Benson and Thurmon, 1979; Riebold et al., 1995; Swindle, 1983).

The two most commonly used benzodiazepine tranquilizers in porcine anesthesia are diazepam, which is fat soluble, and midazolam, which is water soluble. Diazepam (0.5–10 mg/kg im, 0.44–2 mg/kg iv, 1 mg/kg/h iv infusion) provides good hypnosis and sedation for up to 6 hours (Benson and Thurmon, 1979; Thurmon and Tranquilli, 1986). Midazolam (0.1–0.5 mg/kg im or iv, 0.6–1.5 mg/kg/h iv infusion) provides complete sedation for 20 minutes with minimal hemodynamic depression and can be used safely on a daily basis for prolonged periods of time (Ochs et al., 1987; Smith et al., 1991). A combination of azaperone (4 mg/kg im) and midazolam (1 mg/kg im) has been used as a pre-anesthetic prior to propofol induction and inhalation anesthesia (Svendsen and Carter, 1997).

Butyrophenons are usually found in combination with other agents, except for azaperone (2–8 mg/ kg im). It has minimal cardiovascular effects, but provides relatively short immobilization—about 20 minutes (Portier and Slusser, 1985; Riebold et al., 1995; Thurmon and Tranquilli, 1986).

Injectable Anesthetic Agents

Injectable anesthetic agents used in swine include the dissociative anesthetics, barbiturates, opioids, and miscellaneous hypnotic agents. Most of these agents are used in combination with tranquilizers or other agents to provide surgical anesthesia. Unless these agents are meant to provide short-term chemical restraint, they should be administered as continuous iv infusions rather than repeated im or iv injections in the research setting. Experience has shown that continuous iv infusions provide more stable hemodynamics than repeated injections. The iv dosages are variable depending upon the characteristics of the individual animal and the protocol. The dosages cited in this text are guidelines and careful anesthetic monitoring should be used to determine if an adequate plane of anesthesia has been achieved. Agents commonly combined with dissociative agents, such as benzodiazepines, hypnotics, and α-2-adrenergic agonists are discussed with the dissociative agents, because they have little value as sole agents in swine.

Dissociative Agents

Ketamine and the combination agent tiletamine/zolazepam (Telazol) are the two most common injectable anesthetic agents utilized in swine. Usually they are combined with other agents to produce surgical anesthesia and only used as sole agents to provide up to 20 minutes of chemical restraint. They provide poor muscle relaxation but have minimal cardiovascular effects with a single im injection in clinically normal animals (Benson and Thurmon, 1979; Cantor et al., 1981; Smith et al., 1997).

Ketamine (11–33 mg/kg im, 3–10 mg/kg/h iv infusion) does not provide visceral analgesia at any dose. It may be combined with other agents to provide muscle relaxation and analgesia for minor procedures (Benson and Thurmon, 1979; Boschert et al., 1996; Smith et al., 1997; Swindle, 1983). The most commonly used im combinations in research are the following:

ketamine 33 mg/kg and acepromazine 1.1 mg/kg
ketamine 15 mg/kg and diazepam 2 mg/kg
ketamine 33 mg/kg and midazolam 0.5 mg/kg
ketamine 15 mg/kg and azaperone 2 mg/kg
ketamine 20 mg/kg and xylazine 2 mg/kg
ketamine 10 mg/kg and medetomidine 0.2 mg/kg

Only the combination with midazolam provides longer than 20–30 minutes of restraint; however, this combination is profoundly hypothermic. It may last 45–60 minutes and provide sufficient relaxation to perform intubation. Nevertheless, the side effects outweigh the advantages of this combination.

The α-2-adrenergic agonists xylazine and medetomidine are commonly included as combinations with the dissociative agents. The combination with xylazine provides short-term analgesia (5 minutes) but prolonged cardiodepression and heart block, which may be reversed with anticholinergics. Medetomidine has less severe cardiodepression than xylazine (Flecknell, 1997). The combinations with acepromazine, diazepam, and azaperone are similar in action but do not provide enough relaxation to perform intubation or to perform other than minor surgery. They all have the side effect of peripheral vasodilation but not as profoundly as the combinations with xylazine and midazolam. Antipamezole 1 mg/kg im, sc, or iv is a specific antagonist to the α-2-adrenoreceptors (Flecknell, 1997).

Intravenous infusions of ketamine combined with other agents can provide visceral analgesia suitable for major surgical procedures. After induction with a loading dose of the agent, the following infusions can be used: ketamine (1 mg/ml) and xylazine (1 mg/ml) and glycerol guaiacolate (guaifenesin) (5%) mixed in 5% dextrose 1 ml/kg iv followed by 1 ml/kg/h of the mixture, ketamine 8–33 mg/kg/h and midazolam 0.5–1.5 mg/kg/h.

All of these agents as iv infusions can provide a stable plane of anesthesia. The ketamine/xylazine/glycerol guaiacolate (guaifenesin) solution, in particular, causes minimal cardiovascular depression and can be used as a substitute for α-chloralose infusions (Thurmon et al., 1986). Its main disadvantage is the need to mix the combination in the laboratory. The infusion combinations with medetomidine (Vainio et al., 1992) and midazolam are useful for cardiac catheterization protocols but do not provide good muscle relaxation.

The tiletamine/zolazepam (Telazol) combination can provide 20 minutes of immobilization for minor surgery in the commercially available combination (2–8.8 mg/kg im); however, the combination should not be used in animals with cardiovascular compromise because of cardiodepression and hypothermia. In agricultural and pet pig situations, Telazol is combined with xylazine or xylazine and ketamine (Ko et al., 1993; Ko et al., 1997).

All of the combinations are suitable for intubation and short-term anesthesia; however, hemodynamic data have not been published to prove the usefulness of the combinations in research settings. Clinical observation of animals under anesthesia with these combinations has included peripheral cyanosis, hypothermia, and death in animals with cardiovascular compromise. The im combination dosages to provide 20–30 minutes of immobilization are the following:

Telazol 4.4 mg/kg and ketamine 2.2 mg/kg
Telazol 4.4 mg/kg and ketamine 2.2 mg/kg and xylazine 2.2 mg/kg
Telazol 4.4 mg/kg and xylazine 2.2 mg/kg

Barbiturates

Barbiturate anesthesia (Riebold et al., 1995; Smith et al., 1997; Swindle, 1983; Swindle, 1991; Thurmon and Tranquilli, 1986) must be administered iv, usually after induction with one of the dissociative anesthetics to allow the anesthetist to insert an iv catheter. The initial administration of these agents as a bolus will frequently induce apnea which can be overcome by the stimulation of endotracheal intubation. They have a dose-related cardiopulmonary depressant activity that increases over time with repeated iv boluses. The cardiovascular effects can be minimized by using thiobarbiturates, which have minimal hepatic metabolism, as iv infusions. These agents are excreted by the kidneys and can be flushed out of the system with iv fluid administration. Pentobarbital is best reserved for nonsurvival procedures and should be administered as a continuous iv infusion. Dosages of barbiturates are guidelines and may be affected by other drugs and homeostatic factors. They should be given to effect with close monitoring of vital signs. The iv dosages of the most commonly used barbiturates are the following:

thiopental 6.6–30 mg/kg, 3–30 mg/kg/h
thiamylal 6.6–30 mg/kg, 3–30 mg/kg/h
pentobarbital 20–40 mg/kg, 5–40 mg/kg/h

Opioid Infusions

Opioids can be used as iv infusions to provide the primary analgesia for cardiac surgery protocols; however, they have to be combined with other anesthetics, such as the inhalants, during the major manipulative procedures. In general, when isoflurane is used as an adjunct, a level of 0.5% is adequate. They can also be used as low-dose infusions during general surgery to provide balanced anesthesia and analgesia (Ehler et al., 1985; Lunn et al., 1979; Merin et al., 1982; Schumann et al., 1994; Smith et al., 1997; Swindle et al., 1986). The concepts of analgesia with these agents is discussed under analgesics in this chapter.

Opioid infusions have the advantages of not decreasing myocardial contractility and coronary blood flow. They produce a dose-related bradycardia that can be reversed with anticholinergics. They can also be used as stabile iv infusions for taking physiologic measurements for cardiovascular protocols. Hypertension occurs in the higher dose ranges over time. In that situation, the adjunctive anesthetic agents can be eliminated after all of the major surgical manipulations have been performed.

The most commonly used agents for these procedures in swine are fentanyl (30–100 µg/kg/h) and sufentanil (7–30 µg/kg/h). They may be used for induction following placement of an iv catheter or following restraint with midazolam or ketamine. Starting the iv infusion prior to administering an iv bolus to induce anesthesia prevents the animals from exhibiting a sudden onset of bradycardia and muscle rigidity. The iv dosages are as follows:

fentanyl 0.050 mg/kg iv bolus, 0.030–0.100 mg/kg/h iv infusion
sufentanil 0.007 mg/kg iv bolus, 0.015–0.030 mg/kg/h iv infusion

Miscellaneous Agents

Propofol (4–20 mg/kg iv) is an iv hypnotic agent that can be used in combination with other agents to induce anesthesia. It has a relatively narrow therapeutic margin in swine and can produce severe hypotension and apnea. In lower dosages, cardiac output and coronary blood flow is minimally depressed; however, there is also poor analgesia. A continuous infusion rate of 12–20 mg/kg/h can be used to provide stable general anesthesia (Foster et al., 1992; Raff and Harrison, 1989; Ramsey et al., 1993).

Etomidate (4–8 mg/kg iv) is a hypnotic sedative that can be combined with other agents to produce analgesia. The combination of 0.6 mg/kg iv with a ketamine infusion of 10 mg/kg/h iv can be used for anesthesia (Holzchuh and Cremonesi, 1991; Worek et al., 1988).

The agent α-chloralose (55–86 mg/kg iv) has been used for nonsurvival surgery to record physiologic measurements with minimal cardiovascular depression and minimal effects on the baroreceptors and chemoreceptors. It has questionable analgesic value except at the higher dose range, at which time the sparing effects on cardiovascular parameters are lost (Silverman and Muir, 1993; Thurmon and Tranquilli, 1986). It is best replaced by ketamine infusion protocols, opioids, or inhalational anesthesia with isoflurane.

No particular advantage to using these agents or older agents, such as alphaxalone, alphadolone, or etorphine, over other agents in this chapter have been published.

Inhalant Anesthetics

Inhalant anesthetics should be the primary agents considered for general anesthesia in swine (Smith et al., 1997). They provide a better control of the plane of anesthesia and analgesia and have a reduced recovery time over many of the injectable agents. When used in combination with intraoperative analgesics to provide "balanced anesthesia," the anesthetist has the most assurance that the animal is in an appropriate plane of anesthesia for major surgical procedures.

All of these agents should be used in combination with gas scavenging and periodic monitoring of the gas anesthesia machines for leakage, because of the human health problems associated with chronic exposure to low levels of these agents. In particular, the exposure of personnel, especially pregnant women, to waste gases should be avoided with methoxyflurane, halothane, and nitrous oxide. The use of scavenging systems and absorbent filters in combination with closed or semi-closed anesthetic systems should be routine. The gas anesthetic machines should be modern in design and kept in good repair to provide the best assurance that the level of anesthesia indicated by the vaporizer is correct and to prevent personnel exposure to gases leaking from the equipment (Thurmon and Benson, 1996).

The agents that should be considered as the primary choices for use in porcine anesthesia are isoflurane, desflurane, and sevoflurane. Methoxyflurane is difficult to control because of its low potency, and the agent has the possibility of causing nephrotoxicity in humans. Consequently, it is recommended that its use be discontinued along with older agents such as ether. Halothane sensitizes the myocardium to catecholamine-induced arrhythmias and has more severe depressant effects upon the myocardium than the more recently developed agents. These physiologic effects combined with the possibility of hepatotoxicity in humans should preclude its use as an anesthetic in swine. Enflurane is associated with seizure episodes in susceptible animals and does not offer any advantages over the use of other agents (Smith et al., 1997).

Isoflurane, desflurane, and sevoflurane all have similar physiologic effects in swine and are relatively safe for personnel compared to the other inhalants (Weiskopf et al., 1992). The cost differential between isoflurane and the other two agents is significant. Because of the similar physiologic effects of these three agents and the significant difference in cost, isoflurane is recommended as the primary inhalant anesthetic in swine at this time (Smith et al., 1997).

Induction by face mask (Fig. 2.3) followed by endotracheal intubation may be performed with isoflurane without nitrous oxide for protocols in which it is necessary to have a sole agent for anesthesia. The face mask should be free of leaks and the area adequately ventilated. This procedure carries minimal risk for personnel.

All of the inhalant anesthetics increase cerebral blood flow and decrease coronary blood flow in a dose-dependent fashion. These effects are minimized with isoflurane and it may increase coronary blood flow at some dosages. All

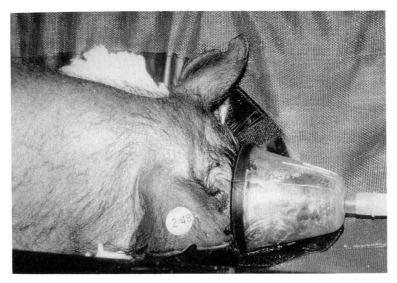

FIGURE 2.3   Yucatan pig in a restraint sling with a face mask for induction of inhalant anesthesia.

produce a dose-related depression in myocardial contractility. Isoflurane, desflurane, and sevoflurane have significantly less deleterious effects on the myocardium than the other agents discussed above (Smith et al., 1997; Weiskopf et al., 1992).

The percentage of the inhalant used for anesthesia may be reduced by the administration of nitrous oxide. Nitrous oxide as a sole agent does not provide visceral analgesia in swine; however, it is effective as an adjunct agent when used in a 1:1 or 2:1 combination with oxygen to deliver the inhalant anesthetic. The combination of isoflurane and nitrous oxide:oxygen 2:1 provides the least myocardial depressant effects of any of the inhalant anesthetic agents and reduces the concentration of isoflurane required by approximately 50%. However, nitrous oxide has the potential of having adverse effects on personnel health and adequate scavenging of waste gases should be assured (Smith et al., 1997).

The mean alveolar concentration (MAC) value is utilized as a measure of an inhalant anesthetics' potency and provides a guideline for the percentage of an anesthetic that should be required for general anesthesia. The MAC value will vary with the age of the animal as well as other variables, such as the delivery system and protocol (Smith et al., 1997). The MAC values (volume %) of these agents in swine are nitrous oxide 195 (Tranquilli et al., 1985), halothane 0.91–1.25 (Eisele et al., 1985; Eisele et al., 1986; Tranquilli et al., 1983), isoflurane 1.2–2.04 (Eger et al., 1988; Eisele et al., 1985; Koblin et al., 1989; Lundeen et al., 1983), and desflurane 8.28–10 (Eger et al., 1988).

The flow rates for anesthetics will vary with the equipment and the procedure, however, a rate of 5–10 ml/kg/min is generally adequate. Anesthetic monitoring procedures described above should be utilized to determine if the anesthetic level and oxygenation are adequate.

Cardiopulmonary Bypass (CPB)

If performed as survival procedures, cardiopulmonary bypass (Fig. 2.4) and extracorporeal membrane oxygenation (ECMO) (Fig. 2.5) in swine are more difficult procedures to perform successfully than in most other species. Difficulties include friability of the atria, postperfusion pulmonary hypertension, cardiac arrhythmias, and edema of visceral tissues (Cameron et al., 1992; Purohit et al., 1993; Qayumi et al., 1992; Smith et al., 1997; Swan and Meaghar, 1971). The methodologies described in this section are derived mainly from the laboratory experiences described by Ehler and Swindle (Ehler et al., 1985; Smith et al., 1997; Swindle et al., 1986). The use of a cooperative team approach

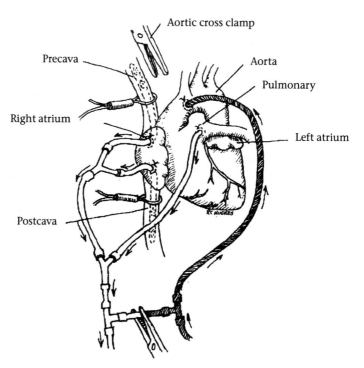

FIGURE 2.4   Catheterization circuit for cardiopulmonary bypass. *Reprinted with permission from Smith et al., 1996, in Anesthesia and Analgesia in Laboratory Animals, D.H. Kohn et al. (eds), New York: Academic Press.*

among the perfusionist, surgeon, anesthetist, and veterinary staff is essential to the success of these protocols.

In its simplest form, blood is collected prior to entering the right side of the heart, circulated through the bypass system for oxygenation and filtering, and then returned to the arterial circulation without passing through the left side of the heart. Many variations to the surgical cannulation are performed depending upon the surgical protocol under investigation. The procedure may be performed with or without the induction of hypothermia and cardioplegia to stop electrical activity and lower myocardial metabolism. In general, the longer the procedure, the more the necessity for those procedures to protect the myocardium. CPB with aortic cross clamp times of less than 30 minutes are more likely to be uneventful in swine. Times of greater than 45 minutes are likely to involve more manipulations during weaning and recovery from CPB.

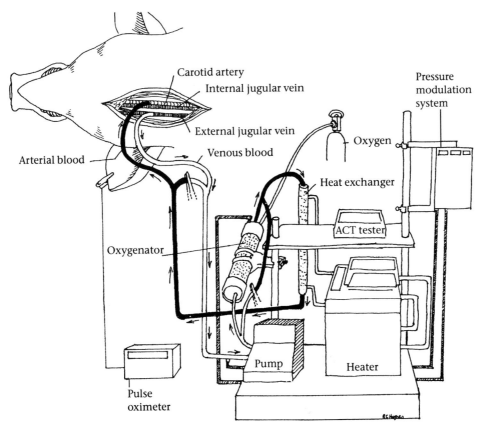

FIGURE 2.5   Extracorporeal membrane oxygenation circuit in swine. *Reprinted with permission from Purohit et al., 1993, Hanford miniature swine model for extracorporeal membrane oxygenation (ECMO). J. Invest. Surg. 6: 503–508.*

Cardiopulmonary Bypass Equipment

Membrane oxygenators are preferred for survival procedures. Generally, the bypass equipment should be a pediatric unit with adequate monitoring devices. Cardiopulmonary monitoring, including ECG, core temperature, arterial blood gases, blood pressure, and serum electrolytes, is essential. Monitoring of activated clotting time (ACT) is essential because of the necessity of systemic heparinization of the animal during the procedure. Monitoring of the hematocrit is also essential.

Surgery

The surgical approach usually is via a median sternotomy (Chapter 9), and the heart is placed in a pericardial cradle. Femoral cutdown is performed for peripheral venous and arterial access during the procedure (Chapter 9). The animal is heparinized with 300 IU/kg. The pre- and postcava are cannulated after an atriotomy is performed in the right atrial appendage. The inserted cannulae are snared around the vessels with umbilical tape or elastic bands. This approach reduces the risk of tearing the friable right atria. Blood is returned to the arterial circulation by implanting a cannula in the aorta distal to the aortic valve and cross clamping of the aorta between the valve and the cannula. Depending upon the procedure, insertion of a cannula to act as a pulmonary arterial vent may be required to provide drainage from the right ventricle and lungs and to manage postperfusion pulmonary hypertension (Horneffer et al., 1986). All of the cannulae are held in place with purse string sutures at their site of entrance into the cardiovascular system. After the cannulae are in place, the aorta may be cross clamped and cardioplegia solution containing potassium is injected into the aortic root. The surgical descriptions for thoracotomy and postoperative considerations discussed in Chapter 9 should be reviewed as they are applicable to CPB procedures.

Monitoring and Perfusionist Parameters

The priming solution should be fresh donor blood to maintain the hematocrit above 25. Blood groups with weak blood group antigens occur in swine; however, cross matching is not usually necessary for a single procedure. Domestic swine may be used as donors for miniature pigs. It is preferred that the last unit of blood collected during terminal collection be discarded because of the potentially high level of catecholamines (Cameron et al., 1992). Crystalloid primes have been associated with visceral edema and colloid solutions should be used if a supplement is required for the whole blood.

Heparinization of the animal should be initiated with 300 IU/kg and the ACT maintained at 180–300 seconds with supplemental dosages in the

100–200 IU/kg range. An ACT of greater than 300 seconds may be required with complex cardiac procedures and the lower range for procedures such as ECMO. These dosages of heparin are usually required approximately every 45 minutes if the higher ACT range is utilized. Unless absolutely essential, protamine should not be used to reverse heparinization at the end of the procedure because of the possibility of adverse reactions which are common in swine. If it is required it is given in a ratio of 1.3:1 protamine:heparin. Control of hemorrhage should be a factor of careful attention to hemostasis by the surgeon rather than drugs.

Arterial pump flow rates are dependent upon the size of the animal and the core temperature. The smaller the animal, the higher the flow rate; and the cooler the temperature, the lower the flow rate. Flow rates for swine range 60–100 ml/kg/min with an average of approximately 75 ml/kg/min. The mean arterial pressure is maintained at 50–60 mmHg with a central venous pressure of 0–5 mmHg during bypass. The systemic vascular resistance is maintained between 800 and 1400 dyne/sec/cm^{-5}. The core temperature is maintained between 15° and 37°C dependent upon the requirements of the protocol. Oxygen delivery is generally 2.2 L/m^2/min or greater.

Other parameters to be monitored by the perfusionist include blood gases and electrolytes. The approximate arterial blood gas parameters to be maintained include: PaO_2 100 mm Hg, $PaCO_2$ 40 mmHg, pH 7.38–7.42, base excess 0 or less. Potassium should be maintained at 4.5–5.5 mmol/L. Venous O_2 saturation is usually 65–75.

Anesthesia

Most anesthetic regimens that have been utilized in swine have been tried during CPB. Isoflurane should be the primary agent of choice unless contraindicated by the protocol or the medical status of the patient. If the animal is in cardiovascular compromise or if malignant hyperthermia is a potential risk, the high-dose opioid infusion protocols described above should be the primary choice. The anesthetist will need to coordinate the procedures closely with the perfusionist. Adjunct agents that may be required include the usual list of emergency drugs listed in the appendix and antiarrhythmic agents such as bretylium. The procedures for administration of these anesthetics as described above should be used.

Weaning from CPB

Most of the problems encountered in CPB in swine will occur within the first 2 hours following termination of the procedure. Weaning from the procedure should be performed slowly and with careful monitoring of the parameters described above. Measurement of CVP and PA pressures should be performed with a Swan–Ganz catheter inserted from the femoral vein.

The right side of the heart is refilled by gradually occluding the venous return from the cannulae after releasing the snares from the caval vessels. The arterial cross clamp is removed and arterial perfusion is gradually stopped. Monitoring of CVP to return to values of 8–15 mmHg is performed. Mean arterial pressure is gradually returned to 90–110 mmHg. Donor whole blood is preferred to reinstitute adequate volume, but colloidal solutions may be administered if necessary. Rewarming should be gradual if hypothermia was used in the procedure.

Careful monitoring to return the animal to homeostasis using the parameters described in this section is essential and demonstration of normative cardiac output should be determined prior to closing the surgical incisions. If the pig is not responding to the weaning procedures, CPB should be reinstituted and the procedure retried after 10–15 minutes. Pulmonary hypertension and acute right-sided heart failure or irreversible ventricular fibrillation are the two most common causes of failure during weaning procedures. Returning to CPB or PA venting should be instituted as an immediate step while controlling this condition. Pulmonary vasoconstriction or clumping of blood products may be involved and should be treated if necessary (Cameron et al., 1992).

Treatment of cardiac arrhythmias may be required and the therapeutic protocols used are the same as for other species, with the exception of the species-specific considerations discussed under arrhythmias. In our experience, prophylactic treatment with bretylium 5 mg/kg iv every 30 minutes during the cardiac manipulations prevents most of the arrhythmias (Horneffer et al. 1986; Schumann et al., 1993; Swindle et al., 1986).

Postoperative Considerations

The postoperative considerations discussed in other sections of this text and for thoracotomies in Chapter 9 are applicable to these procedures. Postoperative recovery and return to homeostasis should be gradual and require at least hourly, if not continuous, monitoring for the first 6–24 hours. Close attention to thermoregulation and analgesia is as important as monitoring of the cardiovascular parameters. The use of intensive care cages with ECG, pulse oximetry, and blood pressure monitoring should be utilized. A team approach to recovery should include a veterinarian with experience in postoperative care for cardiothoracic procedures. Over time, the team members will be able to develop protocols for performing the procedures in their laboratories, and most of these procedures will become routine. Most swine that develop a righting reflex and can be extubated will recover and be able to eat the following day.

Analgesics

The use of analgesics should be routine in porcine surgical protocols. Preoperative or intraoperative use of analgesics prevents the pain reflex from being stimulated and reduces the postoperative recovery times. Combinations of local anesthetics infiltrated along the incision line combined with parenteral opioid analgesics and general anesthesia provide the most comprehensive prophylaxis. Postoperatively, the opioids may be combined with nonsteroidal antiinflammatory drugs (NSAIDs) in cases where the musculoskeletal component of the surgery is extensive. If proactive analgesic regimens are used, it may not be necessary to re-administer postoperative analgesia in cases of minor surgery and only for a few days with major surgical procedures (Jenkins, 1987; Smith and Swindle, 1994; Smith et al., 1997).

Opioids

Most of the opioid analgesics have relatively short half-lives in swine, which limits their usefulness in postoperative protocols (Blum, 1988; Flecknell, 1987; Swindle, 1991). Agents that have half-lives of less than 4 hours include fentanyl (0.05 mg/kg iv or im), sufentanil (0.005–0.010 mg/kg im or iv), meperidine (2–10 mg/kg im), oxymorphone (0.15 mg/kg im), morphine (2.2 mg/kg im), and pentazocine (1.5–3.0 mg/kg im). Morphine has been reported to cause excitement and other adverse behavioral patterns in swine. If these agents are used in opioid infusion protocols as described above, then they may be continued as the postoperative analgesic, as a gradually decreasing infusion. During the withdrawal phase from opioid infusions, some excitement or muscle rigidity may be encountered, which can be reversed by administration of acepromazine (0.5 mg/kg im) or diazepam (2–5 mg/kg im). Fentanyl patches have been tried for postoperative analgesia in swine; however, titration of the dosage may be difficult, and the patches must be secured to the skin with bandages to prevent their ingestion. It is possible to overdose animals with this dosage formulation; therefore, their use is not recommended over other agents discussed in this section.

Butorphanol (0.1–0.3 mg/kg im q.i.d.) and buprenorphine (0.05–0.1 mg/kg b.i.d.) are long acting and have few side effects in swine. Buprenorphine has been extensively used without significant respiratory depression noted in postoperative protocols, including thoracotomies. It should be considered one of the primary opioid analgesics used in porcine protocols (Hawk and Leary, 1995; Hermansen et al., 1986; Swindle, 1991).

NSAIDs

Traditional NSAIDs can be used in combination with opioids for balanced analgesia protocols involving muscular or orthopedic surgery. Some of the newer agents, however, are adequate for postoperative analgesia as sole agents. NSAIDs are associated with fewer platelets, renal function changes, and gastric ulceration. These effects are more pronounced with the older agents such as aspirin.

Phenylbutazone 10–20 mg/kg po b.i.d. and enteric-coated aspirin (10 mg/kg q.i.d.) may be used as adjuncts. Aspirin is also used for anticoagulation in some protocols as a daily dosage. Aspirin should be enteric coated to prevent gastric ulceration with chronic usage.

Ketaprofen (1–3 mg/kg po b.i.d. or t.i.d.) and ketorolac (1 mg/kg im or iv) are newer agents that may have some opioid-receptor activity. They provide adequate analgesia to be used as sole agents.

Local Analgesia

It is possible to use the local anesthetics to provide local, regional, and spinal analgesia. These procedures are not recommended in the research setting unless it is part of the protocol. Rather, they should be used as adjuncts to systemic analgesia. Long-acting agents, such as bupivicaine, can be used as dorsal nerve root blocks in the paravertebral region to provide analgesia for such vertical incisions as lateral thoracotomies. They can also be used to anesthetize the incision site locally or the peritoneum during general surgery in combination with parenteral agents. The difficulties associated with performing epidural blocks in swine (Chapter 10) make it a rarely indicated procedure in the research setting. Topical anesthetic patches have been developed that anesthetize skin as well as mucous membranes. These patches help relieve the distress caused by repeated vascular access needle punctures (Smith et al., 1997; Thurmon and Benson, 1996).

Commonly Recommended Protocols

Some of the commonly recommended protocols that have been routinely used in particular research settings are tabulated in this section. Please refer to more complete information within the description of the surgical procedure and the discussion of the classes of anesthetic agents within this chapter.

Nonsurvival Teaching Protocols

Induction
Ketamine 33 mg/kg im, acepromazine 1.1 mg/kg im, atropine 0.05 mg/kg im.

Maintenance
Thiopental 3–30 mg/kg/h iv infusion or pentobarbital 5–40 mg/kg/h iv infusion.

Comment
This protocol can be used for survival surgery if gas anesthesia is not available. Buprenorphine can be administered intraoperatively at 0.05 mg/kg im; however, it will decrease the amount of barbiturate required by approximately 50%.

General Surgery (without Physiologic Measurements)

Induction
Ketamine 33 mg/kg im, acepromazine 1.1 mg/kg im, atropine 0.05 mg/kg im.

Maintenance
Isoflurane 1.5%–2% in oxygen or 0.5%–1.5% in nitrous oxide: oxygen 2:1.

Comment
This protocol does not allow endotracheal intubation without administration of isoflurane via face mask during induction. Buprenorphine 0.05 mg/kg may be administered intraoperatively and may reduce the percentage of isoflurane required.

General Surgery (with Physiologic Measurements)

Induction
Isoflurane 3%–5% in oxygen via face mask.

Maintenance
Isoflurane 0.5%–1.5% in nitrous oxide:oxygen 2:1.

Comment
This is the simplest protocol that minimizes hemodynamic effects but provides sufficient analgesia and relaxation for major surgery. Following surgical manipulation and closure it is possible to minimize the administration of the inhalant. Buprenorphine 0.05 mg/kg can be administered intraoperatively after the measurements are made.

Cardiothoracic Surgery (with Cardiovascular Manipulations)

Induction
Ketamine 33 mg/kg im, isoflurane 3%–5% in oxygen via face mask.

Maintenance
Isoflurane 0.5%–1.5% in nitrous oxide:oxygen 2:1.

Adjunct Agents
Bretylium 5 mg/kg iv by slow injection every 30 minutes prior and during cardiac manipulation.

Comment
An emergency kit for cardiopulmonary emergencies and a defibrillator should be available.

Cardiothoracic Surgery (with Cardiovascular Compromise)

Induction
Start iv infusion with sufentanil 0.015 mg/kg/h (15 µg). Bolus 0.007 mg/kg (7 µg) iv 5 minutes after infusion is started. If relaxation is required to induce the iv, then administer ketamine 11 mg/kg im first.

Maintenance
Sufentanil 0.015–0.030 mg/kg/h (15–30 µg) iv infusion. Supplement with 0.5% isoflurane in oxygen if required for major surgical manipulations.

Adjunct Agents
Atropine 0.02 mg/kg iv may be required for bradycardia, which can be profound during the induction. Bretylium 5 mg/kg iv every 30 minutes during cardiac manipulation.

Comments
This protocol is useful for cardiopulmonary bypass procedures, especially if there is a predisposition for malignant hyperthermia. It is also useful as anesthesia for endoscopic thoracic surgery or coronary artery surgery in which bradycardia is required. The protocol minimizes the anesthetic effects on coronary blood flow and myocardial contractility. It has a protective antiarrhythmic effect during cardiovascular catheterization and electrophysiology studies. Acepromazine or diazepam may be required during the withdrawal phase of the protocol to counteract muscle tremors and rigidity. Other analgesics should not be administered until the iv infusion is decreased to less than 0.007 mg/kg/h (7 µg). A cardiopulmonary emergency drug kit should be available along with a defibrillator.

Coronary Artery Catheterization

Induction
Ketamine 33 mg/kg im followed by mask induction with isoflurane 3%–5%.

Maintenance
Isoflurane 0.5%–1.5% in nitrous oxide:oxygen 2:1.

Adjunct Agents
The last meal prior to induction of anesthesia animals are administered dilti-

azem 4 mg/kg and aspirin 1 mg/kg po. Bretylium 5 mg/kg iv and heparin 200 IU/kg are administered iv prior to introducing the catheter into the coronary artery. A slow 200-μg infusion of nitroglycerin is administered at the aortic root prior to introducing the catheter.

Comment
If stents are implanted, anticoagulant therapy may have to be administered postoperatively. Buprenorphine 0.05 mg/kg may be administered intraoperatively.

General Physiologic Effects of Anesthetics

The general physiologic effects of common anesthetic agents is summarized below for reference when designing protocols for particular research projects. Combining agents between classes may cause different effects. All effects are dose dependent and may vary among breeds (Benharkate et al., 1993). The information is summarized from Heavner (1994) and Smith et al. (1997). A complete discussion, by multiple authors, of the physiologic effects of anesthetics and analgesics in all laboratory animals is available in Kohn et al. (1997).

Dissociative Agents

Bronchodilation, tachycardia, increased cardiac output, increased blood pressure, increased circulating catecholamines
1. Ketamine
   Prolongs myocardial refractory period, peripheral and coronary vasodilation, increased pulmonary artery vascular resistance, increased cerebral blood flow, poor analgesia
2. Tiletamine/zolazepam (Telazol)
   Mild myocardial depression, respiratory depression, persistent hypothermia, contraindicated in renal disease and cardiovascular compromise, poor analgesia

Barbiturates

1. Thiobarbiturates
   Depressed cardiopulmonary function, decreased cerebral blood flow and intracranial pressure, decreased myocardial contractility, respiratory depression, minimal effects on peripheral vascular resistance, excreted by kidneys
2. Pentobarbital
   Respiratory depression, decreased myocardial contractility and cardiac output, increased peripheral vascular resistance, decreased cerebral blood flow, decreased hematocrit, metabolized by liver

Sedatives

1. Phenothiazines (acepromazine)
   Hypotension, alpha adrenergic blockage, vasodilation, decreased systemic vascular resistance, reduced sensitivity to circulating catecholamines, cardiac output and heart rate not significantly affected
2. Butyrophenones (azaperone, droperidol)
   Extrapyramidal activity due to GABA blockade, hypotension, decreased cardiac output and heart rate, some antiarrhythmic activity
3. Benzodiazepines (zolazepam, diazepam, midazolam)
   Decreased catecholamine release, increased coronary blood flow, slight cardiovascular effects unless combined with opioids (synergistic effect with severe cardiodepression)
4. α-2-adrenergic agonists (xylazine, medetomidine, detomidine)
   Bradycardia, first- to third-degree heart block, decreased cardiac output, increased central venous pressure, hypotension, decreased myocardial contractility, increased susceptibility to catecholamines and arrhythmias, vasoconstriction, transient analgesia

Opioids

Decreased cerebral blood flow, respiratory depression, minimal cardiovascular effects, increased coronary blood flow, slight decrease in peripheral vascular resistance, depressed catecholamine response, bradycardia

Inhalant Anesthetics

All agents increase cerebral blood flow and cerebrospinal fluid, depress ventilation, depress oxygen consumption, produce hypercapnia, induce bronchodilation

1. Isoflurane
   Decreased systemic vascular resistance, little effect on heart rate, unchanged coronary blood flow and cardiac output, little circulating catecholamine sensitivity, least effect on cardiac output, circulating catecholamines, best tissue perfusion
2. Halothane
   Decreased cardiac output, myocardial depression, depressed baroreceptor reflexes, peripheral vascular resistance unchanged, greatest effects on catecholamine sensitivity
3. Enflurane
   Associated with seizures, more cardiodepressant than halothane and isoflurane, decreases blood pressure, decreases cardiac output and decreases systemic vascular resistance

4. Methoxyflurane
   Decreased cardiac output, decreased blood pressure, decreased systemic vascular resistance, most metabolized and most renal effects, most hepatic defluorination
5. Nitrous Oxide
   Unacceptable as sole agent, slight cardiodepression

Drug Dosages of Anesthetic Agents

Miscellaneous Drugs

Antiarrhythmics
   1. Bretylium tosylate 3.0–5.0 mg/kg iv every 30 minutes
   2. Lidocaine 2–4 mg/kg iv 50 µg/kg/min continuous iv infusion

Calcium Channel Blockers
   1. Diltiazem 2–4 mg/kg po t.i.d.
   2. Verapamil 0.15 mg/kg, treat supraventricular tachycardia

Paralytic Agents
   1. Pancuronium 0.02–0.15 mg/kg iv
   2. Vercuronium 1.0 mg/kg iv
   3. Succinylcholine 1.1 mg/kg iv

Coronary Vasorelaxant
   Nitroglycerine 200 µg diluted in 2 ml saline and infused slowly into coronary sinus

Anticholinergic
   1. Treat bradycardia, heart block
   2. Atropine 0.05 mg/kg im, 0.02 mg/kg iv

Malignant Hyperthermia Treatment and Prophylaxis
   Dantrolene 5 mg/kg iv

Ketamine Combinations

   1. Ketamine11–33 mg/kg im
      10–33 mg/kg/h iv infusion
   2. Ketamine 33 mg/kg and acetylpromazine 1.1 mg/kg im
   3. Ketamine 20 mg/kg and xylazine 2 mg/kg im
   4. Ketamine 11 mg/kg and fentanyl/droperidol (InnovarVet) 1 ml/14 kg im
   5. Ketamine 2 mg/kg and xylazine 2 mg/kg and oxymorphone 0.075 mg/kg iv (2× dose for im)

6. Ketamine 15 mg/kg and azaperone 2 mg/kg im
7. Ketamine 20 mg/kg and diazepam 2 mg/kg im
8. Ketamine 33 mg/kg and midazolam 500 μg/kg im
9. Ketamine 33 mg/kg/h and midazolam 1.5 mg/kg/h continuous iv infusion
10. Ketamine 20 mg/kg and climazolam 0.5–1 mg/kg
11. Ketamine 1 mg/ml and xylazine 1 mg/ml and glyceryl guaiacolate (guaifenesin) 5% in 5% dextrose 1 ml/kg iv bolus followed by 1 ml/kg/h
12. Ketamine 1 mg/kg and medetomidine 0.1 mg/kg

Barbiturates

1. Pentobarbital 20–40 mg/kg, 5–40 mg/kg/h iv infusion
2. Thiopental 6.6–30 mg/kg, 3–30 mg/kg/h iv infusion
3. Thiamylal 6.6–30 mg/kg, 3–30 mg/kg/h iv infusion

Miscellaneous Anesthetic Agents

1. α-Chloralose 55–100 mg/kg
2. Etorphine/acetylpromazine (Imobilon) 0.245 mg/10 kg reversed by diprenorphine (Revivon) 0.3 mg/kg
3. Meperidine 1 mg/lb and azaperone 1 mg/lb followed in 20 minutes by ketamine 10 mg/lb and morphine 1 mg/lb
4. Midazolam (Versed) 100–500 μg/kg im or iv; 0.6–1.5 mg/kg/h iv infusion
5. Tiletamine:zolazepam (Telazol) 2–8.8 mg/kg im
6. Telazol 4.4 mg/kg and xylazine 4.4 mg/kg im
7. Telazol 4.4 mg/kg and xylazine 2.2 mg/kg: butorphanol 0.22 mg/kg im
8. Telazol 4.4 mg/kg and xylazine 2.2 mg/kg and azaperone 0.88 mg/kg im
9. Azaperone 2–8 mg/kg im
10. Naloxone 0.5–2 mg/kg iv
11. Diazepam 0.5–10 mg/kg im; 0.44–2 mg/kg iv
12. Brontizolam 1–10 mg/kg po
13. Lorazepam 0.1 mg/kg iv
14. Climazolam 0.5–1 mg/kg im
15. Flurazepam 2 mg/kg iv or po
16. Xylazine 0.2 mg/kg im
17. Etomidate 4–8 mg/kg iv
18. Metomidate 4 mg/kg iv
19. Alphaxolone/alphadolone 6–8 mg/kg im followed by 2–3 mg/kg iv infusion
20. Etomidate 4–8 mg/kg iv/azaperone 2 mg/kg im
21. Etomidate 0.6 mg/kg iv followed by 10 mg/kg/h ketamine iv infusion
22. Atropine 0.05 mg/kg im; 0.02 mg/kg iv
23. Glycopyrrolate 0.004–0.01 mg/kg im

24. Propofol 0.83–1.66 mg/kg iv followed by 14–20 mg/kg/h

Treatment of Intraoperative Cardiac Arrhythmias

Atrial Fibrillation

1. Leads to ventricular tachycardia followed by ventricular fibrillation or standstill
2. Give 2–4 mg/kg bolus of lidocaine without epinephrine followed by continuous iv drip (50 µg/kg/min) if animal has been pretreated with bretylium. This treatment of this transient introperative arrhythmia is to prevent the ventricular complications.

Ventricular Fibrillation or Standstill

1. 10-joule countershock internal paddles/200 joules for external paddles
2. 10–20 mEq bolus of sodium bicarbonate followed by iv drip
3. If no response, 1–2 ml of 1:10,000 epinephrine and lidocaine or bretylium if not pretreated
4. Defibrillator more effective than drugs

Bradycardia

Give atropine .05mg/kg

Prevention of Arrhythmias Associated with Vasoconstriction

1. Calcium channel blocker diltiazem 2–4 mg/kg po t.i.d.
2. Nitroglycerine 200 µg diluted into 2 ml saline iv infusion
3. Bretylium 3.0–5.0 mg/kg iv

Miscellaneous Cardioactive Drugs

1. Aminophylline 5 mg/kg, bronchodilation, tachycardia
2. Digoxin 0.01–0.04 mg/kg, treat atrial arrhythmias, congestive heart failure
3. Dopamine 2–20 µg/kg/min hypotension, cardiogenic shock
4. Dobutamine 12.5–10 µg/kg/min heart failure, cardiogenic shock
5. Epinephrine 0.5–2 ml of 1:10,000 solution, asystole, decreased left ventricular function
6. Propranolol 0.04–0.06 mg/kg, treat uncontrolled tachycardia
7. Isoproterenol 0.01 µg/kg/min, treat AV block, sinus bradycardia, bronchodilator
8. Na Nitroprusside 0.5–0.8 µg/kg/min, treat hypertension

9. Neosynephrine 0.05–0.1 mg/kg iv, treat hypertension with vasocon-striction
10. Warfarin (Coumadin) 0.04–0.08 mg/kg po s.i.d., anticoagulation
11. Indomethacin 50 mg rectal suppository 1–2 s.i.d., prevent platelet clumping after cardiopulmonary bypass (CPB)

Postoperative Analgesia

Signs of pain are incisional pain, abnormal posture, or abnormal behavior.

Drugs
1. Fentanyl 0.02–0.05 mg/kg im (30–100 µg/kg/h iv drip)
2. Sufentanil 5–10 µg/kg im (10–15 µg/kg/h iv drip)
3. Meperidine 10 mg/kg
4. Pentazocine 1.5–3.0 mg/kg im
5. Oxymorphone 0.15 mg/kg im
6. Butorphanol 0.1–0.3 mg/kg im
7. Buprenorphine 0.05–0.1 im every 8–12 hours
8. Continuous iv drip with opioids
9. Local blocks of lateral incisions
10. Aspirin 10–20 mg/kg po q.i.d.
11. Phenylbutazone 4–8 mg/kg po
12. Ketaprofen 1–3 mg/kg b.i.d. po
13. Ketorolac 1 mg/kg im or b.i.d. po

References

Anderson, I.L. 1976. Porcine malignant hyperthermia: Effect of dantrolene sodium on in-vitro halothane-induced contracture of susceptible muscle. Anesthesiology 44(1): 57–60.

Benharkate, M., V. Zanini, R. Blanc, O. Boucheix, F. Coyez, J.P. Genevois, and M. Pairet. 1993. Hemodynamic parameters of anesthetized pigs: A comparative study of farm piglets and Göttingen and Yucatan miniature swine. Lab. Anim. Sci. 43(1): 68–72.

Benson, G.J., and J.C. Thurmon. 1979. Anesthesia of swine under field conditions. J. Am. Vet. Med. Assoc. 174(6): 594–596.

Blum, J.R. 1988. Laboratory animal anesthesia. In Swindle, M.M., and Adams, R.J. (eds), Experimental Surgery and Physiology: Induced Animal Models of Human Disease. Baltimore: Williams and Wilkins, pp. 329–345.

Boschert, K., P.A. Flecknell, R.T. Fosse, T. Framstad, M. Ganter, U. Sjøstrand, J. Stevens, and J. Thurmon. 1996. Ketamine and its use in the pig. Lab. Anim. 30(2): 209–219.

Cameron, D.E., K.M. Tam, W. Cheng, and M. Braxton. 1992. Studies in the physiology of cardiopulmonary bypass using a swine model. In Swindle, M.M. (ed), Swine as Models in Biomedical Research. Ames: Iowa State University Press, pp. 185–196.

Cantor, G.H, D.B. Brunson, and T.W. Reibold. 1981. A comparison of four short-acting anesthetic combinations for swine. Vet. Med. Sm. Anim. Clin. 76(5): 715–720.

Eger, E., B. Johnson, R. Weiskopf, M. Holmes, N. Yasuda, A. Targ, and I. Rampil. 1988.

Minimum alveolar concentration of I-653 and isoflurane in pigs: Definition of a supramaximal stimulus. Anesth. Analg. 67(12): 1174–1176.

Ehler, W.J., J.W. Mack, D.L. Brown, and R.F. David. 1985. Avoidance of malignant hyperthermia in a porcine model for experimental open heart surgery. Lab. Anim. Sci. 35(2): 172–175.

Eisele, P.H., L. Talken, and J.H. Eisele. 1985. Potency of isoflurane and nitrous oxide in conventional swine. Lab. Anim. Sci. 35(1): 76–78.

Eisele, P.H., E.S. Woodle, G.C. Hunter, L. Talken, and R.E. Ward. 1986. Anesthetic, preoperative and postoperative considerations for liver transplantation in swine. Lab. Anim. Sci. 36(4): 402–405.

Flecknell, P.A. 1996. Laboratory Animal Anaesthesia, 2nd ed. New York: Academic Press.

Flecknell, P.J. 1997. Medetomidine and antipamezole: Potential uses in laboratory animals. Lab. Anim. 26(2): 21–25.

Foster, P.S., K.C. Hopkinson, and M.A. Denborough. 1992. Propofol anaesthesia in malignant hyperpyrexia susceptible swine. Clin. Exp. Pharmacol. Physiol. 19(3): 183–186.

Geers, R., C. Decanniere, H. Ville, P. Van Hecke, V. Goedseels, L. Bosschaerts, J. Deley, S. Janssens, and W. Nierynck. 1992. Identification of halothane gene carriers by use of an in vivo 3IP nuclear magnetic resonance spectroscopy in pigs. Am. J. Vet. Res. 53(9): 1711–1714.

Hawk, C.T., and S.L. Leary. 1995. Formulary for Laboratory Animals. Ames: Iowa State University Press.

Heavner, J.E. 1994. Physiologic effects of anesthetic and analgesics. In Smith, A.C., and Swindle, M.M. (eds), Research Animal Anesthesia, Analgesia, and Surgery. Greenbelt, MD: Scientists Center for Animal Welfare, pp. 41–58.

Hermansen, K., L.E. Pedersen, and H.O. Olesen. 1986. The analgesic effect of buprenorphine, etorphine and pethidine in the pig: A randomized double blind crossover study, Acta Pharmacol. Toxicol. 59(1): 27–35.

Holzchuh, M.P., and E. Cremonesi. 1991. Anaesthesia in pigs. Analysis of azaperone and etomidate effects separately and in associations. Utrecht: The Netherlands, Proceedings of the Fourth International Congress of Veterinary Anaesthesia, pp. 197–200.

Horneffer, P.J., V.J. Gott, and T.J. Gardner. 1986. Swine as a cardiac surgical model. In Tumbleson, M.E. (ed), Swine in Biomedical Research, Vol. 1. New York: Plenum Press, pp. 321–326.

Houde, A., S.A. Pomnier, and R. Roy. 1993. Detection of the Ryanodine receptor mutation associated with malignant hyperthermia in purebred swine populations. J. Anim. Sci. 71(6): 1414–1418.

Jenkins, W.L. 1987. Pharmacologic aspects of analgesic drugs in animals: An overview. J. Am. Vet. Med. Assoc. 191(10): 1231–1240.

Ko, J.C.H., B.L. Williams, C.J. McGrath, C.E. Short, and E.R. Rogers. 1997. Comparison of anesthetic effects of Telazol-xylazine-xylazine, Telazol-xylazine-butorphanol, and Telazol-xylazine-azaperone combinations in swine. Contemp. Topics Lab. Anim. Sci. 35(5): 71–74.

Ko, J.C.H., B.L. Williams, V.L. Smith, C.J. McGrath, and J.D. Jacobson. 1993. Comparison of Telazol, Telazol–ketamine, Telazol–xylazine and Telazol–ketamine–xylazine as chemical restraint and anesthetic induction combination in swine. Lab. Anim. Sci. 43(5): 476–480.

Koblin, D.D., R.B. Weiskopf, M.A. Holmes, K. Konopka, I.J. Rampil, E.I. Eger, and L. Waskell. 1989. Metabolism of I-653 and isoflurane in swine. Anesth. Analg. 68(2): 147–149.

Kohn, D.H., S.K. Wixson, W.J. White, and G.J. Benson (eds). 1997. Anesthesia and Analgesia in Laboratory Animals. New York: Academic Press, pp. 313–336.

Lundeen, G., M. Manohar, and C. Parks. 1983. Systemic distribution of blood flow in swine while awake and during 1.0 and 1.5 MAC isoflurane anesthesia with or without 50% nitrous oxide, Anesth. Analg. 62(5): 499–512.

Lunn, J.K. T.H. Stanley, J. Eisele, L. Webster, and A. Woodard. 1979. High dose fentanyl anesthesia for coronary artery surgery: Plasma fentanyl concentrations and influence of nitrous oxide on cardiovascular responses. Anesth. Analg. 58(5): 390–395.

Merin, R.G., P.D. Verdouw, and J.W. deJong. 1982. Myocardial functional and metabolic responses to ischemia in swine during halothane and fentanyl anesthesia, Anesthesiology 56(2): 84–92.

Ochs, H.R., D.J. Greenblatt, W. Eichelkraut, C. Bakker, R. Gobel, and N. Hahn. 1987. Hepatic vs. gastrointestinal presystemic extraction of oral midazolam and flurazepam. J. Pharmacol. Exp. Ther. 243(3): 852–856.

Portier, D.B., and C.A. Slusser. 1985. Azaperone: A review of a new neuroleptic agent for swine. Vet. Med. 80(3): 88–92.

Purohit, D.M., M.M. Swindle, C.D. Smith, H.B. Othersen Jr., and J.M. Kazanovicz. 1993. Hanford miniature swine model for extracoporeal membrane oxygenation (ECMO). J. Invest. Surg. 6(6): 503–508.

Qayumi, A.K., W.R.E. Jamieson, A. Poostizadeh, E. German, and K.D. Gillespie. 1992. Comparison of new iron chelating agents in the prevention of ischemia/reperfusion injury: A swine model of heart–lung transplantation. J. Invest. Surg. 5(2): 115–128.

Raff, M. and G. Harrison. 1989. The screening of propofol in MHS swine. Anesth. Analg. 68(6): 750–751.

Ramsey, D.E., N. Aldred, and J.M. Power. 1993. A simplified approach to the anesthesia of porcine laparoscopic surgical subjects. Lab. Anim. Sci. 43(4): 336–337.

Riebold, T.W., D.R. Geiser, and D.O. Goble. 1995. Large Animal Anesthesia: Principles and Techniques, 2nd ed. Ames: Iowa State University Press.

Schumann, R.E., M. Harold, P.C. Gillette, M.M. Swindle, and C.H. Gaymes. 1993. Prophylactic treatment of swine with bretylium for experimental cardiac catheterization. Lab. Anim. Sci. 43(3): 244–246.

Schumann, R.E., M.M. Swindle, B.J. Knick, C.L. Case, and P.C. Gillette. 1994. High dose narcotic anesthesia using sufentanil in swine for cardiac catheterization and electrophysiologic studies. J. Invest. Surg. 7(3): 243–248.

Silverman, J, and W.W. Muir III. 1993. A review of lab animal anesthesia with chloral hydrate and chloralose. Lab. Anim. Sci. 43(3): 210–216.

Smith, A. C., and M. M. Swindle (eds). 1994. Research Animal Anesthesia, Analgesia and Surgery. Greenbelt, MD: Scientist's Center for Animal Welfare.

Smith, A. C., J.L. Zellner, F.G. Spinale, and M.M. Swindle. 1991. Sedative and cardiovascular effects of midazolam in swine. Lab. Anim. Sci. 41(2): 157–161.

Smith, A.C., W. Ehler, and M.M. Swindle. 1997. Anesthesia and analgesia in swine. In Kohn, D.H., Wixson, S.K., White, W.J., Benson, G.J. (eds), Anesthesia and Analgesia in Laboratory Animals. New York: Academic Press, pp. 313–336

Svendsen, P. and A.M. Carter. 1997. Bloodgas tensions, acid–base status and cardiovascular function in miniature swine anesthetized with halothane and methoxyflurane or intravenous metomiolate hydrochloride. Pharmacol. Toxicol. 64(1): 88–93.

Swan, H., and D.M. Meagher. 1971. Total body bypass in miniature pigs. J. Thorac. Cardiovasc. Surg. 61(6): 956–967.

Swindle, M.M. 1983. Basic Surgical Exercises Using Swine. Philadelphia: Praeger Press.

Swindle, M.M. 1991. Anesthetic and Perioperative Techniques in Swine. Andover, MA: Charles River Laboratories, Inc.

Swindle, M.M., P.J. Horneffer, T.J. Gardner, V.L. Gott, T.S. Hall, R.S. Stuart, W.A. Baumgartner, A.M. Borkon, E. Galloway, and B.A. Reitz. 1986. Anatomic and anesthetic considerations in experimental cardiopulmonary surgery in swine. Lab. Anim. Sci. 36(4): 357–361.

Thurmon, J.C., and G.J. Benson (eds). 1996. Lumb and Jones Veterinary Anesthesia, 3rd ed. Baltimore: Williams and Wilkins.

Thurmon, J.C., and W.J. Tranquilli. 1986. Anesthesia for cardiovascular research. In Stanton, H.C., and Mersmann, H.J. (eds), Swine in Cardiovascular Research, Vol. 1. Boca Raton, FL: CRC Press, pp. 39–59

Thurmon, J.C., W.J. Tranquilli, and G.J. Benson. 1986. Cardiopulmonary responses of swine to intravenous infusion of guaifenesin, ketamine, and xylazine. Am. J. Vet. Res. 47(10): 2138–2140.

Tranquilli, W.J., J.C. Thurmon, G.J. Benson, and E.P. Steffey. 1983. Halothane potency in pigs (*Sus scrofa*). Am. J. Vet. Res. 44(6): 1106–1107.

Tranquilli, W.J., J.C. Thurman, and G.J. Benson. 1985. Anesthetic potency of nitrous oxide in young swine (*Sus scrofa*), Am. J. Vet. Res. 46(1): 58–60.

Vainio, O.M., B.C. Bloor, and C. Kim. 1992. Cardiovascular effects of a ketamine–medetomidine combination that produces deep sedation in Yucatan mini swine. Lab. Anim. Sci. 42(6): 582–588.

Weiskopf, R.B., M.A. Holmes, E.I. Eger II, N. Yasuda, I.J. Rampil, B.H. Johnson, A.G. Targ, I.A. Reid, and L.C. Keil. 1992. Use of swine in the study of anesthetics. In Swindle, M.M. (ed), Swine as Models in Biomedical Research. Ames: Iowa State University Press, pp. 96–117.

Worek, F.S, G. Blumel, J. Zeravik, G.J. Zimmerman, and U.J. Pfeiffer. 1988. Comparison of ketamine and pentobarbital anesthesia with the conscious state in a porcine model of *Pseudomonas aeruginosa* septicemia, Acta Anaesthiol. Scand. 32(7): 509–515.

Addendum to Analgesics

Buprenorphine

Some confusion exists concerning the wide dosage ranges of buprenophine that have been reported as used in swine (0.005–0.1 mg/kg im). In our experience lower dosages (0.005–0.01 mg/kg) do not provide prolonged analgesia for major surgical interventions. The lower dose range may be useful for preemptive analgesia or in combination with other agents. A recent publication indicates that 0.01 mg/kg or higher dosages q 8–12 h provides postoperative analgesia for a significant number of pigs (Rodriguez, et al., 2001).

Fentanyl Transdermal Patches

Experience has demonstrated that transdermal fentanyl patches may be highly variable in their efficacy in swine. Variables include breed, age, site of application, presence of moisture or heat on the patch, and type of procedure. It is possible to overdose swine with these patches, especially if they ingest them. In Yucatan miniature pigs 17–22 kg 100 μg/hr patches provided therapeutic levels, which peaked at 42–48 hours after application. Lower dosages (25–50 μg/hr patches) may be required for farm breeds, which tend to be younger at the same body weight and have thinner skin than minipigs (Wilkinson, et al., 2001). Clinical monitoring for signs of overdosage is essential.

Epidural Morphine

Morphine epidural solution 0.1 mg/kg administered preoperatively is effective for analgesia for abdominal procedures.

Carprophen

Carprophen 2–3 mg/kg PO, BID may be used for post operative analgesia.

Additional References

Rodriguez, N.A., D.M. Cooper, J.M. Risdahl. 2001. Antinociecptive activity of and clinical experience with buprenorphine in swine. Contemporary Topics in Lab. Anim. Sci. 40(3): 17–20.

Wilkinson A.C., M.L. Thomas III, B.C. Morse. 2001. Evaluation of a transdermal fentanyl system in Yucatan miniature pigs. Contemporary Topics in Lab. Anim. Sci. 40(3): 12–16.

3 WOUND CLOSURE AND INTEGUMENT

General Principles and Surgical Preparation

The pig is a relatively hairless animal with a fixed skin that is tightly attached to the subcutaneous tissues similar to that in humans. The cutaneous blood supply and sequence of events in wound healing are also similar to that in humans. However, the skin of the pig is thicker and less vascular overall than human skin. There are also differences in the accessory tissues, such as the lack of apocrine sweat glands and the presence of an intrafollicular muscle in swine (Fig. 3.1).

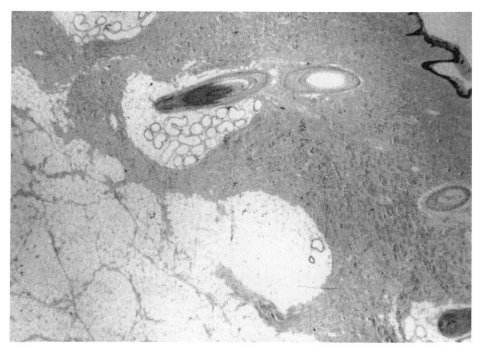

FIGURE 3.1   Histologic section of normal pigskin (×100, Hematoxylin and Eosin stain).

The pig has been used extensively as a model for superficial and deep wound healing and plastic surgical techniques, and it has been developed as a model of dermal toxicity (Bolton et al., 1988; Chvapil and Chvapil, 1992; Kerrigan et al., 1986; Mertz et al., 1986; Riviere et al., 1986; Monteiro-Riviere, 1986; Monteiro-Riviere and Riviere, 1996; Ordman and Gillman, 1966).

Any standard method of aseptic preparation of the skin for humans or other species may be applied to the pig. None of these methods ensures a completely sterile environment on the skin, and, consequently, skin contact with other organs and tissues should be minimized when performing surgery in body cavities. The methodology preferred in the author's laboratories is described here.

Swine are cleaned of gross contamination from the total body in a separate surgical prep room for animals. The area of surgical intervention is clipped with electric clippers and in some cases is shaved. The skin is scrubbed three times with iodine surgical scrub and rinsed with alcohol. The animal is then transported to the operating room where a sterile preparation of iodine prep solution is applied using sponge forceps and sterile sponges. In most cases, the iodine solution is removed with alcohol and the skin dried with sterile gauze sponges. A transparent iodine-impregnated adhesive drape is applied over the dry skin. If the iodine-impregnated drape is not used, as for some minor procedures, the last solution of iodine remains on the skin. The adhesive iodine-impregnated drapes work well on swine and provide protection from contamination of tissues and organs by the skin after the incision is made because they adhere to the edges of the incision if the skin preparation has been performed as described above (Fig. 3.2).

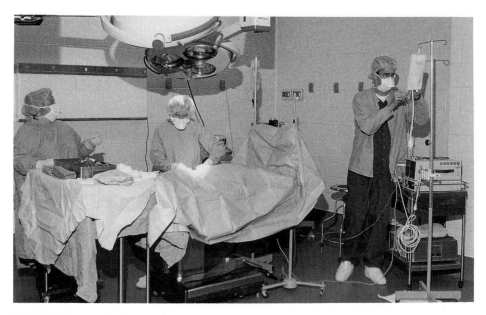

FIGURE 3.2   Pig draped for aseptic surgery.

The principles of surgery are the same for swine as they are for other species. Careful attention to hemostasis, atraumatic handling of tissues, proper use of surgical instruments, closure of dead space and aseptic technique will minimize complications associated with surgery (Ethicon, 1988; Swindle, 1983).

Suture Selection for Wound Closure

Selection of the appropriate size and type of suture material is important for the prevention of postoperative complications. In general, the suture material should not cause reactions that may impede healing and should be of the smallest appropriate size to provide appropriate wound closure. If too many sutures are placed or if the suture is much larger than necessary, it overloads the region with foreign material and may cause regional ischemia or create an inappropriate foreign body reaction. These generalities depend upon the region in which the suture is implanted and the type of suture material. It is beyond the purpose of this text to provide an instruction manual for beginning techniques in surgery or for a discussion of all of the aspects of suture selection. However, a technical training book is available detailing beginning surgical techniques in swine (Swindle, 1983), and a complete discussion of the principles of suture selection and wound healing are also available (Ethicon, 1988).

Selection of the appropriate-sized suture material is subjective and depends upon the experience of the surgeon. Several examples based upon experience may be of value in that selection and are listed here. When closing incisions in 25-kg swine, the selection of 2/0 suture for closure of the muscle layers and 3/0 suture for closure of the subcutaneous, subcuticular or skin layers works well. If closing the same incision in 50-kg swine, selection of 0 or 1 suture for the muscle layers, 2/0 suture for subcutaneous layers, and 3/0 suture for the subcuticular or skin layer would be appropriate.

One way of classifying suture material is whether the material is absorbable or nonabsorbable. Another classification would be whether the suture is manufactured from synthetic or natural materials. Other classifications based upon manufacturing techniques include braided or monofilament and coated or noncoated. Generally sutures that are braided are manufactured to provide greater strength, and ones that are coated materials are to prevent reactions and to delay absorption. Selection of the type of material and the intended usage will also dictate the number of throws required in the surgical knot, with the coated or monofilament sutures usually requiring more than three throws (Ethicon, 1988).

Synthetic sutures of either absorbable or nonabsorbable material work well depending upon the surgical incision that is being closed. Silk, linen, cotton, and gut are natural materials that should not be routinely used to close surgical wounds in swine. All of these materials are reactive and may lead to inappropriate bodily responses, such as seromas, which may impede wound healing. Use of these materials should be a special circumstance dictated by the protocol.

Absorbable materials that have been routinely used without complications include the following synthetics: polydiaxonone, polyglycolic acid, polyglactin 910, polyglyconate, lactomer 9-1. Nonabsorbable materials routinely used have included nylon, polyester, polypropylene, polyamide, polytetraflurethylene, polyglecaprone 25, stainless steel. This list is not all inclusive, and, as a general rule, the synthetic manufactured materials developed in recent years have all proved to be safe and effective.

Both absorbable and nonabsorbable surgical staples have been developed, and staple surgical techniques greatly increase the speed of wound closure. These devices are essential in endoscopic surgical techniques. However, closure of the skin of animals with staples provides some opportunities for complications that are not as likely to occur with suture materials. Staples may be caught on cages and may hold contaminants, such as hair or feces, close to the skin incision more readily than some suturing techniques. These problems can be minimized by caging and bandaging procedures; however, the surgeon should be aware of their potential occurrence prior to selecting staples for skin closure.

Wound Closure and Bandaging Techniques

The same suture patterns and techniques that are used for wound closure for other species are applicable to the pig. Bandaging techniques are somewhat species specific and will be described in this section with a brief review of wound closure techniques (Smith and Swindle, 1994). Specific closures for areas, such as the abdomen or thorax, and suture techniques for visceral organs are discussed in the appropriate chapters of this text.

Closure of a wound should be performed in anatomically correct layers. Either simple interrupted or continuous sutures can be used on internal layers, such as peritoneum, muscle, and subcutaneous tissues (Figs. 3.3 and 3.4). Simple interrupted sutures provide more security but increase the foreign material load that is implanted and may provide uneven tension in a given layer because of variability between the individual sutures. Care must be taken when using continuous sutures to close these layers, because an improperly tied knot at either end of the suture line can lead to dehiscence of the wound. The distance between the suture insertions will depend upon the type of tissue, type of suture, and skill of the surgeon. Generally speaking, the suture placement should approximate the edges of the wound in an anatomically correct fashion without placing undue tension on the suture line and while making sure that the closure does not leave dead space that may lead to seromas or pockets of infection.

Thin muscle layers can be closed with a suture pattern that penetrates the full thickness of the muscle. Thick muscles can be closed with the external fascia only, as that is the layer that provides the strength for holding the sutures. Fat does not hold sutures and must be approximated with the subcutaneous

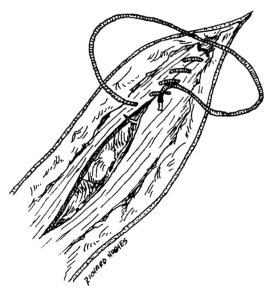

FIGURE 3.3   Closure of muscle layers for an abdominal incision.

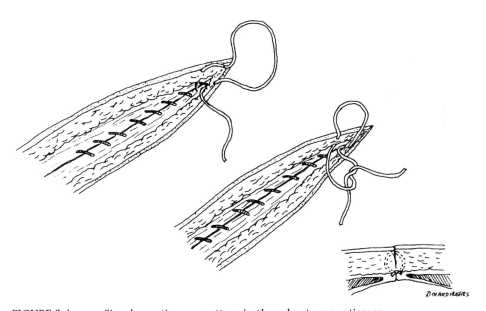

FIGURE 3.4   Simple continuous pattern in the subcutaneous tissues.

layers. The subcutaneous layers are generally closed with a continuous suture pattern. In addition to closing dead space, this layer reduces the tension that must be applied to the skin sutures (Figs. 3.3 and 3.4).

Problems with closure of abdominal or subcutaneous incisions may be encountered in large swine because of excess fat deposition. Use of a rubber surgical retractor (surgical fish) to hold abdominal tissues in situ during closure of the peritoneal and initial muscle layers is recommended. These devices can be removed through the small opening when the last few sutures are ready to be placed. Fat deposition also makes the area greasy and suture materials difficult to tie. Horizontal mattress sutures may have to be placed in the muscle layers of large animals for tension relief on the suture line.

The skin must be approximated with a minimal amount of tension, because it swells during the healing process; too tight a closure will cause irritation and secondary cutting of the skin. The ideal closure for pigskin is subcuticular suture with buried knots using 3/0 absorbable synthetic suture (Fig. 3.5). If the knot is buried at both ends, it provides a cosmetic closure with minimal complications. Simple interrupted sutures (Fig. 3.6) may be used to close the skin

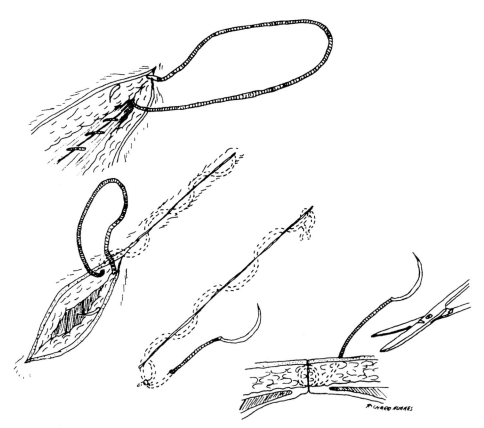

FIGURE 3.5   Subcuticular suture pattern with the knot buried at both ends.

using 3/0 synthetic nonabsorbable suture. As a general rule, simple interrupted sutures should be placed 5 mm from the skin edges with approximately 5–10 mm between sutures. Horizontal mattress sutures (Fig. 3.7) may be used outside the suture line as tension-relief sutures on long incision lines, but should not be used as the primary skin closure pattern. Vertical mattress sutures (Fig. 3.8) can be used to give a secure cosmetic closure if an eversion pattern is desired. Skin staples can be problematic for the reasons described above. Continuous suture patterns are best not used for routine closure of skin, but may be acceptable in some situations related to the research (Fig. 3.9).

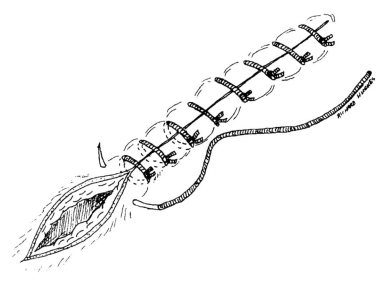

FIGURE 3.6   Simple interrupted skin suture pattern.

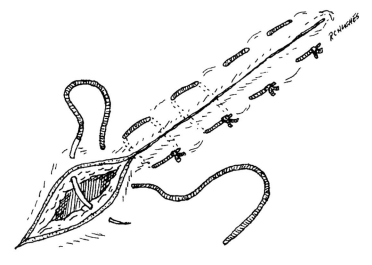

FIGURE 3.7   Horizontal mattress suture pattern in the skin.

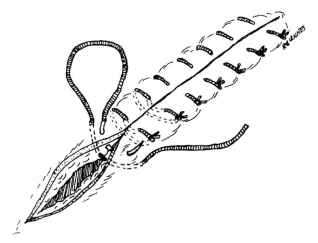

FIGURE 3.8   Vertical mattress suture pattern in the skin.

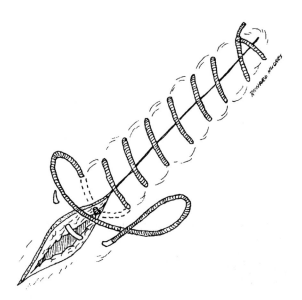

FIGURE 3.9   Continuous suture pattern in the skin.

If the skin closure is not anatomically correct, and there is an eversion or outpouching of the skin at the end of the suture line due to uneven closure, corrective measures should be taken. Cutting through the outpouching at a 45-degree angle and placing a few simple interrupted sutures will usually correct most situations. The suture line should not be placed over subcutaneously implanted devices. It is best to have the suture line either caudal or cranial to the device rather than dorsal or ventral. This prevents undue tension on the suture line from the weight or pressure of the device.

Bandaging of the incision may be indicated in some situations, including large incisions under tension, implantation of subcutaneous devices, suture lines that are likely to be contaminated from urine or feces, and incisions that are placed in areas that the animal is likely to irritate. The use of topical spray bandages provides a short-term seal of the skin incision and is a good idea for most incisions. Bandages should be changed every 1–2 days or if they become contaminated with moisture, urine, or feces.

The pig should be bandaged in a circumferential fashion for incisions on the trunk and neck. Nonadhesive self-adhering bandage material can be used after placing sterile gauze pads to protect the suture line; however, these are easily removed by the animal after recovery. If they are used, the cranial and caudal ends of the bandage should be held in place with adhesive bandage material that includes the bare skin with the edge of the bandage material. Orthopedic stockinette can be used for a total body bandage after cutting out leg holes (Fig. 3.10). This will provide a loose covering for wound-healing studies without directly applying pressure to the wound. Both the cranial and caudal ends of the stockinette should be secured with adhesive tape as described above. Porous elastic adhesive tape in wide widths functions better than ordinary white bandage tape in swine, because it provides a better contour fit and can be secured more tightly.

Bandaging of the extremities and difficult areas, such as the perineum, requires some creativity. The same principles that apply to other animals apply to the pig. Use of skin adhesives may be necessary to provide additional security for the tape. Some of the plastic skin drape material used during surgery can be used for the short term; however, this material is nonporous and will keep the wound moist and impair healing if used for long-term bandaging.

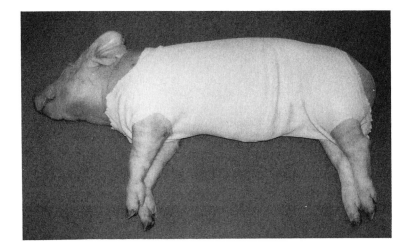

FIGURE 3.10   Orthopedic stockinette bandage of the trunk of a pig.

Tether and harness systems can be designed to maintain chronic catheterization models (see Chapter 8, Fig. 8.10). Jacket systems have also been designed for swine and are commercially available. Care must be taken to have different-sized jackets available for chronic models, because small swine will tend to outgrow them in a few weeks (Davies and Henning, 1986; Smith and Swindle, 1994; Swindle et al., 1996).

Skin Flaps and Grafts

Swine have been important models in the study of skin flaps and grafts and a technical manuscript reviewing the various types of flaps has been published (Kerrigan et al., 1986). Swine have also been used for burn studies for both techniques and as a replacement for human skin, cutaneous pharmacology and toxicology, wound healing and surgical techniques (Daniel et al., 1981; McGraft and Hundahl, 1982; Riviere et al., 1986; Sasaki and Pang, 1984; Shircliffe et al., 1974). The porcine skin has a cutaneous blood supply similar to humans because it is a fixed skin animal unlike most animal species (Forbes, 1969).

The classification of flaps described by Kerrigan et al. (1986) will be used here (Figs. 3.11–3.13). Experimentally, the lengths of the flaps are longer than the described survival length to ensure a zone of necrosis. The zone of necrosis is the region generally studied for techniques and agents that enhance survival. If a zone of necrosis is not required, then the length of the flap is reduced to ensure that adequate blood supply to the flap remains intact.

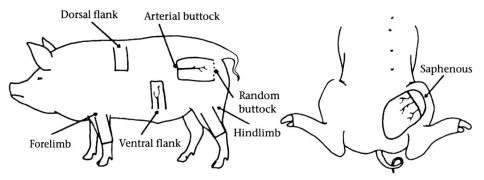

FIGURE 3.11   Location of the sites of various skin flaps and grafts. *Reprinted with permission from Kerrigan et al., 1986, The pig as an experimental animal in plastic surgery research for the study of skin flaps, myocutaneous flaps and fasciocutaneous flaps, Lab. Anim. Sci. 36: 408–412.*

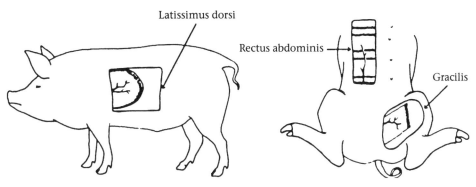

FIGURE 3.12 Location of myocutaneous flaps. *Reprinted with permission from Kerrigan et al., 1986, The pig as an experimental animal in plastic surgery research for the study of skin flaps, myocutaneous flaps and fasciocutaneous flaps, Lab. Anim. Sci. 36: 408–412.*

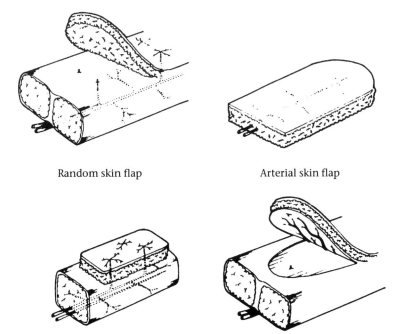

Random skin flap   Arterial skin flap

FIGURE 3.13 Location of fasciocutaneous flaps. *Reprinted with permission from Kerrigan et al., 1986, The pig as an experimental animal in plastic surgery research for the study of skin flaps, myocutaneous flaps and fasciocutaneous flaps, Lab. Anim. Sci. 36: 408–412.*

Random Skin Flaps

Random skin flaps include the dorsal flank flap, the random buttock flap, and the random limb flap. The dorsal flank flap is raised 4 cm ventral to the midline. The survival length of a 4-cm-wide flap is 6.75 cm. The full thickness flap is raised and elevated to its dorsal base. The length of the flap is varied depending upon the experimental parameters. Random buttock flaps are raised over the lateral thigh and will be free of panniculus carnosus, unlike the flank flap. Survival flaps are 10 cm in width and 4.6 cm in length. The flap is incised on three sides, raised to its dorsal margin and sutured upon itself. The length of the flap is varied as required. Random skin flaps are used on both the forelimb and hindlimb and are elevated in the subcutaneous tissues as before. Survival lengths for forelimb flaps are 7.2 cm and for hindlimb are 6.7 cm.

Arterial Skin Flaps

Arterial skin flaps include an arterial pedicle. The ventral flank flap is raised with the base 4 cm lateral to the nipple line and has a branch of the intercostal artery as its vascular branch. The survival length of a 4-cm-wide flap is 8.6 cm. A buttock arterial flap may be raised using the superficial circumflex iliac artery as the vascular pedicle. The 10-cm-wide flap is raised over the cranial dorsal iliac spine with a survival length of 13.3 cm. Because the lateral femoral cutaneous nerve is included in this flap, it also qualifies as a neurovascular pedicle. The saphenous flap uses the saphenous artery as its vascular pedicle and is located on the medial aspect of the hindlimb. The location of the flap is its main disadvantage, and, because of the vascular supply, there is not a defined survival length.

Myocutaneous Flaps

Myocutaneous flaps include the underlying muscle and a vascular supply. The latissimus dorsi flap is most commonly used and the large thoracodorsal artery provides predictable survival. A flap of 10×16 cm starting at the caudal border of the shoulder is predictably survivable. The latissimus dorsi muscle is dissected and isolated relatively easily compared to other models. The gracilis myocutaneous flap is raised on the medial hindlimb and includes the deep femoral artery as its arterial pedicle. The flap usually measures 10×20 cm and is one of the few areas where a skin flap can be raised on the contralateral side for comparison. Its main disadvantage is its location and the relative difficulty in dissection. A rectus abdominus muscle may be raised on the ventral surface of the abdomen using the cranial epigastric artery. Two sized flaps are used: 5×5 cm and 6.5×18 cm. No predictable survivable flap size has been described. Besides location, there are differences in classification of the three muscles. The latissimus dorsi is a Type V, the gracilis is a Type II, and the rectus abdominus is a Type III. Trapezius, pectoralis profundus ascendens, and biceps femoris myocutaneous flaps have found less usage and are not as well defined as these models because of the differences in conformation between swine and humans.

Fasciocutaneous flaps have been raised on the forelimb and hindlimb to include the skin and deep fascia. The forelimb flap is raised 5 cm wide over the lateral condyle of the humerus at the juncture of the lateral head of the triceps and the extersor carpi radialis. The survival length of the flap is 8.2 cm. The hindlimb flap is raised on the lateral aspect one-half to two-thirds of the distance between the major trochanter of the femur and the calcaneus. A 5-cm-wide flap has a survival length of 7.9 cm.

Skin flaps in swine can be problematic if multiple flaps are performed on the animal at the same time. If the suturing technique is adequate to prevent mobility of the flap, then problems of acute surgical pain can be largely avoided. If flaps are designed to have a zone of necrosis, then the animals should be monitored closely for signs of discomfort and infection. Use of stockinette bandages, as described above, can protect the wound from contamination. The use of analgesics and antibiotics should be considered strongly unless they are contraindicated by the protocol.

Wound-Healing Models

The pig has been used for both superficial and deep wound-healing studies (Bolton et al., 1988; Chvapil and Chvapil, 1992; Mertz et al., 1986; Ordman and Gillman, 1966). Epidermal and dermal repair models have been standardized in the pig and in many other protocols, such as those involving skin flaps, described above, wound healing is a part of the protocol. Swine have also been used for cutaneous toxicologic research (Riviere et al., 1986). Differences in rates of wound healing may be noted between breeds, possibly due to age and genetic differences when comparing animal studies (Chvapil and Chvapil, 1992). Using multiple wounds on the same animal provides the ability to have the animal serve as its own control.

Epidermal wound healing is studied to evaluate pharmaceutical and bandaging interventions and their effects on epidermal regeneration. The pig has been evaluated both as a model of epidermal migration (Chvapil and Chvapil, 1992; Mertz et al., 1986) and as a model of epidermal proliferation (Winter, 1972). The method of wounding may vary slightly between studies but basically involves infliction of multiple epidermal wounds of the same size and depth bilaterally using a keratome. A common configuration involves excision of 16–24 wounds 2.2 × 2.2 cm and 0.04 cm deep.

In contrast to the superficial wounds described above, deep wounds heal by scarring rather than regeneration. Dermal wounds may involve the use of skin flaps, described above, simple full thickness incisions or excised full thickness wounds. A size of 3 × 5 cm and 0.8–1.5 cm deep has been standardized for excision wounds in the miniature pig (Chvapil and Chvapil, 1992).

In the case of both split thickness and full thickness wounds, the pig may experience postoperative discomfort. It is advisable to use the orthopedic stockinette bandaging technique described above. The use of antibiotics and analgesics is strongly advised unless contraindicated by the research protocol.

References

Bolton, L.L., E. Pines, and D.T. Rovee. 1988. Wound healing and integumentary system. In Swindle, M.M., and Adams, R.J. (eds), Experimental Surgery and Physiology: Induced Animal Models of Human Disease, Baltimore: Williams and Wilkins, pp. 1–9.

Chvapil, M., and T.A. Chvapil. 1992. Wound healing models in the miniature Yucatan pig. In Swindle, M.M. (ed), Swine as Models in Biomedical Research. Ames: Iowa State University Press, pp. 265–288.

Daniel, R.K., D.L. Priest, and D.C. Wheatley. 1981. Etiological factors in pressure sores: An experimental model. Arch. Phys. Med. Rehabil. 62(10): 492–498.

Davies, A.S., and M. Henning. 1986. Use of swine as a model of musculoskeletal growth in animals. In Tumbleson, M.E. (ed), Swine in Biomedical Research, Vol. 2. New York: Plenum Publishers, pp. 839–848.

Ethicon. 1988. Wound Closure Manual. Sommerville, NJ: Ethicon, Inc.

Forbes, P.D. 1969. Vascular supply of the skin and hair in swine. In Montagna, W., and Dobson, R.L. (eds), Advances in Biology of the Skin. New York: Pergamon.

Kerrigan, C.L., R.G. Zelt, J.G. Thomson, and E. Diano. 1986. The pig as an experimental animal in plastic surgery research for the study of skin flaps, myocutaneous flaps and fasciocutaneous flaps. Lab. Anim. Sci. 36(4): 408–412.

McGraft, M.H., and S.C. Hundahl. 1982. The spatial and temporal quantification of myofibroblasts. Plast. Reconstr. Surg. 69: 975–983.

Mertz, P.M., P.A. Hebda, and W.H. Eaglstein. 1986. A porcine model for evaluation of epidermal wound healing. In Tumbleson, M.E. (ed), Swine in Biomedical Research, Vol. 1. New York: Plenum Press, pp. 291–302.

Monteiro-Riviere, N.A. 1986. Ultrastructural evaluation of the porcine integument. In Tumbleson, M.E. (ed), Swine in Biomedical Research, Vol. 1. New York: Plenum Press, pp. 641–655.

Monteiro-Riviere, N.A., and J. Riviere. 1996. The pig as a model for cutaneous pharmacology and toxicology research. In Tumbleson, M.E., and Schook, L.B. (eds), Advances in Swine in Biomedical Research, Vol. 2. New York: Plenum Press, pp. 425–458.

Ordman, L.J., and T. Gillman. 1966. Studies in the healing of cutaneous wounds. III. A critical comparison in the pig of the healing of surgical incisions closed with sutures or adhesive tape based on tensile strength and clinical histological criteria. Arch. Surg. 93(6): 911–928.

Riviere, J.E., K.F. Bowman, and N.A. Monteiro-Riviere. 1986. The isolated perfused porcine skin flap: A novel animal model for cutaneous toxicologic research. In Tumbleson, M.E. (ed), Swine in Biomedical Research, Vol. 1. New York: Plenum Press, pp. 657–666.

Sasaki, G.H., and C.Y. Pang. 1984. Pathophysiology of skin flaps raised on expanded pig skin. Plast. Reconstr. Surg. 74(1): 59–67.

Shircliffe, A.C., P.M. James, and J.H. Meredith. 1974. Technique for obtaining porcine heterografts for use on burned patients. J. Trauma 14(2): 168–174.

Smith, A.C., and M.M. Swindle. 1994. Post surgical care. In Smith, A.C., and Swindle, M.M. (eds), Research Animal Anesthesia, Analgesia and Surgery. Greenbelt, MD: SCAW, pp. 167–170.

Swindle, M.M. 1983. Basic Surgical Exercises Using Swine. New York: Praeger Publishers.

Swindle, M.M., D.B. Wiest. S.S. Garner, A.C. Smith, and P.C. Gillette. 1996. Pregnant Yucatan miniature swine as a model for investigating fetal drug therapy. In Tumbleson, M. and Schook, L. (eds), Advances in Swine in Biomedical Research, Vol. 2. New York: Plenum Press, pp. 629–635.

Winter, G.D. 1972. Epidermal regeneration in the domestic pig. In Maibach, H.I., Rovee, D.T. (eds), Epidermal Wound Healing. Chicago: Year Book, pp. 71–112.

4 GASTROINTESTINAL PROCEDURES

General Principles of Abdominal Surgery

Swine need to be fasted prior to surgery in order to facilitate the approach to the organs and to prevent vomiting, which rarely occurs. Unless a gastrotomy is to be performed, it is not necessary to withhold water. It is advisable to fast swine if the intestines are to be exteriorized for major abdominal surgery, because it decreases the edematous response. Gastrointestinal (GI) transit time varies with the breed, diet, and size of the pig; however, the stomach and small intestine may generally be considered to be emptied by a 12-hour fast. The large intestines, including the spiral colon and cecum, generally require 48 hours to empty. Use of hypertonic osmotic purgative solutions (i.e., Golytely) will provide a more thoroughly cleansed intestinal tract; however, these solutions must be administered by stomach tube. Approximately 1 liter/25 kg is required for purgation. Use of enemas and stimulant purgatives is discouraged because of the difficulty of administration, discomfort to the animal, and the associated messiness of the procedure; however, they are effective. Bedding must be removed from the cages of fasted swine, because they will readily consume it, as well as any other foreign material that is available in the absence of food. Pigs will readily consume commercially available glucose/electrolyte solutions (i.e., Gatorade) or protein supplements (i.e., Ensure). These can be given to pigs during the prolonged 48-hour fasts necessary for some procedures without increasing residue in the gastrointestinal tract. It may also be useful in postoperative care situations in which the pig cannot be given solid food for a prolonged period of time. Prophylactic antibiotics preoperatively and intraoperatively are indicated if the intestines are to be entered surgically (Becker et al., 1992; Swindle, 1983).

Prior to surgically preparing the male pig for any type of abdominal surgery, the preputial diverticulum must be expressed as described for the urinary system in Chapter 7.

Following laparotomy, it is advisable to use saline-wetted laparotomy sponges to keep the tissue at the edges of the incision moist (Fig. 4.1). Also, the use of sponges facilitates collection of the inadvertent spillage of gastrointestinal contents in order to minimize contamination of the abdominal cavity during enterotomy. Gentle handling of the intestines with wetted sponges and atraumatic instrumentation is essential to minimize the complications associated with postoperative adhesions. The mesentery of the pig is very friable and prone to edema following prolonged manipulation. As for contaminated surgery in other species, it may be necessary to copiously flush the abdomen with isotonic solutions containing antibiotics, although this is not necessary as a routine. If only regional contamination occurs, then the flushing should only be performed in the area affected.

Closure of abdominal incisions is best accomplished in layers using synthetic absorbable sutures in either a simple interrupted or a continuous pattern. Closure of the peritoneum as an individual layer is not always possible in younger animals or in the caudal abdomen. In fact, closure of the peritoneum as a separate layer is unnecessary. Muscle fascia should be included in the sutures in order to bring the layers into proper apposition. Suturing of the skin is easily accomplished with subcuticular sutures, and this pattern is less likely to

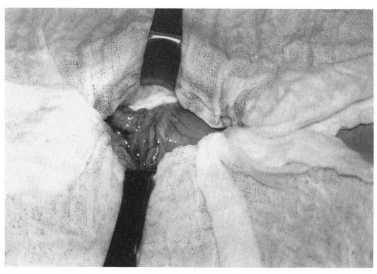

FIGURE 4.1   Celiotomy incision with wetted laparotomy sponges in place.

have localized wound inflammation than external suture patterns or staples.

All of the GI procedures can be performed using staple surgery technologies at least in part. Also most of the procedures can be approached using laparoscopic or endoscopic surgical techniques rather than open surgical procedures. These techniques have been shown to be equivalent for wound-healing characteristics when compared to open techniques. For simplicity, the manual suturing techniques are described in this textbook (Kopchok et al., 1993; Noel et al., 1994; Olson et al., 1995). The unique anatomic features of the gastrointestinal tract are outlined in Chapter 1. Photos of the abdominal viscera are included for reference when planning celiotomies (Figs. 4.2–4.4). Methods of closing intestines and other hollow viscous organs are illustrated (Figs. 4.5–4.8).

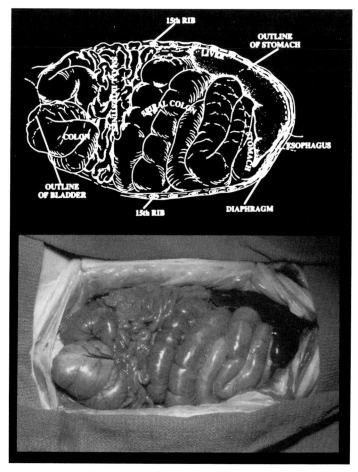

FIGURE 4.2 Ventral view of abdominal viscera. *Reprinted with permission from Shantz et al., 1996, Essentials of Experimental Surgery: Gastroenterology, Netherlands: Harwood Academic Publishers.*

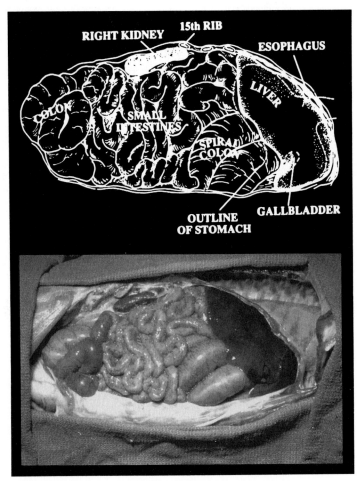

FIGURE 4.3   Right lateral view of abdominal viscera. *Reprinted with permission from Shantz et al., 1996, Essentials of Experimental Surgery: Gastroenterology, Netherlands: Harwood Academic Publishers.*

Gastrotomy/Gastrostomy Techniques

The stomach is best approached from an upper midline incision from the xiphoid cartilage to the umbilicus. Following laparotomy, the stomach may be retracted gently out of the abdomen and the edges of the incision are packed off with wetted laparotomy sponges. The gastrotomy incision is made in the avascular plane of the greater curvature after stabilization of the plane with Babcock forceps or stay sutures. Closure of the gastrotomy is performed with either staple surgical techniques or a two-layer inverting closure technique. The preferred suturing technique uses synthetic absorbable sutures in a Cushing pattern oversewn with a Lembert. The stomach should be thoroughly rinsed with saline prior to replacing it in the abdomen.

Gastrostomy tubes, ports, or cannulae may be sewn in place for gastric access using the same principles of surgery. Exteriorization of the devices is best

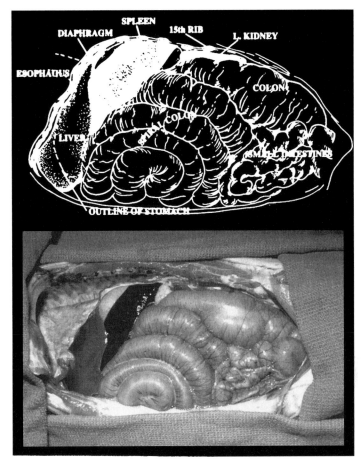

FIGURE 4.4   Left lateral view of abdominal viscera. *Reprinted with permission from Shantz et al., 1996, Essentials of Experimental Surgery: Gastroenterology, Netherlands: Harwood Academic Publishers.*

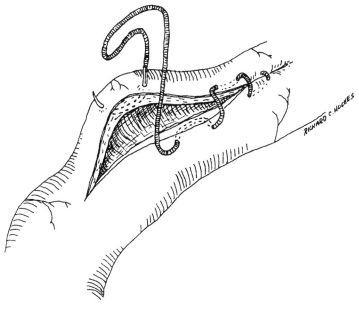

FIGURE 4.5   Closure of an intestinal incision with a Cushing pattern.

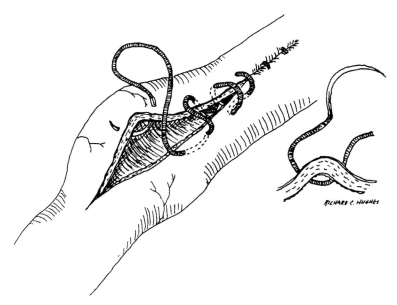

FIGURE 4.6   Closure of an intestinal incision with a Connell pattern (suture enters lumen).

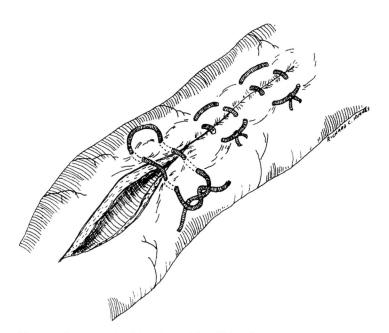

FIGURE 4.7   Closure of an intestinal incision with a Halsted pattern.

performed on the lateral abdominal wall dorsal to the lateral border of the mammary glands or preferably on the dorsum of the flank. This prevents irritation of the exteriorized device when the pig is recumbent or rubs itself on the cage (Hennig et al., 1980; Pekas, 1983).

Heidenhein pouches (Fig. 4.9) may be utilized in the pig in the same manner as originally described for other species to collect gastric secretions without

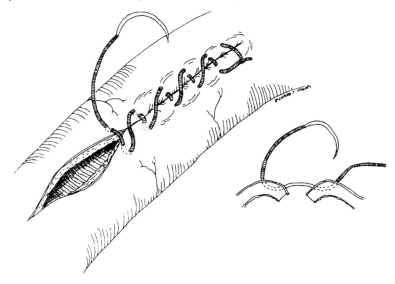

FIGURE 4.8   Closure of an intestinal incision with a Lembert pattern.

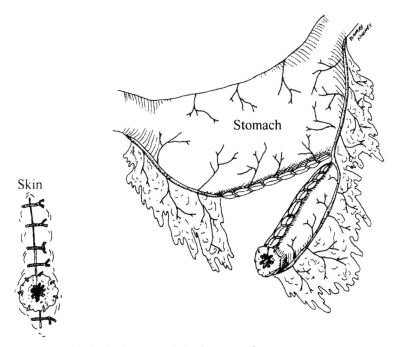

FIGURE 4.9   Creation of a Heidenhein pouch in the stomach.

gastric contents (Markowitz et al., 1964). For this procedure, a sleeve of the stomach is isolated from the body along the greater curvature while maintaining the blood supply of the gastroepiploic artery. The body of the stomach and the sleeve are sutured with a double row of inverting sutures. The isolated gastric pouch may be cannulated to the outside on the lower abdomen. In performing this procedure the branches of the vagus nerve are sacrificed. A Pavlov pouch maintains the integrity between the cranial portion of the pouch with the body of the stomach, thus preserving innervation at that end. The distal end of the pouch is fistulated to the outside.

Gastrojejunostomy techniques may also be utilized in swine. The jejunum is located by finding the root of the mesentery, which is caudal to the stomach and associated with the cranial mesenteric vessels. Care should be taken to ensure that there is not torsion of the mesentery and that the caudal direction of the peristalsis remains intact. A side-to-side surgical anastomosis is performed using standard techniques. Single-layer closure using either interlocking or simple continuous sutures is generally acceptable. Using two-layer inverting closure techniques may be necessary in large animals or in the case of existing pathology (Swindle, 1983).

A model of gastroesophageal reflux has recently been described (Schopf et al., 1997). This model is created by performing a longitudinal myectomy 3 cm proximal and distal to the gastroesophageal junction using a ventral midline incision from the xiphoid to the umbilicus. The approach and dissection is similar to the one described for vagotomy in this chapter. The myectomy must be performed carefully to avoid incising the mucosal layer, similar to the dissection described for pyloroplasty in this chapter. However, the myectomy incision is not closed, and, postoperatively, the animal should be kept on a liquid diet for 3 days. Otherwise, the abdominal incision is closed routinely, and postoperative care is routine. This procedure results in a chronic reflux esophagitis within days if the procedure is technically successful.

Pyloroplasty

The pylorus may be approached either through a midline or right paramedian incision. If the paramedian incision is used it is made along the lateral aspect of the mammary glands from the last rib to the level of the umbilicus. The pylorus is identified by palpation and must be differentiated from the muscular torus pyloricus. The pylorus is exteriorized through the incision and stabilized by an assistant with wetted gauze sponges. A linear incision is made along the longitudinal plane of the stomach and duodenum in an avascular area. Repeated gentle incisions are made until all layers of the muscularis mucosa have been incised, and the submucosa bulges from the incision. At this point, the axis of the completed incision is changed at a right angle and the incision is closed using Lembert sutures. The net effect of the procedure is to enlarge the opening of the pylorus by incising the musculature and by reversing the plane of the incision (Fig. 4.10). Care should be taken to not incise the submucosa or

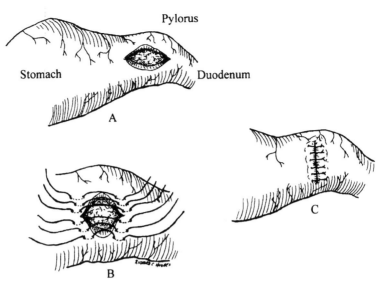

Pylorus

Stomach   Duodenum

A

C

B

FIGURE 4.10   Closure of a pyloroplasty at right angles to the surgical incision.

mucosa; if this occurs, however, the closure of the incision described above will repair the defect (Swindle, 1983).

Enterotomy/Intestinal Fistulation

The small intestine (Fig. 4.11) can be surgically entered using standard techniques (Swindle, 1983; Swindle et al., 1998). The duodenum can be approached by either a cranial midline incision or a right paramedian incision lateral to the mammary glands. The ileum is best approached through the cranial midline incision as for the proximal duodenum. The majority of the small intestinal mass, including most of the jejunum is in the right mid and caudal areas of the abdomen. It may be readily approached from the midline in females; however, a right paramedian incision in the caudal quadrant of the abdomen lateral to the mammary glands is preferable in males. This incision can be made through relatively thin abdominal musculature with minimal vasculature requiring ligation in this region.

Prior to enterotomy, the area of interest is brought out through the abdominal incision and the area is packed off with wetted laparotomy sponges. A longitudinal incision is made along the antimesenteric border of the intestine in an avascular plane. If a catheter or other fistula device is to be inserted, then a stab incision may be made in the same plane with a no. 11 blade. It is not necessary to cross clamp the intestine in most cases if the animal has been properly fasted. An assistant can preclude intestinal contents from entering the incision by pinching off the lumen at either end of the enterotomy incision. Following enterotomy, the incision may be closed using simple interrupted sutures with synthetic absorbable suture material.

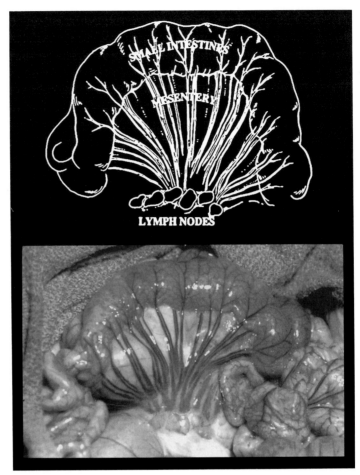

FIGURE 4.11   Photograph and illustration of a loop of small intestine.

For intestinal infusions, vascular access ports (Access Technologies, Skokie, IL) have been modified to function as intestinal access ports. A 9-Fr silicone catheter with the end hole closed and four side slits approximately 1 cm in length has been found to be useful. The catheter has a bead preplaced 1 cm distal to a silicone flange that has been preplaced to provide an anchor for sutures to the intestinal serosa (Fig. 4.12). The access port may either be sutured to the skin on the outside or implanted subcutaneously in the flank or over the rib cage. The site of entrance into the intestine is closed between the bead and the flange with a purse-string suture. The flange is sutured to the intestine with two to four simple interrupted sutures.

The small intestine may also be fistulated as a Thiry fistula or Thiry–Vella loop (see below). When either of these procedures are performed, then the fistula is best exteriorized on the lateral portion of the right flank in order to min-

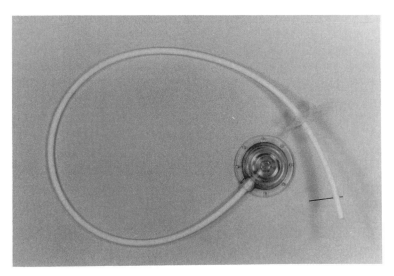

FIGURE 4.12   Intestinal access port for chronic infusion of the intestine. *Photo courtesy of Access Technologies, Inc.*

imize tension on the isolated intestinal loop. Ports may be placed at the site of the fistulation to minimize contamination and inflammation of the exit site.

Intestinal Anastomosis

The intestine may be approached surgically through any of the incisions described above for enterotomies (Swindle, 1983). The small intestine may be anastomosed by either end-to-end, end-to-side or side-to-side techniques. The main variation between the pig and other species relates to the formation of the vascular arcades of the mesenteric vessels in the subserosa of the intestine rather than in the mesentery. The peculiar fanlike arrangement of the mesenteric vessels also necessitates a change in techniques to suture the mesentery (Schantz et al., 1996).

When performing an intestinal anastomosis, the vascular supply to the intestine that is to be removed is ligated at its base close to the root of the mesentery. The line of demarcation of the blood supply in the intestine should be closely observed in order to ensure that all infarcted nonviable intestine is removed. The intestine should be cross clamped with intestinal forceps along the line of demarcation to ensure that the line of incision will be at the junction of viable and infarcted intestine. This line will be at an oblique angle to the long axis of the intestine. The angle will approximate the angle of the mesenteric arterial supply to the region. The section of intestine that has been ligated and its associated mesentery is excised after placing a second set of intestinal forceps at either end of the viable intestine to prevent contamination of the surgical site with reflux of intestinal contents. This pair of forceps should be applied atraumatically with the minimal amount of pressure required to prevent the movement of intestinal contents into the area of the incision. The intestinal forceps should be either linen or rubber shod to prevent cutting of the tissue by the metal forceps. Alternatively, an assistant may use digital pressure to pinch off the lumens of the viable intestine at either end of the incision. These proximal and distal clamps should be placed so that the excised ends of the remaining intestine are long enough for the edges to be sutured.

The intestinal anastomosis may be closed with simple interrupted sutures using synthetic absorbable sutures. This suture pattern enters the lumen and is pulled tightly enough when tying the knots to cut through the mucosa and become embedded in the intestinal wall. This is applicable to most small swine; however, in larger animals, either a continuous pattern or a two-layer closure of continuous sutures oversewn with inverting sutures may be required. Single-layer closure is usually indicated except in the case of larger animals or potential contamination that may impair healing. Regardless of which suturing technique is chosen, the sutures must be meticulously placed in order to provide for correct anatomic alignment and to provide a suture line without leakage. As a general rule, the sutures for this anastomosis should be approximately 5 mm from the edges of the incision and 5–10 mm between sutures. The remaining clamps should be removed and the incision line checked for leakage. In some cases, the intestinal lumen along the lines of excision may not be the same size, and it might require additional trimming of the tissue edges. Any leaks may be closed by the addition of simple interrupted or inverting sutures.

The mesenteric incision will need to be sutured to prevent bowel torsion and stricture. In most cases the edges of mesentery will retract to the adjacent mesenteric vessels and the mesenteric tissue adjacent to the incision will become edematous. If the edges of the mesentery are readily identifiable, then the incision may be closed with simple interrupted or continuous sutures using absorbable synthetic suture material. However, this will not be the case in most animals. In those animals in which the edges of the mesentery are not readily identifiable, a series of horizontal mattress sutures are placed on the proximal and distal sides of the first viable set of mesenteric vessels at either end of the excised intestines (Fig. 4.13). This pattern will close the mesenteric rent without occluding the blood supply to the remaining intestine.

The anastomosed intestine should be rinsed copiously with isotonic saline solution prior to replacing it in the abdomen. If contamination is suspected, then rinsing of the abdomen with antibiotic-containing saline solution may be indicated.

Intestinal Diversion/Intestinal Bypass

Various techniques are used to perform small intestinal diversion or bypass in the experimental setting (Assimos et al., 1986; Fleming and Arce, 1986; Hand

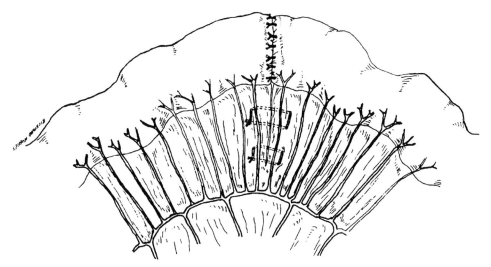

FIGURE 4.13   Closure of the mesentery with horizontal mattress sutures and an intestinal anastomosis with simple interrupted sutures.

et al., 1981; Markowitz et al., 1964; Swindle et al., 1998; Turner and Mellwrath, 1982). These would include such techniques as the Thiry fistula, Thiry–Vella fistula, and jejunoileal bypass. The techniques for suturing the intestine are the same as those discussed for intestinal anastomosis. In this section, a review of some of the types of procedures that are possible in swine is provided. Examples of the specific porcine anatomic features that must be considered are provided.

The Thiry fistula (Fig. 4.14) is performed by isolating a segment of small intestine with the vascular and nerve supply intact, closing one end by oversewing the stump, and exteriorizing the open end. The intestine from which the segment is isolated is closed using an end-to-end anastomosis. Peristalsis may either be directed into the abdomen or out of the fistulated abdominal wall depending upon the goals of the experiment. The Thiry–Vella loop (Fig. 4.15) is isolated in the same manner as the Thiry fistula, except that both ends of the intestine are exteriorized. When the intestinal segment is selected it should be a section that will not have tension on the mesenteric attachment after isolation. The isolated segment should be flushed copiously with warm saline to minimize contamination of the abdomen and the exteriorization incision. Prophylactic antibiotics are indicated with this procedure (Markowitz et al., 1964).

The most appropriate place to exteriorize the intestine is on the right flank in a dependent portion. The thick musculature of the dorsal and lateral flank in larger swine will cause intestinal ischemia in the segment passing through the muscle. Toward the ventral portion of the abdominal wall, the muscle becomes much thinner. This problem is negated if the intestine is isolated in this area. The skin and muscle are incised, and the open end of the intestine is

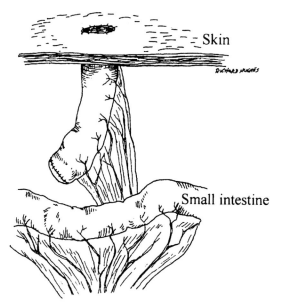

FIGURE 4.14   Thiry fistula.

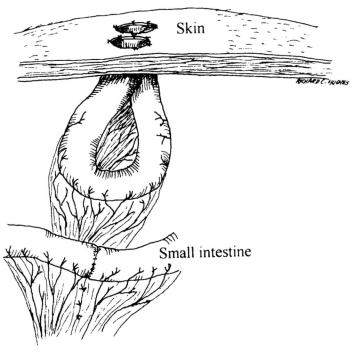

FIGURE 4.15   Thiry–Vella fistula.

passed through the incision, while taking care to avoid spilling intestinal contents into the musculature. This can be facilitated by clamping the open end with atraumatic intestinal forceps. The end of the intestinal loop is sutured to the subcuticular layer of the skin using simple interrupted sutures with a monofilament nonabsorbable suture. Instead of exteriorizing the end of the intestine, it may be cannulated and left in the abdomen with only the prosthetic port exteriorized.

A model of jejunoileal bypass has been developed in swine to study nutritional complications associated with the procedure (Assimos et al., 1986). The intestine is divided caudal to the duodenum. The junction of the duodenum and jejunum is indistinct; however, it is generally considered to be caudal to the loop of the duodenum that passes cranially and then laterally from the caudal end of the body of the pancreas. The cranial end of the jejunum is oversewn and sutured to the cranial abdominal wall to prevent intussusception. The ileum is transected close to the ileocecal junction. The end of the duodenum is sutured end-to-end to the distal end of the transected ileum. The transected proximal end of the ileum is sutured end-to-side to the ventrolateral portion of the spiral colon. This results in almost complete bypass of the jejunum and ileum. Postoperatively, swine continue to maintain their weight with few gastrointestinal complications.

Potential methods of bypassing and fistulating the intestine are almost limitless. These more traditional procedures were chosen to illustrate specific surgical considerations in swine.

Colonic Anastomosis and Fistulation

The procedures described for anastomosis and fistulation of the small intestine may be applied to the large intestine after taking consideration of the unique anatomy in the pig, especially the spiral colon (Swindle et al., 1998). The spiral colon, which contains the cecum and ascending colon, is approached through a cranial midline incision and in larger animals, may have to be extended caudal to the umbilicus. The short transverse colon can be approached through the same incision. The descending colon may either be approached through a caudal midline incision in females or a left paramedian incision in males similar to the approach described above for the jejunum.

Anastomosis of the descending colon may be performed in a similar manner as described for the small intestine; however, it is necessary to close the colon with two layers of sutures, preferably synthetic absorbables. The internal suture pattern should be continuous or simple interrupted. The outer layer should be closed with simple inverting Lembert sutures. It is essential to prevent contamination of the abdomen with colonic contents by careful packing of the colon prior to incising it and copious flushing of the finished incision.

The spiral colon is not amenable to anastomosis using standard techniques because of its unique anatomy (Fig. 4.16). In the research setting, anastomosis is not likely to be attempted. However, the use of fistulas for the study of colonic contents, transport mechanisms, or infusion of pharmacologic agents may be indicated. In this case, the area of the colon to be fistulated may be readily identified by its gross anatomic characteristics. The spiral colon lies in the left upper quadrant of the abdomen and contains the cecum and the majority of the ascending colon in an outer centripetal coil and an inner centrifugal coil. The cecum is located in the caudal aspect and is joined by the ileum at the base of the spiral colon dorsally adjacent to the left kidney and pancreas. A vermiform appendix is not present. The outer coil continues ventrally in a clockwise pattern (from the dorsal perspective) to form the apex. The outer coil contains two tenia. The inner centrifugal coil does not contain tenia and progresses dorsally until it exits cranially at the base of the spiral colon. The transverse colon is short and quickly turns caudally to form the descending colon. A true sigmoid flexure, analogous to humans, is not present prior to its transformation into the rectum in the pelvic cavity (Schantz et al., 1996).

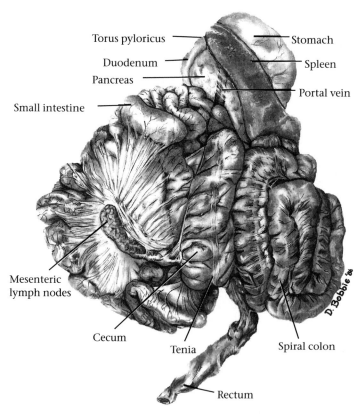

FIGURE 4.16   Intestinal viscera depicting the structure of the spiral colon. *Reprinted with permission from Swindle, 1984, Comparative Anatomy of the Pig, Charles River Technical Bulletin, Charles River Laboratories, Inc.*

Fistulas and ports may also be created in the same manner as for the small intestine. For the cecum and large intestine, however, they need to be exteriorized on the left flank. If functional ostomies, such as colostomies, are performed then they are best exteriorized on the thin-walled dependent portion of the abdomen in order to minimize skin contact with the excreta.

Total Colectomy

A total colectomy may be performed in the pig. In the experimental setting this would usually be performed to simulate the conditions of colectomy following necrotizing enterocolitis or trauma. The bowel prep should include hypertonic purgatives and antibiotics preoperatively. The ileum should be transected at the ileocecal junction and the spiral colon retracted caudally to expose the branches of the cranial mesenteric artery that provide blood supply to the structure. The dissection is continued caudally while ligating the arterial and venous branches supplying the mesocolon. The arterial branches are major subdivisions of the cranial and caudal mesenteric arteries, but the mesenteric veins have to be ligated separately. The transected ileum can be anastomosed using an end-to-side or side-to-side anastomosis technique to the rectum. Prior to transection of the large bowel, it should be ascertained that the ileum can be stretched to reach the area of transection.

The major postoperative complication will be diarrhea and nutritional deficiencies related to the shortened bowel. This surgery creates a similar condition as that which occurs with short bowel syndrome in humans (Dudgeon et al., 1988).

Rectal Prolapse

Rectal prolapse is a clinical condition that may result secondarily to any condition that results in rectal straining such as diarrhea. It can also be produced experimentally by surgically prolapsing the rectum through the anus from a laparotomy.

Primary treatment should be targeted at reducing the swelling due to vascular congestion and edema prior to replacement of the prolapsed segment into the pelvic cavity. If necrosis has already occurred, then the prolapsed segment must be amputated and a colonic resection performed.

If the prolapsed segment is healthy, then swelling can be reduced by rinsing with hypertonic solutions such as 50% glucose. The segment should be lubricated with a water soluble lubricant and replaced by gentle digital manipulation. A purse-string suture can be placed around the rectum temporarily to help prevent recurrence while the swelling is reduced and the condition is stabilized. A variety of prostheses have been developed to place into the rectum during this phase.

If the rectum must be amputated, then it is best accomplished with surgical staples. However, the prolapsed section of the rectum may be surgically amputated to the level of normal tissue and manually sutured using an interlocking continuous suture with synthetic absorbable sutures. In young animals, prostheses may be placed in the rectum and rubber bands applied over the prostheses to cause necrosis of the prolapsed section of the rectum. This technique is employed in agricultural situations in the field and should generally not be used in laboratory settings where there is availability of general anesthesia and surgical technologies (Bollwahn, 1992; Kjar, 1976; Turner and Mellwrath, 1982).

Recurrence is likely if the primary cause of the prolapse is not treated.

Intestinal and Multivisceral Transplantation

Heterotopic and orthotopic transplantation of small bowel has been described in swine. They have also been used as a model of multivisceral transplantation. Both models are performed from a ventral midline incision that may extend the complete length of the abdomen in a complex model such as multivisceral en bloc transplantation (Podesta et al., 1994; Pritchard and Kirkman, 1988; Pritchard et al., 1986; Ricour et al., 1983).

An isolated loop of small intestine from the jejunum to the ileum is isolated and divided between intestinal clamps as described above for an intestinal anastomosis. The mesentery is divided, and the segment of the cranial mesenteric artery and vein are identified supplying the graft. In this region, the vessels will have the largest diameter. The donor is heparinized, and the segment of the artery and vein are divided. The graft is flushed with chilled heparinized crystalloid solution, and the donor is sacrificed.

Using a ventral midline incision, the recipient's infrarenal aorta and vena cava are isolated. The graft is placed transversely into the abdomen and the cranial mesenteric artery and vein are sutured end-to-side in turn to the aorta and vena cava using Satinsky clamps. The transplanted graft is placed carefully to avoid torsion of the stump. The ends of the graft are isolated as stomas in the ventral abdomen as described above for Thiry–Vella loops (Fig. 4.17).

For orthotopic transplant, the terminal ileum is used, allowing the surgeon to use the most accessible vessels supplying the graft. The segment of bowel is isolated as described above, except that only a branch of the mesenteric vessels supplying the segment is divided. Consequently, this may be done as a survival procedure for the donor, because the rest of the bowel is not devascularized as described for the heterotopic transplant. A reciprocal transplant may be performed with the recipient of this graft as well, if the experimental design allows it. The graft is sutured end-to-end to the recipient's mesenteric vessels after a similar segment of small bowel has been extricated.

Multivisceral transplantation of the liver, stomach, duodenum, pancreas,

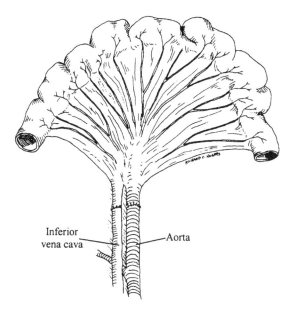

FIGURE 4.17   Segmental intestinal transplant with fistulated ends.

small intestine, and a portion of the large intestine has been developed in swine (Fig. 4.18). The donor is prepared in a standard fashion for a ventral midline incision from the xiphoid process to the pubis. The aorta and vena cava are isolated cranial to the liver and extending caudally to the kidneys ensuring that the celiac, cranial mesenteric, and caudal mesenteric vessels are retained intact, but ligation of the lumbar branches is necessary. The esophagus is clamped and divided at its junction with the stomach, and the descending colon is divided distal to the major blood supply of the caudal mesenteric artery. The vessels supplying the kidneys, adrenals, and mesentery are sacrificed so that only the three major vessels listed above remain. The ligaments of the liver are divided so that all the en bloc viscera is mobilized.

Cannulae are placed in the proximal and terminal aorta, and cold perfusion is initiated after heparinization. The perfusate is removed using suction in the right atrium. After perfusion is underway, then the remaining attachments are divided, and the block of viscera is transferred to a bowl of cold perfusate and preservation solution. The proximal end of the aorta is oversewn.

The recipient is prepared in a similar manner to the donor. A veno–veno bypass is prepared between the external jugular vein and the femoral vein. The colon and stomach are transected leaving a portion of the antrum of the stomach intact. The abdominal aorta is preserved in its entirety, including the kidneys. The vena cava remains intact, except for the portion that is intrahepatic.

The vessels are transected starting with the liver, and veno–veno bypass is

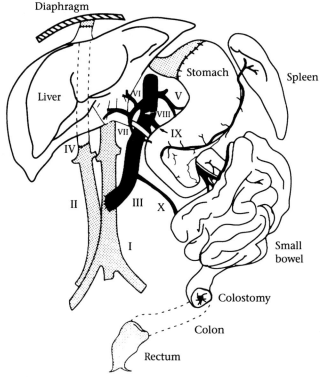

FIGURE 4.18   Diagram of multivisceral transplantation. *Reprinted with permission from Podesta et al., 1994, Multivisceral transplantation in the pig, in C.V. Cramer et al. (eds), Handbook of Animal Models in Transplantation Research, Boca Raton: CRC Press.*

initiated at the time that the celiac trunk and the cranial mesenteric artery are divided. This is the last step prior to removal of the organs.

The vessels of the donor organs are anastomosed into the recipient in the following order: suprahepatic vena cava, infrahepatic vena cava, and distal donor aorta to recipient infrarenal aorta in an end-to-side pattern. At this time, the aortic clamp is removed and the reperfusion process is initiated including removal of the veno–veno bypass. The intestinal tract continuity is re-established in a standard fashion by sewing the donor stomach to the recipient stomach cuff in an end-to-side pattern and re-anastomosing the colon in an end-to-end pattern.

Intraoperative monitoring and homeostasis control is a substantial task with this type of surgery and hemodynamic control is of prime importance. Postoperative monitoring and reinitiation of oral nutrition is also a substantive issue. The list of complications to be considered in addition to the issues of graft versus host disease and rejection include hemorrhage, ascites, thrombo-

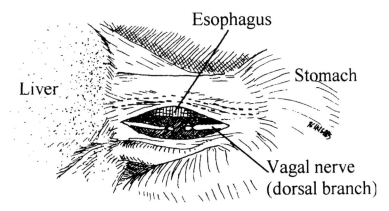

FIGURE 4.19   Technique of truncal vagotomy.

sis, infection, and malabsorption. This type of study should include a multi-disciplinary team approach to these issues.

Vagotomy

The vagus nerve may be transected intra-abdominally as the branches of the nerve traverse along the esophagus cranial to the esophageal sphincter at the cardia of the stomach (Fig. 4.19). Using a midline approach the stomach can be retracted caudally and the liver cranially to expose the caudal esophagus. The fascia over the esophagus is opened with scissors and the branches of the vagus nerve can be observed along the ventral border on either side of the esophagus. The nerves can be transected with scissors and the fascia re-sutured. A section of the nerve can be removed to ensure that the transection remains permanent (Josephs et al., 1992; Swindle, 1983).

Selective vagotomy can be performed by tracing branches of the nerve as they are associated with the blood vessels supplying the lesser curvature of the stomach. In a similar fashion to the truncal vagotomy described above, each nerve branch is isolated and severed. Manipulation of the vagus nerve has been associated with bradycardia and cardiac arrest in some cases. It is best to keep the animal atropinized during manipulation of the main branches of this nerve (Josephs et al., 1992).

References

Assimos, D.G., W.H. Boyce, M. Lively, N. Weidner, J.C. Lewis, G. Howard, E. Furr, M. Sorrell, D.L. McCullough, B.C. Bullock, and T.E. Palmer. 1986. Porcine urologic models including jejunoileal bypass. In Tumbleson ME (ed), Swine in Biomedical Research, Vol. 1. New York: Plenum Press, pp. 399–424.

Becker, B.A., Y. Niwano, and H.D. Johnson. 1992. Physiologic and immune responses associated with 48-hour fast of pigs. Lab. Anim. Sci. 42(1): 51–53.

Bollwahn, W. 1992. Surgical procedures in boars and sows. In Leman, A.D., Straw, B.E., Mengeling, W.L., D'Allaire, S., and Taylor, D.J. (eds.), Diseases of Swine, 7th ed. Ames: Iowa State University Press, pp. 782–793.

Dudgeon, D.L., T.R. Gadacz, H.E. Gladen, K.D. Lillemoe, and M.M. Swindle. 1988. Alimentary tract and liver. In Swindle, M.M., Adams, R.J. (eds.), Experimental Surgery and Physiology: Induced Animal Models of Human Disease. Baltimore: Williams and Wilkins, pp. 217–257.

Fleming, S.E., and D. Arce. 1986. Using the pig to study digestion and fermentation in the gut. In Tumbleson ME (ed), Swine in Biomedical Research, Vol. 1. New York: Plenum Press, pp. 123–134.

Hand, M.S., R.W. Phillips, C.W. Miller, R.A. Mason, and W.V. Lumb. 1981. A method for quantitation of hepatic, pancreatic and intestinal function in conscious Yucatan miniature swine. Lab. Anim. Sci. 31(6): 728–731.

Hennig, U., B. Idzior, J. Wunsche, and H.D. Bock. 1980. Fistulation technique for the digestive tract of swine for the examination of protein metabolism. Arch. Exp. Veterinarmed. 34(3): 325–331.

Josephs, L.G., J.H. Arnold, and J.L. Sawyers. 1992. Laparoscopic highly selective vagotomy. J. Laparoendoscopic Surg. 2(3): 151–153.

Kjar, H.A. 1976. Amputation of prolapsed rectum in young pigs. J. Am. Vet. Med. Assoc. 168(3): 229–230.

Kopchok, G.E., D.M. Cavaye, S.R. Klein, M.P. Mueller, J.L. Lee, and R.A. White. 1993. Endoscopic surgery training: Application of an in vitro trainer and in vivo swine model. J. Invest. Surg. 6(4): 329–337.

Markowitz, J., J. Archibald, and H.G. Downie. 1964. Experimental Surgery, 5th ed. Baltimore: Williams and Wilkins.

Noel, P., H. Fagot, J.M. Fabre, C. Mann, F. Quenet, F. Guillon, H. Baumel, and J. Domergue. 1994. Resection anastomosis of the small intestine by celioscopy in swine. Comparative experimental study between manual and mechanical anastomosis. Ann. Chir. 48(10): 921–929.

Olson, K.H., E.G. Balcos, M.C. Lowe, and M.P. Bubrick. 1995. A comparative study of open, laparoscopic intracorporeal and laparoscopic assisted low anterior resection and anastomosis in pigs. Am. Surg. 61(3): 197–201.

Pekas, J.C. 1983. A method for direct gastric feeding and the effect on voluntary ingestion in young swine. Appetite 4(1): 23–30.

Podesta, L., D.V. Cramer, L. Makowka, and M. Nores. 1994. Multivisceral transplantation in the pig. In Cramer. D.V., Podesta, L., Makowka, L. (eds), Handbook of Animal Models in Transplantation Research. Boca Raton, FL: CRC Press, pp. 231–242.

Pritchard, T.J., and R.L. Kirkman. 1988. Transplantation of the gastrointestinal tract: Small intestine. In Swindle, M.M., and Adams, R.J. (eds), Experimental Surgery and Physiology: Induced Animal Models of Human Disease. Baltimore: Williams and Wilkins, pp. 291–293.

Pritchard, T.J., W.A. Kottun, and R.L. Kirkman. 1986. Technical aspects of small intestinal transplantation in young pigs. In Tumbleson, M.E. (ed), Swine in Biomedical Research, Vol. 1. New York: Plenum Press, pp. 391–398.

Ricour, C., Y. Revillon, F. Arnaud-Battandier, D. Ghnassia, P. Weyne, A. Lauffenburger, J. Jos, J.L. Fontaine, P. Gallix, and M. Vaiman. 1983. Successful small bowel allografts in piglets using cyclosporine. Transplant. Proc. 15(Suppl. 1–2): 3019–3026.

Schantz, L.D., K. Laber-Laird, S. Bingel, and M. Swindle. 1996. Pigs: Applied anatomy of the gastrointestinal tract. In Jensen, S.L., Gregersen, H., Moody, F., and Shokouh-Amiri, M.H. (eds.), Essentials of Experimental Surgery: Gastroenterology. New York: Harwood Academic Publishers, pp. 2611–2619.

Schopf, B.W., G. Blair, S. Dong, and K. Troger. 1997. A porcine model of gastrointestinal reflux. J. Invest. Surg. 10(2): 105–114.

Swindle, M.M. 1983. Basic Surgical Exercises Using Swine. Philadelphia: Praeger Press.

Swindle, M.M., A.C. Smith, and J.G. Goodrich. 1998. Chronic cannulation and fistulization techniques in swine: A review and recommendations. J. Invest. Surg. 11(1): 4–14.

Turner, A.S., and C.W. Mellwrath. 1982. Techniques in large animal surgery. Philadelphia: Lea and Febiger, pp. 309–317.

5 LIVER AND BILIARY SYSTEM

General Principles of Surgery

From a surgical standpoint, the liver and gallbladder of the pig have relatively few differences from those of humans (Figs. 5.1 and 5.2). The bile duct of the pig enters the duodenum separately from the pancreatic duct. The sizes of the bile duct and Sphincter of Oddi are variable depending upon the size and breed of the pig (Table 5.1). The diameter of the bile duct seems to vary substantially even in the same size and breed of pig; however, it readily dilates when catheterized. Normal pressure in the common bile duct is usually less than 10 cm H_2O. The liver contains six lobes: the left lateral, the left medial, the quadrate, the right medial, the right lateral, and the caudate, which contains a caudate process partially surrounding the caudal vena cava. The gallbladder is located in a fossa formed by the left and right medial and quadrate lobes in the right upper quadrant of the abdomen. Bile production is variable depending upon the weight and breed of the pig, as well as diet, and normals must be established for each laboratory. The size and volume of the gallbladder is also variable, but, in a sexually mature animal, it measures approximately 3 cm wide by 5 cm long at the maximum points and contains about 25 ml of bile in a fasted animal at surgery. The hepatic artery and the portal vein enter the liver in close approximation to the common bile duct. Lymph nodes and fascia in the area make the dissection of these structures difficult. The liver of the pig is friable, but contains fibrous septations between lobules, which can be readily noted histologically (Fig. 5.3) (Schantz et al., 1996).

The metabolic functions of porcine liver are more similar to humans than even most species of primates. Consequently, interest in xenografic procedures has increased as immunosup-

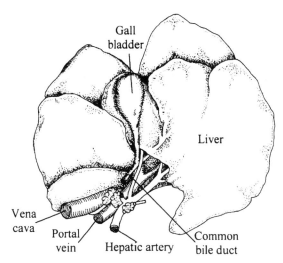

FIGURE 5.1   View of the diaphragmatic surface of the liver.

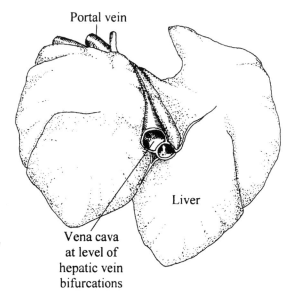

FIGURE 5.2   View of the visceral surface of the liver.

pressive and transgenic technologies have improved (Institute of Medicine, 1996; Ryabinin, 1996). A porcine model of acute and chronic hepatic hemodynamics and metabolism of glucose, lactate, alanine, and glycerol was developed and validated because of its similarities to human metabolism (Drougas et al., 1996). The cytochrome P450 system in swine has similar enzymatic activity to humans except for the absence of CYP2C19 and CYP2D6. Females have higher levels of enzymes than males (Skaanild and Friis, 1997).

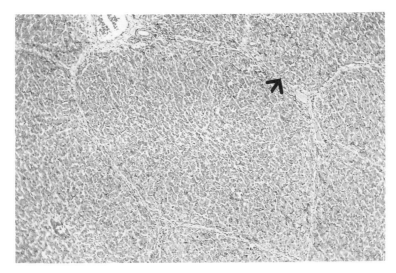

FIGURE 5.3   Histology of the porcine liver illustrating fibrous septae (*arrow*) (×100, Hematoxylin and Eosin stain).

Table 5.1.   Sample sizes of common bile duct based upon measurements

Breed	Weight (kg)	Bile duct diameter ID (mm)
Yucatan	29	3.0
	52	2.7–3.7
Yorkshire	16	3.0
	20	2.3
Landrace	47	2.7
	70	8–12

NOTE: ID, inside dimension.

Cholecystectomy

The gallbladder can be approached with a right paramedian celiotomy incision lateral to the mammary glands, starting cranially at the caudal border of the last rib. The length of the incision will be variable depending upon the size of the pig. Care should be taken to avoid the cranial epigastric vessels in the same area. The area of interest can be isolated with either laparotomy sponges or self retaining retractors. The ventral tip of the gallbladder should be grasped with gallbladder forceps and gentle finger dissection can be used to separate it from the liver. The technique involves applying gentle pressure caudally with the forceps while making gentle side to side movements with the tip of the finger. Experience has shown that only in larger adult swine is it necessary to use other surgical instruments either to cut or cauterize during the dissection. Rupture of the gallbladder is rare if gentle handling and atraumatic forceps are used. The cystic duct is cross clamped with two pairs of right-angle forceps and cut between them following the gallbladder dissection. A double ligature with synthetic absorbable sutures is applied to the stump of the duct. Hemostasis in the gallbladder fossa is usually achieved by packing the area with gauze sponges for 3–5 minutes. Oxycellulose sponges may be placed in the fossa for extra security against hemorrhage. Prior to closure of the incision, any bile that has leaked into the peritoneal cavity should be removed by flushing and suction. The peritoneum, muscle layers, and skin are closed routinely (Swindle, 1983).

Cannulation or Constriction of the Common Bile Duct

Reentrant cannulation of the common bile duct may be achieved with reasonable success if close attention is paid to the design of the cannula (Fig. 5.4). Generally this procedure is performed simultaneously with a cholecystectomy in order to ensure that the bile sample collected is freshly produced by the liver and stored in the gallbladder. The size of the bile duct will vary substantially, even at similar weights within the same breed. However, most swine greater than 15 kg will accommodate at least a 5-Fr catheter, and adult pigs can be cannulated with much larger catheters (Table 5.1).

Complete ligation of the common bile duct without cholecystectomy will result in great dilatation of the gallbladder and ductal system within a few

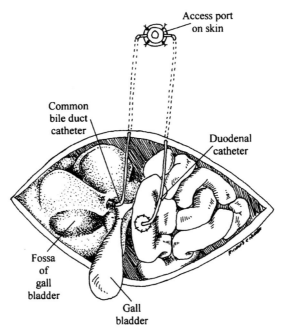

FIGURE 5.4   Reentrant cannulation of the bile duct.

hours. The common and cystic ducts will be impressively dilated with an accompanying increase in intraductal pressure. In spite of the amount of dilatation, the onset of clinical symptoms of biliary stricture is delayed and variable between breeds and sizes of swine. As a general rule, however, swine will become symptomatic 3–4 weeks following surgery. Cholecystectomy at the time of placing the stricture will result in a more rapid onset of symptoms.

Total ligation or constriction of the bile duct should be performed close to the Sphincter of Oddi at the distal end of the duct. The ligature can be made to include a premeasured rod laid along the bile duct. After the ligature is placed, the rod can be removed to achieve a stricture instead of a total blockage.

If cannulation of the duct is to be performed, then it should be a reentry cannulation unless the procedure is to be performed acutely or the animal supplemented orally with bile salts. The general principle of reentry cannulation involves placing a small catheter proximally into the common bile duct, exteriorizing it with a port or valve on the skin to collect samples, and then returning the bile via another catheter into the duodenum. There are insignificant differences between having the intestinal catheter enter through the Sphincter of Oddi or another location in the proximal duodenum.

In order to perform a reentry cannulation of the biliary system, a midline celiotomy incision is performed from the xiphoid process to the umbilicus. The liver is retracted cranially and the intestinal mass caudally. Use of a Balfour retractor and laparotomy sponges greatly facilitates the exposure. The externalized port or valve is located on the surface of skin over the last two ribs on the right ventrolateral region of the abdomen. The cannulae for the bile duct and the reentry cannula for the duodenum are passed into the cranial abdomen through separate puncture or trochar incisions. The position of the externalized collection device must be ventral to the bile duct in order to facilitate biliary flow.

The bile duct is ligated at the entrance to the duodenum. This will result in dilation of the common bile duct, which can then be partially transected using iris scissors. The biliary catheter is advanced into the bile duct toward the liver using a vein pick to facilitate the opening of the lumen. The tip of the catheter should be advanced to the area of the edge of the hepatic lobe. It is sutured in place with a ligature, and it is helpful if retention beads have been affixed to the catheter in order to facilitate its retention in the short common bile duct. This catheter should be composed of a firm material, such as polypropylene, in order to prevent the ligature from occluding the lumen. The catheter should also be transparent so that the movement of bile can be observed. The remainder of the catheter can be silicone. Catheters are designed to have the smaller polypropylene portion inside a larger silicone catheter except for the portion that is actually cannulated inside the bile duct (Access Technologies, Skokie, IL). This provides a stiff portion of the catheter inside the bile duct with a flexible catheter inside the abdominal cavity. The patency of the catheter should be verified, and it should be repositioned if necessary. If the procedure requires that bile samples from the gallbladder be excluded from the collection, then a cholecystectomy is performed. A cholecystectomy increases the pressure in the duct and facilitates biliary flow.

The reentrant catheter can be placed into the proximal duodenum, taking care not to disturb the pancreas or pancreatic duct. As per the description of the cannula for an intestinal access port (Chapter 4), the catheter can be placed into the lumen of the duodenum after making a stab incision. This portion of the catheter should be silicone. The catheter should be open ended instead of slitlike as per the previous discussion of intestinal access ports. This modification is necessary because of the low pressure in the biliary system. The catheter can be sutured into the intestine with a purse-string suture.Preferably, a retention bead should be affixed to the catheter to ensure its retention in the lumen. A cuff can also be placed on the catheter and sutured to the surface of the intestine using simple interrupted stay sutures. Patency of the catheter should be rechecked and biliary flow observed as soon as this procedure is finished. Ascending infections from the intestine to the biliary system and kinking of the catheter resulting in biliary stasis and liver failure are two potential complications of this procedure.

The abdomen is closed after sutures are placed in the peritoneum at the entrance of the two cannulae into the abdominal cavity to prevent a possible dehiscence. The midline incision is closed in a routine manner as described previously (Hand et al., 1981; Swindle, 1983; Terblanche and Van Horn-Hickman, 1978).

Partial Hepatectomy/Liver Biopsy/Intrahepatic Cannulation

Liver biopsies and partial lobectomies can be performed in swine using the same surgical techniques as for other species. The tip of a lobe can be removed by applying a suture ligature circumferentially around a small segment, referred to as the guillotine technique. Alternatively, a larger segment can be removed by cross clamping with noncrushing intestinal clamps and placing overlapping mattress sutures or staples in the viable segment to provide hemostasis. Oxycellulose sponges may be applied to the cut edges to provide additional hemostasis. Percutaneous needle biopsies may be performed by using truecut biopsy needles passed caudomedially through either the 10th or 11th right intercostal spaces in the dorsal half of the lateral wall (Swindle, 1983).

Intrahepatic veins and ducts may be cannulated by modification of the procedure described above. After cross clamping the left lobe of the liver, an incision is made from the edge into the parenchyma until a central vein is transected. The vein may be cannulated with an appropriate catheter. Biliary structures may also be cannulated. The incision is closed as described above with suturing of oxycellulose sponges over the incision. The cannula can be externalized after surgical fixation in the abdominal cavity (Svendsen, 1997).

Complete lobectomies may be performed by modification of the techniques described above for larger segments. The left lateral is the most easily removed lobe. Its excision is discussed under liver transplantation below (Camprodon et al., 1977; Kahn et al., 1994; Procaccini et al., 1994).

Liver Transplantation

Orthotopic, heterotopic, and xenografic transplantations have all been studied in this species. Hepatic transplantation in swine was developed because of the anatomic and physiologic similarities of the porcine liver to human liver, notably because of its ability to withstand total portal vein occlusion for up to 10 minutes, resistance to hepatic venous sphincter vasospasm, and its relative resistance to immunologic rejection posttransplantation. This last characteristic may be due to the use of related individuals from linebred herds of swine, rather than other characteristics of its immune system. Allografts, autografts, and segmental and auxiliary liver grafts have all been described in detail. Multivisceral transplantation including the liver has been previously described (see Chapter 4, Fig. 4.18) (Calne et al., 1967; Dent et al., 1971; Flye, 1992; Gadacz, 1988; Hickman et al., 1971; Kahn et al., 1994; Mizrahi et al., 1996; Oldhaufer et al., 1993; Pennington and Sarr, 1988; Procaccini et al., 1994; Ryabinin, 1996; Sika et al., 1996; Terblanche and Van Horn-Hickman, 1978; Terblanche et al., 1967).

For swine in all phases of the surgery, the mean arterial pressure should be maintained at 60–70 mmHg, and swine should be kept normothermic with adequate perfusion with maintenance fluids. Animals need to be fasted from solids for 48 hours to empty the bowel. Intestines may be packed off from the hepatic region with wetted laparotomy sponges or placed in a plastic bowel bag. Anesthesia, maintenance of homeostasis, and appropriate perioperative care are as essential to the success of this procedure as performing the surgery (Eisele et al., 1986; Mizrahi et al., 1996; Stump et al., 1986).

Donor Liver

Swine are anesthetized, and a midline celiotomy incision is made from the xiphoid process to the pubis. For the donor procedure, the sternum should be split for greater exposure. The falciform, left triangular, and gastrohepatic ligaments are divided. The porta hepatis is dissected free from the peritoneum to the level of the pancreas. This will expose the portal vein and hepatic artery. The caudal vena cava is dissected free of its peritoneal attachments from the level of the adrenal glands cranially through the diaphragm. Generous lengths of these vessels should be dissected in order to have adequate vessel length for reanastomoses during reimplantation. Consequently, their branches are ligated. At the time of harvest, the common bile duct, hepatic artery, portal vein, and vena cava are ligated and divided. The donor liver is cooled and flushed with crystalloid solution and/or a preservation solution. The perfusion is performed through the portal vein during harvesting. Harvesting of the donor liver should be timed closely to the preparation of the recipient for transplantation. Prior to implantation, the excess tissue is trimmed from the liver. Blood from the donor pig should be collected by exsanguination and used postoperatively as required in the recipient pig.

Allograft and Autograft Implantation

The recipient for whole-organ transplant is prepared in a manner similar to the preparation of the donor animal. An external jugular vein cutdown is performed to facilitate the bypass technique. A catheter is inserted into the splenic vein proximally in the heparinized recipient, and the primed catheter is placed into the external jugular vein to provide a passive bypass. If circulatory function is not adequate, then mechanical pumping may have to be provided. The same structures listed above for the donor organ are transected after initiation of bypass and clamping of vessels with vascular clamps. Vascular suture in a continuous pattern is used to reanastomose the vessels in this order: the prehepatic caudal vena cava, 90% of the infrahepatic vena cava, the portal vein, completion of the infrahepatic caudal vena cava, and the hepatic artery. After anastomosing the first two vessels, the liver is allowed to distend with blood by clamping the donor infrahepatic caudal vena cava prior to completing the anastomosis of the two segments of the vessel. Prior to tying the last knot of the anastomosis, the bypass segment is clamped, and the incomplete vascular connection is used as a vent and checked to ensure that air is not present, to remove 50–100 ml of waste blood after reperfusing the liver, and to see that the portal and vena caval circulations are restored. The hepatic artery is reanastomosed in a routine end-to-end manner, or, if a Carrell patch was taken during harvesting of the donor organ, it is reanastomosed to the aorta. The bile duct is the last connection and may be sutured using an intraluminal stent to guide the anastomosis (Fig. 5.5).

Also, an auxiliary liver transplant can be performed by implanting the second liver into the right renal fossa of a recipient following excision of the kidney. The vascular anastomoses are hepatic artery or donor aorta to infrarenal aorta, hepatic vein, or infrahepatic caudal vena cava to infrarenal caudal vena cava, oversewing of the suprahepatic vena cava, portal vein to superior mesenteric vein, and common bile duct to a Roux-en-Y limb of small bowel (Kahn et al., 1994).

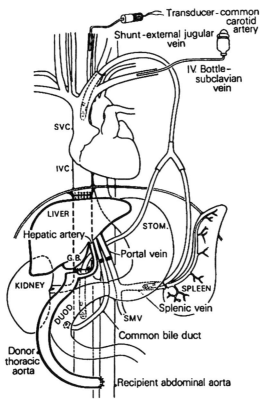

FIGURE 5.5   Orthotopic liver transplantation in the pig. *Reprinted with permission from Flye, 1992, Orthotopic liver transplantation in outbred and partially inbred swine, in M.M. Swindle (ed), Swine as Models in Biomedical Research, Ames: Iowa State University Press, pp. 44–56.*

Segmental Liver Grafts

A living donor may be used to transplant the left lateral lobe of the liver into a recipient. Approximately 10 g/kg body weight of liver tissue is necessary to provide normal metabolic functions. The segmental graft is harvested by incising the capsule and finger fracturing the parenchyma along the fissure of the lobe. The branches of the hepatic artery, hepatic vein, and portal vein are ligated, and the graft is treated as described above. The recipient liver is excised leaving the vena cava intact and veno–veno bypass is instituted as described above. Reimplantation is made into the site of the excised liver by anastomosing the hepatic veins followed by the portal vein, the hepatic artery and the bile duct (Camprodon et al., 1977; Procaccini et al., 1994).

Postoperatively, care must be taken to provide adequate fluid therapy intravenously and to avoid solid food for 24–48 hours postoperatively. Aspirin po may be given as an anticoagulant depending upon the size of the vascular anastomoses. Systemic antibiotics are indicated. Immunosuppressive agents may be given depending upon the protocol.

Hepatic Xenoperfusion

Porcine liver has been utilized clinically as a bridge to transplantation in an effort to prevent fatal levels of ammonia and other toxic metabolites from accumulating in the patient with minor success in the past (Norman et al., 1966). A renewed interest in the procedure has developed because of the possibility that transgenic manipulation of the donor swine will result in an increased success rate (Adham et al., 1996; Argibay et al., 1996; Collins et al., 1994; Mizrahi et al., 1996; Pohlein et al., 1996; Terajima et al., 1996; Terajima et al., 1997; Travis et al., 1996).

The liver may be harvested following the procedure for donor liver harvesting discussed under liver transplantation. Female swine, 20–30 kg body weight, are preferred for the procedure because of the size of the liver and vessels. If the system is to be used for clinical xenoperfusion, then the infectious disease precautions in Chapter 14 should be followed. Modifications to the dissection technique that may be applicable have been described by Mizrahi et al. (1996) and Travis et al. (1996).

The modifications of Mizrahi et al. (1996) include approaching the portal vein through the splenic vein for cannulation and not occluding the inflow or outflow vessels of the liver during cold perfusion. The technique also involves placing the gastrointestinal viscera in a sterile plastic bag to facilitate manipulation during the dissection.

Travis et al. (1996) also recommended adrenalectomy to prevent catecholamine production in the development of an isolated perfusion model for the study of pharmacologic agents. Their system provides an in situ functioning liver (Fig. 5.6).

When the system is to be used clinically for xenoperfusion, the isolated liver is kept in a sterile pan of iced saline and perfused through an extracorporeal system. The system involves shunting the human blood through the portal vein and suprahepatic vena cava to provide inflow and outflow lines. The hepatic artery is used in addition to the portal vein for infusion. Separate infusions with oxygenated blood are required. Using a two-pump system, the blood is circulated from the femoral vein of the patient through the liver and back into the venous system of the patient. The liver must be flushed with saline to exclude all porcine hematogenous products prior to connecting to the circuit. Hepatic hemodynamics in the isolated liver must be monitored during this procedure. Flow rates of approximately 1 ml/g of liver per minute have been recommended for the portal vein and approximately 25% of that rate for the hepatic artery (Terajima et al., 1997).

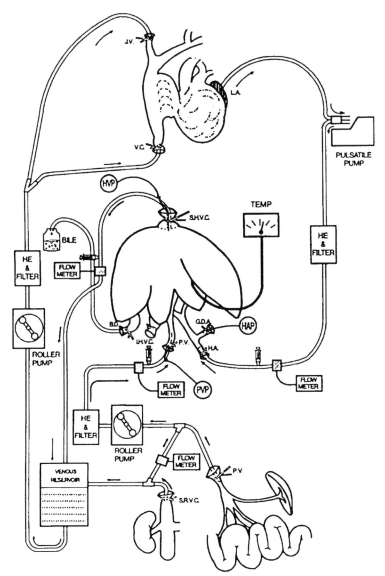

FIGURE 5.6   Isolated in situ liver perfusion system. *Reprinted with permission from Travis et al., 1996, Development of an in situ isolated porcine liver perfusion model for tightly controlled physiologic and pharmacologic studies, J. Invest. Surg. 9(2): 131–147.*

Liver function is monitored by measuring bile production, oxygen consumption, and by clinical observation of the organ for changes in color and consistency. These techniques are still experimental and will undoubtedly undergo further modification.

References

Adham, M., S. Peyrol, M. Vernet, C. Bonnefont, C. Barakat, D. Rigal, M. Chevallier, I. Berger, M. Raccurt, C. Ducerf, J. Baulieux, and M. Pouyet. 1996. Functional and immunological study of isolated liver xenoperfusion. Transplant. Proc. 28(5): 2852-2853.

Argibay P., J. Vazquez, P. Barros, D. Verge, F. Nunez, H. Garcia, J. Pekolj, and E. De Santibanes. 1996. Extracorporeal auxiliary xenoperfusion: Animal model of support in fulminant liver failure. Transplant. Proc. 28(2): 749-750.

Calne, R.Y., H.J.O. White, and D.E. Yoffa. 1967. Observations of orthotopic liver transplantation in the pig. B. M. J. 2(1): 478.

Camprodon, R., J. Solsona, J.A. Guerrero, C.G. Mendoza, J. Segura, and J.M. Fabregat. 1977. Intrahepatic vascular division in the pig: Basis for partial hepatectomies. Arch. Surg. 112(1K0): 38-40.

Collins, B.H., R.S. Chari, J.C. Maggee, R.C. Harland, B.J. Lindman, J.S. Logan, R.R. Bollinger, W.C. Meyers, and J.L. Platt. 1994. Mechanisms of injury in porcine livers perfused with blood of patients with fulminant hepatic failure. Transplantation 58(11): 1162-1171.

Dent D.M., R. Hickman, C.J. Uys, S. Saunders, and J. Terblanche. 1971. Natural history of liver allo and auto transplantation in the pig. Br. J. Surg. 58(6): 407-413.

Drougas JG, S.E. Barnard, J.K. Wright, M. Sika, R.R Lopez, K.A. Stokes, P.E. Williams, and C.W. Pinson. 1996. A model for the extended studies of hepatic hemodynamics and metabolism in swine. Lab. Anim. Sci. 46(6): 648-655.

Eisele, P.H., E.S. Woodle, G.C. Hunter, L. Talken, and R.E. Ward. 1986. Anesthetic, preoperative and postoperative considerations for liver transplantation in swine. Lab. Anim. Sci. 36(4): 402-405.

Flye, M.W. 1992. Orthotopic liver transplantation in outbred and partially inbred swine. In Swindle, M.M. (ed), Swine as Models in Biomedical Research. Ames: Iowa State University Press, pp. 44-56.

Gadacz, T.R. 1988. Portal hypertension. In Swindle, M.M., Adams, R.J. (eds), Experimental Surgery and Physiology: Induced Animal Models of Human Disease. Baltimore: Williams and Wilkins, pp. 250-253.

Hand, M.S., R.W. Phillips, C.W. Miller, R.A. Mason, and W.V. Lumb. 1981. A method for quantitation of hepatic, pancreatic and intestinal function in conscious Yucatan miniature swine. Lab. Anim. Sci. 31(6): 728-731.

Hickman R., W.A. van Hoorn, and J. Terblanche. 1971. Exchange transplantation of the liver in the pig. Transplantation 24(2): 237.

Institute of Medicine. 1996. Xenotransplantation: Swine, Ethics and Public Policy, Washington, DC: National Academy Press.

Kahn, D., R. Hickman, H. Pienaar, and J. Terblanche. 1994. Liver transplantation in the pig. In Cramer, D.V., Podesta, L., and Makowka, L. (eds), Handbook of Animal Models in Transplantation Research. Boca Raton: CRC Press, pp. 75-86.

Mizrahi, S.S., J.W. Jones, Jr., and F.R. Bentley. 1996. A facilitated technique for hepatectomy of porcine liver. J. Invest. Surg. 9(3): 393-398.

Norman, J.C., C.A. Saravis, M.E. Brown, and W.V. McDermott, Jr. 1966. Immunochemical observations in clinical heterologous (xenogeneic) liver perfusions. Surgery 60(1): 179-190.

Oldhafer K. J., J. Hauss, G. Gubernatis, R. Pichlmayr, and H. U. Spiegel. 1993. Liver transplantation in pigs: A model for studying reperfusion injury. J. Invest. Surg. 6(5): 439-450.

Pennington, L., and M.G. Sarr. 1988. Liver transplantation. In: Swindle, M.M., and

Adams, R.J. (eds), Experimental Surgery and Physiology: Induced Animal Models of Human Disease. Baltimore: Williams and Wilkins. pp. 294–295.

Pohlein C., A. Pascher, P. Bauman, D. Abendroth, M. Jochum, D.J. White, and C. Hammer. 1996. Transgenic porcine livers reduce liberation of humoral mediators during xenoperfusion with human blood. Transplant. Proc. 28(2): 772–774.

Procaccini, E., R. Ruggiero, R. Rea, G. Boccia, G. Varletta, and C. Saccone. 1994. Segmental liver transplantation. Experimental studies in swine. Ann. Ital. Chir. 65(1): 125–129.

Ryabinin, V.E. 1996. Swine liver usage in extracorporeal detoxification. In Tumbleson, M.E., and Schook, L.B. (eds), Advances in Swine in Biomedical Research, Vol. 2. New York: Plenum Press, pp. 475–483.

Schantz, L.D., K. Laber-Laird, S. Bingel, and M. Swindle. 1996. Pigs: Applied anatomy of the gastrointestinal tract. In Jensen, S.L., Gregersen, H., Moody, F., and Shokouh-Amiri, M.H. (eds), Essentials of Experimental Surgery: Gastroenterology. New York: Harwood Academic Publishers, pp. 2611–2619.

Sika, M., J. G. Drougas, Y. T. Becker, W. C. Chapman, J. K. Wright, K. L. Donovan, V. J. Striepe, D. B. H. Van Buren, K. A. Stokes, S. E. Barnard, K. T. Blair, K. Jabbour, P. E. Williams, C. W. Pinion. 1996. Porcine model of orthotopic liver transplantation for chronic studies, In Tumbleson, M. E. and Schook, L. B. (eds), Advances in Swine in Biomedical Research, Vol 1. NY: Plenum Press, pp. 171–187.

Skaanild, M.T., and C. Friis. 1997. Characterization of the P450 System in Göttingen minipigs. Pharmacol. Toxicol. 80(Suppl. II): 28–33.

Stump, K.C., L.R. Pennington, J.F. Burdick, T. Hoshino, and M.M. Swindle. 1986. Practical anesthesia for orthotopic liver transplantation in swine. In Powers, D.L. (ed). Proceedings of the Second Annual Meeting of the Academy of Surgical Research. Clemson, SC: Clemson University Press, pp. 10–12.

Svendsen, P. 1997. Anesthesia and basic experimental surgery of minipigs. Pharmacol. Toxicol. 80(Suppl. II): 23–26.

Swindle, M.M. 1983. Basic Surgical Exercises Using Swine. Philadelphia: Praeger Press.

Terajima H., Y. Shirakata, T. Yagi, S. Mashima, H. Shinohara, S. Satoh, Y. Arima, T. Gomi, T. Hirose, I. Ikai, T. Morimoto, T. Inamoto, and Y. Yamaoka. 1996. Long-duration xenogeneic extracorporeal pig liver perfusion with human blood, Transpl. Int. 9(Suppl.)1: S388–S391.

Terajima H., Y. Shirakata, T. Yagi, S. Mashima, H. Shiohara, S. Satoh, Y. Arima, T. Gomi, T. Hirose, R. Takahashi, I. Ikai, T. Morimoto, T. Inamoto, M. Yamamoto, and Y. Yamaoka. 1997. Successful long-term xenoperfusion of the pig liver: Continuous administration of prostaglandin E1 and insulin, Transplantation 63(4): 507–512.

Terblanche J., and R. Van Horn-Hickman. 1978. The prevention of gastric ulceration by highly selective vagotomy in a new peptic ulcer experimental model, the bile duct-ligated pig. Surgery 84(2): 206–211.

Terblanche J., J.H. Peacock, K.E. Hobbs, A.C. Hunt, J. Bowes, and E.J. Tierris. 1967. Orthotopic liver homotransplantation: Experimental study in the unmodified pig. S. Afr. Med. J. 42(20): 486–497.

Travis, D.L., A.W. Paulsen, and Y. Genyk. 1996. Development of an in situ isolated porcine liver perfusion model for tightly controlled physiologic and pharmacologic studies. J. Invest. Surg. 9(2): 131–147.

6 PANCREAS AND SPLEEN

General Principles of Surgery

The pancreas of the pig is extensive, and the tail follows the lesser curvature of the stomach from the spleen and left kidney to a position along the proximal duodenum. The body of the pancreas encircles the portal and superior mesenteric veins and extends dorsally to the region of the left kidney. The pancreatic duct is composed of two separate ducts draining the tail and body. They anastomose to form the common pancreatic duct immediately prior to the pancreatic sphincter. The pancreatic duct enters the duodenum caudal to and separate from the bile duct in the proximal duodenum (Fig. 6.1; see also Chapter 1, Fig. 1.21). Surgically, it may be readily identified as a firm, whitish structure along the caudal third of the portion of the pancreas that is associated with the duodenum. There is usually a single pancreatic artery supplying the tail of the pancreas as a branch of the splenic or common hepatic artery. The pancreatoduodenal artery courses between the duodenum and the pancreas along its joint border and supplies both from a series of small branches. Venous drainage is through the splenic vein. Histologically (Fig. 6.2), the pancreatic islet cells are relatively indistinct, but functionally similar to humans (Hand et al., 1981; Koyama et al., 1986; Schantz et al., 1996; Stump et al., 1988).

The spleen is a pedunculated organ that is elongated in shape and located in close apposition to the greater curvature of the stomach in the left upper quadrant of the abdomen. It extends from the left kidney ventrally to the midline. There are three main vascular supplies to the organ. These are located in the splenic ligament: the left gastroepiploic, the splenic, and the short gastric arteries and veins. The vascular supply enters the organ from the head to one-half the distance to the tail of the spleen (Getty, 1975; Swindle, 1983).

119

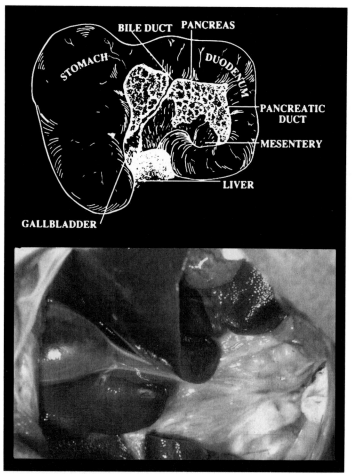

FIGURE 6.1   Illustration of the relationship between the common bile duct and the
                    pancreatic duct. The stomach and duodenum are retracted laterally.
                    *Reprinted with permission from Schantz et al., 1996, Pigs: Applied anatomy of
                    the gastrointestianl tract, in S.L. Jensen et al., (eds), Essentials of Experimental
                    Surgery: Gastroenterology, Netherlands: Harwood Academic Publishers.*

Pancreatectomy

A total pancreatectomy can be performed without compromise or removal of
the duodenum (Stump et al., 1988). With the pig in dorsal recumbency, a midline incision is made from the xiphoid cartilage to at least the umbilicus. In
larger animals, the incision may have to be extended caudally. Balfour retractors and laparotomy sponges are utilized to pack off the spiral colon and small
intestinal mass in order to see the tail of the pancreas. In larger animals, solid
food should be withheld for 48 hours to empty the spiral colon.

Using gentle dissection, the retroperitoneal portion of the pancreatic tail is

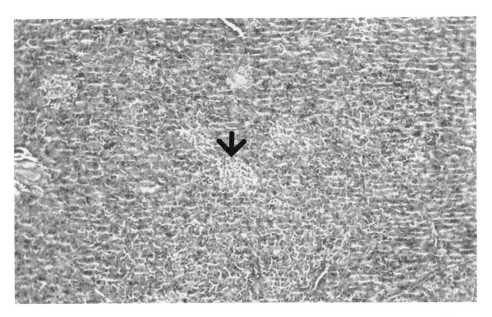

FIGURE 6.2   Histology of the pancreas illustrating the indistinct islets of Langerhans
                 (*arrow*) (×100, Hematoxylin and Eosin stain).

dissected free, and, using gentle retraction, the dissection is continued until the pancreatic artery is encountered. After ligation and transection of the artery, the pancreas is dissected to the level of the pylorus. At this point the dissection turns caudally, and the branches of the pancreatoduodenal artery supplying the pancreas are ligated as they are encountered. This dissection is more easily performed in the pig than in many other species because of the relatively loose connection between this artery and the pancreatic body. When the pancreatic duct is encountered, it is also ligated.

At this point, the dissection becomes more difficult. The major portion of the pancreatic body is deep and surrounds the portal vein and cranial mesenteric vessels. In order to perform this dissection, an assistant is required to perform additional retraction with hand-held ribbon retractors. It is best to continue the dissection dorsally from the duodenum. The pancreas has to be split in order to dissect it from the portal vein. Care should be taken to minimize spillage of pancreatic enzymes and the area should be flushed with saline following removal of the pancreas. The abdomen is closed in a routine manner.

A chemical ablation of the islet cells may be performed by injecting alloxan, 200 mg/kg iv, or streptozotocin, 140–150 mg/kg, as an iv infusion over 5 minutes (Mullen et al., 1992).

Diet and insulin control of glucose levels is difficult in swine. An amount of feed equivalent to 4% of the body weight of the pig is provided as a starter ration. If pancreatectomy is complete, then oral pancreatic exocrine enzymes should be added to the food. In this species as a general rule, elevations in blood glucose and glucosuria are moderate, and ketonuria and acidosis are not encountered. Swine die within 10 days if not treated with insulin. The goal of an experimental study requiring pancreatectomy is likely to be either treatment with various insulin protocols or islet cell transplantation. A detailed discussion of the monitoring and treatment of hyperglycemia is available (Mullen et al., 1992; Stump et al., 1988). Normals for insulin levels and protocols for conducting both oral and intravenous glucose tolerance tests have been published (Mullen et al., 1992; Stump et al., 1988). There are variations among breeds and ages within the breed, consequently, it is appropriate to establish normals for each laboratory experiment. As a generality, swine may be monitored for weight loss and glucose for several days prior to initiating insulin replacement. When they are treated with insulin, the total amount may generally be reduced after the dosage is stabilized for 3–4 weeks. Hypoglycemia can be treated by glucose infusion. Atherosclerotic complications of diabetes are a possibility in this species, because they develop both spontaneous and experimental atherosclerosis. Analgesics and iv infusions of fluids and nutritional solutions should be provided for 1–3 days postoperatively (Laber-Laird et al., 1992; Mullen et al., 1992; Sasiki et al., 1984; Stump et al., 1988).

Segmental Pancreatectomy/Pancreatic Transplant

Most of the swine used in pancreatic transplantation are used for islet cell transplantation techniques after pancreatectomy, digestion of the organ for purification, and isolation of the beta cells. Much of the research in this arena is directed toward preservation of the function of the cells and methods of delivery as xenografic transplants to humans. Fetal pancreases are frequently harvested and used in these procedures. Swine have also been used as a model in segmental pancreatic transplant using the tail of the organ (Koyama et al., 1986; Mullen et al., 1992; Pennington and Sarr, 1988; Sasaki et al., 1984).

The same midline incision described for the total pancreatectomy (above) is used for this procedure. Starting at the tail and extending to the distal body near the duodenum, the organ is mobilized using gentle dissection. The tail is the ventral strip of the pancreas. It contains the main portion of the pancreatic duct and has a single arterial blood supply. It is this section of the pancreas that is harvested as a segmental donor organ (Fig. 6.3). The short gastric and left gastric vessels are ligated, and the origin of the pancreatic blood supply is identified. It may branch off of either the common hepatic artery or the splenic artery. The common hepatic artery and splenic artery are transected distant from the branch supplying the tail of the pancreas in order to leave the celiac artery intact and to have ample distance to avoid damaging the pancreatic

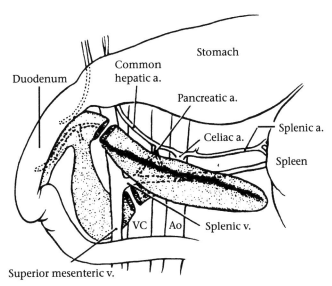

FIGURE 6.3   Harvesting the pancreas for a segmental pancreatic transplant with
                  Roux-en-Y intestinal loop. *Reprinted with permission from Koyama et al.,*
                  1986, Pancreatic allotransplantation with Roux-en-Y jejunal diversion in
                  swine: Its technical aspects, in M.E. Tumbleson (ed), Swine in Biomedical
                  Research, Vol. 1, New York: Plenum Press, pp. 385-389.

artery. The pancreatic vein is transected as it enters the splenic vein, and the
tail of the organ is transected from the distal body of the pancreas at the level
of the cranial mesenteric vein, which represents its narrowest section. The
celiac artery is cannulated and transected, and the organ is perfused with cold
perfusate and heparin.

The recipient animal has a left nephrectomy performed from a ventral midline celiotomy as described. End-to-end anastomosis is performed with the
donor splenic vein to the renal vein and the donor celiac artery to the renal
artery. A Roux-en-Y loop is isolated in the recipient jejunum by transecting a
section of the jejunum and performing an end-to-side anastomosis of the
proximal segment to the distal segment. A 40-cm section of the loop is isolated
and flushed free of intestinal contents. An invaginated section of the pancreas
is anastomosed into the proximal end of the loop in order to provide exocrine
duct entrance into the gastrointestinal tract without contamination by intestinal contents of the anastomotic site (see Chapter 7, Fig. 7.2). The abdominal incision is closed in a routine manner.

Postoperative care should include systemic antibiotics, immunosuppressive
therapy, and analgesics. Animals receive fluid and nutrition by a continuous iv
infusion for 3 days prior to starting solid food.

Pancreatic Duct Ablation/Cannulation/Pancreatitis

It is more difficult to induce acute and chronic pancreatitis in swine than in other species. The pancreatic duct is readily identifiable at its entrance into the duodenum from the distal portion of the body. It is palpable as a firm tubular structure with a grayish white appearance. Its entrance into the duodenum is distal from that of the bile duct (Engelhardt et al., 1982; Sarr, 1988; Thorpe and Frey, 1971).

Acute pancreatitis has been produced by the injection under pressure of bile incubated with active trypsin. The lesions are much milder in the pig than in other species (Sarr, 1988; Thorpe and Frey, 1971).

A model of chronic pancreatitis can be produced by ligation of the duct and creation of ischemia by ligating the branches of the pancreatoduodenal artery supplying the body of the pancreas. The blood supply to the tail is left intact. Lesions of chronic inflammation and fibrosis appear within weeks of the ductal ablation. Pseudocysts may also be present. There is exocrine deficiency with weight loss and gastrointestinal signs, but no signs of diabetes (Pitkaranta et al., 1989).

The pancreatic duct can be cannulated for short-term collection of pancreatic enzymes; however, animals will die of electrolyte imbalances and inability to digest nutrients in approximately a week. These problems can be alleviated by using reentry cannulation of the duodenum after exteriorizing the catheter on the abdominal wall to partially return pacreatic secretions. The catheter is passed into the main pancreatic duct and ligated in place. The catheter is exited through the ventral abdominal wall to the collection device and then reentered into the abdomen and the proximal duodenum. Suture retention beads should be used inside the pancreatic duct and the duodenum to avoid dislodgement. Alternatively, side entrance catheters can be used in the accessory duct or T-tubes in the main duct if only partial collection of the pancreatic secretions is desired (Niebergall-Roth et al., 1997; Swindle et al., 1998).

Splenectomy and Splenic Vascular Catheterization

The spleen is approached using a paracostal incision with the pig in dorsal recumbency. The incision starts from the lateral margin of the mammary glands at the halfway point between the first and second nipple on the left side. The incision parallels the caudal margin of the caudal edge of the rib line and extends caudolaterally to approximately the level of the third nipple. The splenectomy may also be performed from a midline incision; however, dissection of the short gastric vessels is more difficult (Swindle, 1983).

After celiotomy, the tail of the pancreas is retracted out of the abdomen. The vessels supplying the splenic hilus are clamped, transected, and ligated in this order: left gastroepiploic, splenic, and short gastric artery and veins. The arteries and veins may be ligated together. The short gastric vessels are deep in the abdomen and in close proximity to the stomach. They generally are ligated in situ and then transected. While dissecting this vessel, care should be taken to avoid damage to the underlying pancreas (Fig. 6.4).

The splenic vessels may also be used to catheterize the portal system with or without splenectomy. The surgical exposure for this procedure is easier than the exposure described for the portal vein catheterization in Chapter 9; however, the location of the tip of the catheter is not as readily discernable and catheters made of nonflexible materials may penetrate into the abdomen at the entrance of the vessel into the portal vein. Sacrifice of a single vessel or pair of vessels in the spleen for this procedure does not cause a problem because of the extensive collateral circulation.

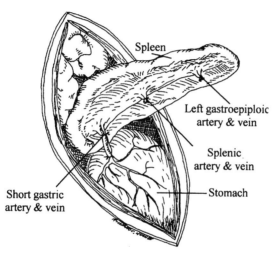

FIGURE 6.4   Ligation of the vessels of the splenic hilus for splenectomy.

References

Engelhardt, W., P.O. Schwille, C. Gebhardt, M. Stolte, and H. Zirngibl. 1982. Pancreatic tissue hormones and molar insulin glucagon ratio in portal and peripheral blood of the minipig—Influence of pancreatic duct occlusion. Eur. Surg. Res. 14(2): 97–100.

Getty, R. (ed) 1975. Sisson and Grossman's the Anatomy of the Domestic Animals—Porcine, Vol. 2. Philadelphia: W.B. Saunders, pp. 1215–1422.

Hand, M.S., R.W. Phillips, C.W. Miller, R.A. Mason, and W.V. Lumb. 1981. A method for quantitation of hepatic, pancreatic and intestinal function in conscious Yucatan miniature swine. Lab. Anim. Sci. 31(6): 728–731.

Koyama, I., L.R. Pennington, M.M. Swindle, and G.M. Williams. 1986. Pancreatic allo-transplantation with Roux-en-Y jejunal diversion in swine: Its technical aspects. In Tumbleson, M.E. (ed), Swine in Biomedical Research, Vol. 1. New York: Plenum Press, pp. 385–390.

Laber-Laird, K., A.C. Smith, M.M. Swindle, and J. Colwell. 1992. Effects of isoflurane anesthesia on glucose clearance in Yucatan minipigs. Lab. Anim. Sci. 42(6): 579–581.

Mullen, Y., Y. Taura, M. Nagata, K. Miyazawa, and E. Stein. 1992. Swine as a model for pancreatic beta-cell transplantation. In Swindle, M.M. (ed), Swine as Models in Biomedical Research. Ames: Iowa State University Press, pp. 16–34.

Niebergall-Roth E., S. Teyssen, and M.V. Singer. 1997. Pancreatic exocrine studies in intact animals: Historic and current methods. Lab. Anim. Sci. 47(6): 606–616.

Pennington, L., and M.G. Sarr. 1988. Pancreas transplantation. In Swindle, M.M., and Adams, R.J. (eds), Experimental Surgery and Physiology: Induced Animal Models of Human Disease. Baltimore: Williams and Wilkins, pp. 296–297.

Pitkaranta, P., L. Kivisaari, S. Nordling, A. Saari, and T. Schroder. 1989. Experimental chronic pancreatitis in the pig. Scand. J. Gastroenterol. 24(8): 987–992.

Sarr, M.G. 1988. Pancreas. In Swindle, M.M., and Adams, R.J. (eds), Experimental Surgery and Physiology: Induced Animal Models of Human Disease. Baltimore: Williams and Wilkins, pp. 204–216.

Sasaki, N. K. Yoneda, C. Bigger, J. Brown, and Y. Mullen. 1984. Fetal pancreas transplantation in miniature swine. Developmental characteristics of fetal pig pancreases. Transplantation 38(4): 335–340.

Schantz, L.D., K. Laber-Laird, S. Bingel, and M. Swindle. 1996. Pigs: Applied anatomy of the gastrointestinal tract. In Jensen, S.L., Gregersen, H., Moody, F., and Shokouh-Amiri, M.H. (eds), Essentials of Experimental Surgery: Gastroenterology. New York: Harwood Academic Publishers, pp. 2611–2619.

Stump, K.C., M.M. Swindle, C.D. Saudek, and J.D. Strandberg. 1988. Pancreatectomized swine as a model of diabetes mellitus. Lab. Anim. Sci. 38(4): 439–443.

Swindle, M.M. 1983. Basic Surgical Exercises Using Swine. Philadelphia: Praeger Press.

Swindle, M.M., A.C. Smith, and J.A. Goodrich. 1998. Chronic cannulation and fistulization procedures in swine: A review and recommendations. J. Invest. Surg. 11(1): 1–8.

Thorpe, C.D., and C.F. Frey. 1971. Experimental pancreatitis in pigs. Arch. Surg. 103(6): 720–723.

7 URINARY SYSTEM AND ADRENAL GLANDS

___

General Principles of Surgery

The urinary system of the pig is anatomically similar to that of most species. The left kidney is more cranial than the right kidney and its cranial pole is located at approximately the 13th rib. The renal artery and vein branches into two branches close to the renal hilus. The blood supply is divided into cranial and caudal segments rather than into longitudinal halves as in other species. This means that the avascular plane of the kidney is transverse rather than longitudinal (Fig. 7.1). The ureters extend caudoventrally to the dorsolateral aspect of the neck of the urinary bladder. The urinary bladder is large and thin walled but typical in morphology. It receives its innervation from S2 to S4. The urethra courses along the pelvic floor into the penis. The tip of the penis is located on the ventral abdominal wall in a preputial diverticulum. The external opening of the preputial diverticulum is located immediately caudal to the umbilicus. The contents of this structure must always be expressed prior to performing abdominal surgery in male swine. The desquamated cells and urine in the preputial diverticulum are foul smelling and contaminated. Gloves should be worn during the expression of this material (Hodson, 1986; Russell et al., 1981; Swindle, 1983; Swindle and Olson, 1988; Terris, 1986).

The adrenal glands are associated with the medial surface toward the cranial pole of each kidney. The right adrenal gland is tightly adhered to the caudal vena cava. The arterial supply of the glands is from either the aorta or branches of the lumbar arteries, and the venous drainage is into either the vena cava or the renal veins (Fig. 7.1) (Venzke, 1975; Swindle and Smith, 1998).

Catheterization of the urinary bladder through the penis is difficult to impossible depending upon the size of the animal

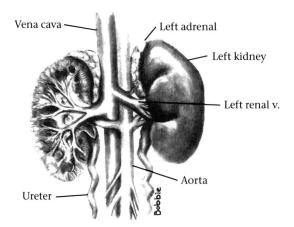

FIGURE 7.1   Illustration of the renal internal and surface anatomy. *Reprinted with permission from Swindle, 1984, Comparative Anatomy of the Pig, Charles River Technical Bulletin, Charles River Laboratories, Inc.*

and the breed because of the male anatomy. Consequently, the urinary bladder can be emptied by manual expression in small animals or via needle aspiration. Needle aspiration should be performed very carefully because the bladder is relatively thin walled and tears easily. The male urethra may be entered percutaneously with an intracath needle as it courses ventrally over the pubis in the perineum. It may be palpated on the midline. This catheterization procedure can be readily performed with practice. The female urethra may be catheterized conventionally and may be entered on the floor of the vagina approximately one-quarter to one-third of the distance to the cervix (Swindle, 1983).

Nephrectomy

Nephrectomy can be performed either through a ventral midline approach or a retroperitoneal approach through the flank. The flank approach is the approach of choice if only one kidney is involved in the surgical procedure (Swindle, 1983; Webster et al., 1992).

The flank approach is performed with the pig in ventral or lateral recumbency. A curved linear incision is made caudal to the last rib following its contour approximately one-quarter to one-third of the distance ventrally from the lateral aspect of the vertebral wings to the midline. The muscle layers are either cut or bluntly divided and retracted until the peritoneum is exposed. Using manual manipulation, the peritoneum is retracted ventrally after peeling it from the dorsal aspect of the abdominal musculature and the kidney. When performed properly the kidney is exposed without entering the abdominal cavity and having the resulting interference with the abdominal viscera.

If bilateral renal procedures are to be performed or if other abdominal procedures are involved in the protocol, then a ventral midline incision is the preferred approach. The spiral colon will interfere with observation of the kidneys, especially the left one, if it has not been emptied preoperatively. This may be performed either by a 48-hour fast from solid foods or by administering hypertonic saline cathartics, as previously described. The ventral midline incision is initiated at the xiphoid process and extends caudally beyond the umbilicus. Balfour retractors and laparotomy sponges are required to retract the viscera for surgical exposure of the kidneys. The intestinal mass should not be exteriorized to enhance exposure because of the complications of edema and ischemia, to which the pig is highly susceptible.

The renal artery is bluntly dissected and ligated first. A branch of the suprarenal artery supplying the adrenals will have to be ligated in some cases, especially on the left kidney. This is followed by isolation and ligation of the renal vein and then the ureter. From the flank approach, it is helpful to make a sling of surgical gauze around the cranial and caudal poles of the kidney. This aids in the manipulation of the organ to enhance retraction and exposure. When dissecting in the midline region, care should be taken to avoid damaging the lymphatics. They can usually be seen; and should be ligated, if damaged, to avoid chyloperitoneum.

Following removal of the kidney, the incision is closed in a routine manner. When closing a flank incision, it is not necessary to suture the retracted peritoneum back in place. The muscle layers are closed in anatomically correct layers by suturing the fascia. The skin and subcutaneous tissues are closed in a routine fashion.

Partial Nephrectomy/Intrarenal Surgery

The branches of the renal artery supplying the kidney divide the blood supply transversely rather than longitudinally. The avascular plane of the kidney may be readily demonstrated by temporarily occluding the blood supply of one of the branches of the renal artery in the hilus of the kidney (Russell et al., 1981; Swindle and Olson, 1988).

If a surgical approach to the renal pelvis is indicated, then this avascular plane forms the line of incision into the kidney parenchyma. The capsule of the kidney is incised with a scalpel, and the incision may be continued either with a scalpel or bluntly with a surgical spatula. The kidney is surgically repaired with mattress sutures of synthetic absorbable or nonabsorbable sutures, which occlude the edges of the incision and provide hemostasis. In heminephrectomy, this technique of closure will occlude most of the blood supply, but it may be necessary to provide additional hemostasis with oxycellulose sponges (Russell et al., 1981; Swindle and Olson, 1988).

The blood supply to the kidney may be reduced by either surgical imbrication, inflatable circumferential cuffs or Goldblatt clamp techniques that occlude the renal blood flow. This procedure is performed usually to produce a model of renal hypertension. In order to produce the model surgically, it is necessary to remove one kidney and significantly reduce the blood supply to the remaining kidney. The exception to this is the 2-kidney deoxycorticosterone acetate (DOCA) salt model in Yucatan miniature swine (O'Hagan and Zambraski, 1986; Swindle and Olson, 1988).

In order to produce the model of hypertension, the left kidney is surgically removed as described above. The right kidney, which has a longer artery than the left, is the kidney to which the blood supply is reduced. In our laboratories, a reduction of approximately 75% of the renal blood flow will produce chronic hypertension. An acute hypertensive episode may be initiated by challenge with 0.9% NaCl at a rate of 20 ml/kg iv as a bolus and maintenance infusion. An increase of 20% above baseline arterial pressure is considered significant.

Renal Transplant

The pig has been used in renal transplantation research to study organ preservation, rejection phenomena, and surgical procedures including allographic, xenografic, heterotopic, and orthotopic techniques. In addition to the anatomic characteristics of the kidneys described above, it is important to use anesthetic and perioperative techniques that maintain adequate blood pressure to ensure tissue perfusion (>50 torr) and avoid vasospasm (Howard et al., 1994; Kirkman et al., 1979; Pennington, 1992; Sachs, 1992; Williams, 1988).

Selection of the donor and recipient breeds will be determined by the longevity of the experiment and the type of experiment being performed. For example, if the recipient is to be another pig and the experiment is meant to be longer than 3 weeks in length, then one of the miniature breeds should be considered because of the difficulty in maintaining large farm pigs postsurgically. Differences will be noted in the histocompatibility complex among breeds as well. Many sources of farm and miniature pigs will have closely related individuals in the herd even if they are not littermates.

The surgical approach to the kidneys and the general perioperative procedures, such as fasting, are the same as the ones noted for nephrectomy. The midline incision is preferred because of the increased surgical exposure. The flank approach may be preferred if the donor animal is expected to survive the experiment, especially if a future reimplantation procedure is anticipated using the midline approach.

In a nonsurvival donor procedure to harvest the kidneys, the aorta and vena cava are isolated cranial and caudal to the renal vessels, and the kidneys are harvested en bloc. This procedure will involve ligation of the dorsal lumbar branches of the aorta and careful dissection to avoid blood loss. The aorta and vena cava are ligated proximally and distally after heparinization of the animal. A sufficient length of ureter to ensure successful reimplantation without stretching should be simultaneously harvested.

In a survival procedure, a decision has to be made concerning which kidney is to be harvested. For the left kidney, the renal artery will be shorter and the renal vein longer. For the right kidney, the opposite is true, and the adrenal gland is closely associated with the junction of the renal vein and vena cava. If using a flank approach, the left kidney is generally the kidney of choice to remove. When a single kidney is harvested, it is best to use a Satinsky clamp to isolate the renal vessels and harvest them using a Carrel patch technique. Reimplantation of the renal vessels is greatly enhanced when such a patch is available. It also minimizes the manipulation of the renal artery, which is very prone to vasospasm. Care should be taken to avoid damaging the lymphatics in a survival procedure, because the accumulation of lymph in the abdominal cavity will result in a postoperative complication. They may either be ligated or cauterized. The donor kidney should be perfused with a cold preservation solution and kept in a chilled preservation solution or isotonic iced slurry until reimplantation.

The midline approach is preferred for reimplantation of the kidneys. A prolonged fast (24–48 hours) ensures that the colon will be emptied, which aids both the surgical exposure and the prevention of edema postsurgically following manipulation of the intestinal mass. The kidney is usually implanted into the distal aorta and vena cava or the iliac vessels in order to minimize the length of ureter that has to be reimplanted (Fig. 7.2); and thus minimize the chances of ischemic necrosis of the structure. After heparinizing the recipient, a Satinsky clamp is applied to the artery and a longitudinal incision made. The cranial and caudal ends of the Carrel patch are sutured with 6/0 nonabsorbable cardiovascular suture, and the patch is anastomosed with a simple continuous pattern. The same procedure is performed for the renal vein, and blood reperfusion is allowed by removing first the venous, then the arterial clamps. The kidney is observed to return to a normal color following the presence of blood flow through the vessels.

The ureter is trimmed to reach the dorsal surface of the bladder without stretching, and the end is spatulated. By opening the tip of the urethra longitudinally, the lumen of the anastomosed ureter is increased in size. A silicone tube or stent may be passed into the ureter to ensure that the lumen is not sutured closed. Simple interrupted sutures of 6/0 nonabsorbable cardiovascular suture are preplaced and the luminal tube removed prior to closure.

Postimplantation, the animal should be flushed with iv fluid at a rate of 10–20 ml/kg/h and an infusion of 50 ml of 50% mannitol or glucose. An iv injection of methylene blue may be used to check for leaks in the ureteral anastomosis. Closure of the surgical incision is routine, and the postoperative recovery procedures should be aimed toward maintenance of adequate fluid levels and normal body temperature. Use of postoperative analgesics, antibiotics, and other therapeutic agents depends upon the experimental protocol.

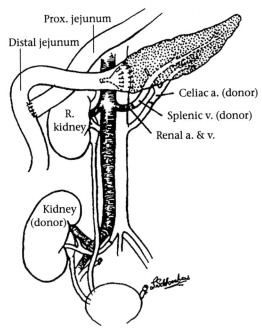

Prox. jejunum
Distal jejunum
Celiac a. (donor)
R. kidney
Splenic v. (donor)
Renal a. & v.
Kidney (donor)

FIGURE 7.2   Orthotopic transplantation of the kidney in conjunction with segmental pancreatic transplant. *Reprinted with permission from Koyama et al., 1986, Pancreatic allotransplantation with Roux-en-Y jejunal diversion, in M.E. Tumbleson (ed), Swine in Biomedical Research, Vol. 1, New York: Plenum Press, pp. 385-389.*

Cystotomy/Ureteral Diversion

The bladder of the pig is thin walled and difficult to catheterize (see above). Consequently, it may be desirable to suture a catheter in place during abdominal surgery in some experimental models. In the pet pig population, urolithiasis is also a problem, and cystotomy may be part of the indicated treatment.

The surgical approach is via a ventral midline incision in females and a paramedian incision lateral to the penis in the male. The bladder is usually drained carefully using a needle and syringe in the male because of the difficulty in catheterization. The surgical approach may be made in any avascular portion of the bladder after packing it away from the viscera with wetted gauze sponges.

Implantation of a Foley catheter may be used for urine collection after it is sutured in place with a purse-string suture in the perineum. If a cystotomy is performed to remove uroliths, the area is copiously flushed with saline prior to suturing the incision closed. The bladder is too thin walled for a double suture layer closure except in larger animals. Any type of suture pattern that achieves a waterproof seal is appropriate. These would include a two-layer pattern of Cushing oversewn with Lembert sutures, simple interrupted, or continuous patterns using synthetic nonabsorbable sutures. The abdominal incision may be closed using a standard technique (Swindle, 1983).

Urinary Tract Obstruction/Reflux Nephropathy/ Hydronephrosis

Swine are the preferred model for the study of lower and upper urinary tract obstruction and the resulting complications because of the similarities of their internal renal anatomy to that of humans. Models have been created in various ages of swine to study the different effects of maturity. Swine less than 1 month of age are similar to neonatal humans in development of the urinary tract and swine 5–6 months of age are similar to adults. Most of the pediatric models have been studied in 8- to 12-week-old pigs. Swine can have a spontaneous occurrence of both vesico-ureteral reflux and hydronephrosis and should be screened prior to surgery (Constantinou et al., 1986; Djurhuus et al. 1976; Jørgensen and Djurhuus, 1986; Jørgensen et al., 1983; Jørgensen et al., 1984a,b; Melick et al., 1961).

A model of intrarenal reflux may be produced by surgically reimplanting the ureters. This is performed using the same ventral midline incision described for cystotomy. The intravesical ureteral roof is excised along with a small wedge of ipsilateral trigonal muscle. The ureteral roof is reimplanted at an angle in order to straighten the juxtavesicular portion of the ureter after performing a ventral cystotomy. The relaxation and changed angle of the ureteral orifice reliably produces vesico-ureteral reflux. This is an improvement over a previous model of cutting the lower 3–4 mm of the wall of the ureteric orifice following a cystotomy. Intrarenal reflux will not occur with this model unless there is a pressure increase secondary to lower urinary tract obstruction. This is performed by partially obstructing the ureter at the neck of the bladder with a wire or plastic ring. The amount of constriction is variable depending upon the age and breed of the pig; however, reports range from 3- to 6-mm diameters for the rings. Reflux starts to occur at a bladder pressure of approximately 10 cm H_2O in operated animals compared to a pressure of greater than 20 cm H_2O in nonoperated animals. Infection may be studied as a complication in either of these models. The progression of the syndrome depends upon the length of time of the extravesicular obstruction as well as the degree of constriction. This procedure may lead to renal failure (Jørgensen and Djurhuus, 1986; Jørgensen et al., 1984a,b).

Hydronephrosis and hydroureteronephrosis may also be produced surgically. The left ureter is primarily studied because of the increased incidence of left sided involvement clinically in humans. The surgical approach is retroperitoneal through the flank as described for the nephrectomy (above). The ureter is identified as it progresses caudomedially to the caudal pole of the kidney in the retroperitoneal space. Complete obstruction is performed by ligating the ureter. This will lead to a rapid dilation of the kidney within hours, after which the kidney then shrinks and develops a progressive nephropathy over months (Constantinou et al., 1986; Djurhuus et al., 1976).

Partial obstruction results in more progressive changes over a period of 3–4 months. Partial obstruction may be produced by partial occlusion with cuffs or sutures tied over a premeasured rod or catheter. However, a model of progressive chronic hydronephrosis can be consistently produced by implanting a 1- to 2-cm length of the ureter into the psoas muscle caudal to the kidney. For this model, the fascia of the psoas muscle is incised, and the muscle fibers are split in a curved fashion medially toward the midline in the body of the muscle. The ureter is gently placed into the psoas muscle without torsion or kinking (Fig. 7.3). The sheath and ventral edge of the muscle are loosely approximated with simple interrupted sutures. This will lead to a progressive syndrome of chronic hydronephrosis secondary to obstruction within weeks.

The abdominal incision is closed in a routine manner.

Perineal Urethrostomy/Urinary Diversion

In cases of urolithiasis or trauma in males, it may be necessary to permanently divert the urinary outlet to the perineum or ventral midline. In experimental

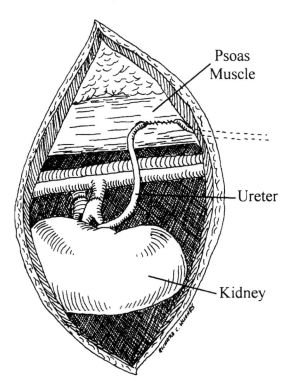

FIGURE 7.3.   Suturing the urethra into the psoas muscle from a flank approach.

models it may be necessary to perform these procedures to facilitate chronic urine collection (Noordhuizen-Stassen and Wensing, 1983; Swindle, 1983; Tscholl, 1978).

The urethra may be palpated by using a rolling movement with the fingers on the brim of the pubis in the perineal region. If percutaneous catheterization (see above) is not achieved or desired, then a perineal urethrostomy may be performed. A dorsal to ventral midline incision approximately 1–2 cm in length is made through the skin and subcutaneous tissue in the dependent portion of the perineum dorsal to the scrotum. The urethra and base of the penis can be identified between the crura and ischiocavernosus muscles and isolated in the subcutaneous tissue. The penis and urethra are ligated ventrally, and, using iris scissors, the urethra is split dorsally for a distance of at least 1 cm. Care should be taken to avoid trauma to this tissue by using atraumatic instruments, such as Debakey forceps, when handling the urethra. Complete hemostasis in the subcutaneous tissue is essential for the success of this procedure. After splitting the urethra, it is sutured to the skin using a simple interrupted pattern with synthetic absorbable or monofilament nonabsorbable sutures. This will result in a dorsal oval-shaped entrance into the urethra with a ventral rectangular shaped apron. The skin is closed with simple interrupted sutures (Fig. 7.4).

If urine collection is the goal of this surgery, pediatric adhesive urine collection bags may be attached to the skin over the incision site. The skin must be prepped with alcohol in order to achieve adhesion with these bags, and stay sutures may be required. The main complication encountered postoperatively

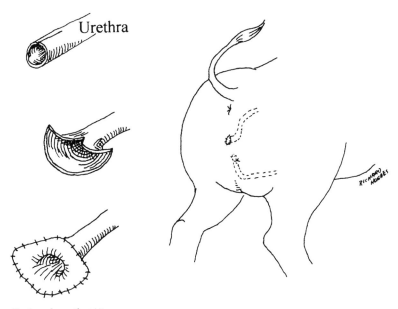

FIGURE 7.4   Perineal urethrostomy.

will be urine scalding, especially if the pig is uncastrated and the scrotum is prominent. This complication requires the use of topical antiinflammatory and/or antibiotic ointments on a chronic basis if it occurs. Simultaneous castration may help relieve this complication by making the scrotum less prominent. Another complication to be considered is contamination with feces in this area. Alternatively, a Foley catheter may be placed into the incised urethra and directed caudally into the plastic adhesive pouch. In this case, the incision is closed with a purse-string suture.

If long-term maintenance of the animal is indicated, then it may be preferable to perform urinary diversion by performing a urethrostomy with the urethra directed ventrally cranial to the scrotum on the ventral midline.

Preputial Diverticulum Ablation

The preputial diverticulum may be surgically ablated to reduce the odor of male pigs and to relieve infection of the structure. The structure should be manually expressed and flushed with saline and dilute Betadine solution prior to surgery. There are two lateral epithelial-lined pouches within the structure. These are exteriorized one at a time by inserting Allis or Babcock forceps into the preputial opening and directing them laterally. After grasping the lining of the structure with the forceps, the lining is steadily pulled out of the opening. This process is then repeated on the opposite side. Any visible blood vessels are cauterized or ligated, and the structure is excised. The resected pockets are packed with umbilical tape or gauze for 5–10 minutes to provide hemostasis. After the gauze is removed, the structure is examined for hemorrhage and repacked if necessary.

The surgery may also be performed by an open technique. With this technique, the diverticular pouches are packed with umbilical tape or gauze to identify them, and a skin incision is made over each structure. The pouches are then dissected free from the subcutaneous tissue. The surgical wound is closed with subcuticular sutures (Bollwahn, 1992; Dutton et al., 1997; Kross et al., 1982; Lawhorn et al., 1994).

Adrenalectomy

The surgical approaches to the adrenal gland are the same as for midline, flank, and retroperitoneal approaches to the kidney described above for nephrectomy. The surgical anatomy of the adrenal glands is depicted in Figures 1.22 (Chapter 1) and 7.1. Indications for adrenalectomy in swine will most likely involve the creation of a model of adrenal insufficiency and thus will probably be bilateral. If a unilateral adrenalectomy is indicated, the left adrenal gland is more readily removed (Dougherty, 1981).

Regardless of the surgical approach, the adrenal glands are readily mobilized by blunt dissection. In older animals, they will probably be covered with perirenal fat. After identification of the arterial branches, the branches are ligated and transected. Variations in the blood supply to both glands may be encountered and care should be taken not to damage the renal vessels during the dissection. Careful dissection is required to separate the right adrenal gland from the wall of the caudal vena cava and to ligate the venous drainage. Removal of this gland may require repair of the vessel wall. After the adrenalectomy is performed, the abdominal incision is closed in a routine fashion.

Intraoperative and postoperative care is directed toward controlling the effects of glucocorticoid and mineralocorticoid insufficiency. In a bilateral procedure, these complications can rapidly lead to death from electrolyte imbalances. Unilateral procedures may induce adrenocortical insufficiency, which may require supplementation until the remaining adrenal gland hypertrophies and restores function. Monitoring of serum electrolytes, especially potassium, and glucose is essential. Fluid therapy and glucocorticoid administration, with such agents as prednisolone, will be necessary to restore imbalances. With a bilateral adrenalectomy, the exogenous maintenance therapy is permanent. Otherwise, postoperative care is routine for celiotomies and laparotomies.

References

Bollwahn, W. 1992. Surgical procedures in boars and sows. In Leman, A.D., Straw, B.E., Mengeling, W.L., D'Allaire, S., and Taylor, D.J. (eds), Diseases of Swine, 7th ed. Ames: Iowa State University Press, pp. 782–793.

Constantinou, C.E., J.C. Djurhuus, L. Vercesi, A.J. Ford, and J.D. Meindl. 1986. Model for chronic obstruction and hydronephrosis. In Tumbleson, M.E. (ed), Swine in Biomedical Research, Vol. 3. New York: Plenum Press, pp. 1711–1724.

Djurhuus, J.C., B. Nerstrom, N. Gyrd-Hansen, and H. Rask-Anderson. 1976. Experimental hydronephrosis. Acta. Chir. Scand. 472(Suppl.): 17–28.

Dougherty, R.W. 1981. Experimental Surgery in Farm Animals. Ames: Iowa State University Press.

Dutton, D.M., B. Lawhorn, and R.N. Hooper. 1997. Ablation of the cranial portion of he preputial cavity in a pig. J. Am. Vet. Med. Assoc. 211(5): 598–599.

Hodson C.J. 1986. The pig as a model for studying kidney disease in man. In Tumbleson, M.E.(ed), Swine in Biomedical Research, Vol. 3. New York: Plenum Press, pp. 1691–1704.

Howard, T., C.A. Cosenza, D.V. Cramer, and L. Makowka. 1994. Kidney transplantation in Yucatan miniature swine. In Cramer, D.V., Podesta, L., and Makowka L. (eds), Handbook of Animal Models in Transplantation Research. Boca Raton: CRC Press, pp. 19–28.

Jørgensen, T.M., and J.C. Djurhuus. 1986. Experimental vesicoureteric reflux in pigs. In Tumbleson, M.E.(ed), Swine in Biomedical Research, Vol. 3. New York: Plenum Press, pp. 1737–1751.

Jørgensen, T.M., J.C. Djurhuus, H.S. Jorgensen, and S.S. Sorensen. 1983. Experimental bladder hyperreflexia in pigs. Urol. Res. 11(5): 239–240.

Jørgensen, T.M., J. Mortensen, K. Nielsen, and J.C. Djurhuus. 1984a. Pathogenetic factors in vesico-ureteral reflux. A longitudinal cystometrographic study in pigs. Scand. J. Urol. Nephrol. 18(1): 43–48.

Jørgensen, T.M., S. Olsen, J.C. Djurhuus, and J.P. Norgaard. 1984b. Renal morphology in experimental vesicoureteral reflux in pigs. Scand. J. Urol. Nephrol. 18(1): 49–58.

Kirkman, R.I., R.B. Colvin, M.W. Flye, G.S. Leight, S.A. Rosenberg, and G.M. Williams. 1979. Transplantation in miniature swine: VI. Factors influencing survival of renal allografts. Transplantation 28(1): 18–23.

Kross, S.B., N.K. Ames, and C. Gibson. 1982. Extirpation of the preputial diverticulum in a boar. Vet. Med. Sm. Anim. Clin. 77(4): 549–553.

Lawhorn, B., P.D. Jarrett, and G.F. Lackey. 1994. Removal of the preputial diverticulum in swine. J. Am. Vet. Med. Assoc. 205: 92–96.

Melick, W.F., J.J. Naryka, and J.H. Schmidt. 1961. Experimental studies of ureteral peristaltic patterns in the pig. Similarity of pig and human ureter and bladder physiology. J. Urol. 85(1): 145–148.

Noordhuizen-Stassen, E.N., and C.J. Wensing. 1983. The effect of transection of the main vascular and nervous supply of the testis on the development of spermatogenic epithelium in the pig. J. Pediatr. Surg. 18(5): 601–606.

O'Hagan, K.P., and E.J. Zambraski. 1986. Kidney function in deoxycorticosterone acetate (DOCA) treated hypertensive Yucatan miniature swine. In Tumbleson, M.E. (ed), Swine in Biomedical Research, Vol. 3. New York: Plenum Press, pp. 1779–1787.

Pennington, L.R. 1992. Renal transplantation in swine. In Swindle, M.M. (ed), Swine as Models in Biomedical Research. Ames: Iowa State University Press, pp. 35–43.

Russell, J.M., R.T. Webb, and W.H. Boyce. 1981. Intrarenal surgery. Animal model I. Invest. Urol. 19(2): 123–125.

Sachs, D.H. 1992. MHC-homozygous miniature swine. In Swindle, M.M. (ed), Swine as Models in Biomedical Research. Ames: Iowa State University Press, pp. 3–15.

Swindle, M.M. 1983. Basic Surgical Exercises Using Swine. Philadelphia: Praeger Press.

Swindle, M.M., and J. Olson. 1988. Urogenital system. In Swindle, M.M., Adams, R.J. (eds), Experimental Surgery and Physiology: Induced Animal Models of Human Disease. Baltimore: Williams and Wilkins, pp. 42–73.

Swindle M.M., and A.C. Smith. 1998. Comparative anatomy and physiology of the pig. Scand. J. Lab. Anim. Sci. 25(Suppl 1): 1-10.

Terris, J.M. 1986. Swine as a model in renal physiology and nephrology: An overview. In Tumbleson, M.E. (ed), Swine in Biomedical Research, Vol. 2. New York: Plenum Press, pp. 1673–1690.

Tscholl, R. 1978. Urinary diversion. Urol. Res. 6(1): 59–63.

Venzke, W.G. 1975. Porcine endocrinology. In Getty, R. (ed), Sisson and Grossman's The Anatomy of the Domestic Animals—Porcine, Vol. 2. Philadelphia: WB Saunders, pp. 1304-1305.

Webster, S.K., M.A. Deleo, and K.E. Burhop. 1992. The anephric micropig as a model for peritoneal dialysis. In Swindle, M.M. (ed), Swine as Models in Biomedical Research. Ames: Iowa State University Press, pp. 64–73.

Williams, G.M. 1988. Renal transplantation. In Swindle, M.M., and Adams, R.J. (eds), Experimental Surgery and Physiology: Induced Animal Models of Human Disease. Baltimore: Williams and Wilkins, pp. 298–299.

8 REPRODUCTIVE SYSTEM

General Principles of Surgery

The reproductive tract of the female is typical of that of a bicornuate species that produces litters. The ovaries are located caudal to the kidneys and are only loosely attached by a thin ovarian ligament and suspended within the broad ligament of the uterus. The ovarian vessels are the last branches of the aorta and vena cava prior to the iliac bifurcation at approximately L5–L6. The fallopian tubes are long and tortuous and typically form coils in the caudal abdominal cavity (Fig. 8.1). The fallopian tubes of an 80- to 100-kg pig approximate the diameter of those of an adult human (Rock et al., 1979). The uterine horns are long and curve cranially from the ovaries and then reverse direction to form the body of the uterus at approximately the same region of the ovaries in the midsagittal plane. The cervix is thick and has a curved cervical canal. The vagina extends caudally in the pelvic cavity and contains the urethral orifice on the ventral floor at approximately the level of the caudal edge of the pubic bone. The pig has an epitheliochorial placentation with drug transport and metabolic mechanisms similar to humans (Swindle and Bobbie, 1987; Swindle et al., 1996; Wiest et al., 1996).

The male reproductive system is typical of domestic animals in location; however, there are several variations in anatomy that are important surgically. The scrotum and testicles are located in the perineal region and may be of considerable size in adult males. The spermatic cord passes through each inguinal ring in the caudal abdomen. The spermatic vessels branch off the aorta and vena cava just cranial to the iliac bifurcation. Each ductus deferens enters the urethra independently on the dorsal surface at the neck of the bladder. The accessory sex glands are similar to humans except for the prominence of the various structures. The paired vesicular glands are large and lo-

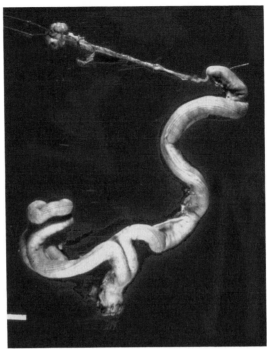

FIGURE 8.1   Anatomy of the female reproductive tract. The fallopian tube is fully extended on one horn.

cated on either side along the neck of the bladder. The prostate is small and located on the dorsal surface of the urethra at the entrance of the ductus deferens. Paired bulbourethral glands extend along the dorsolateral surface of the urethra starting at the caudal brim of the pubis and may extend the entire length of the pubis in intact adults. The crus of the penis and the ischiocavernosus muscles form at the caudal surface of the pubis with the base of the penis. The penis extends ventrally and cranially forming a fibromuscular sigmoid flexure as it curves from the perineum to the ventral surface of the abdomen. The penis extends almost to the umbilicus before terminating in the preputial diverticulum in a corkscrew shape. The preputial diverticulum is described additionally with the urinary system; however, it is important to restate that it must be cleaned prior to surgically preparing the abdomen and that gloves should be worn to avoid contamination with the foul-smelling fluid contents. The tip of the penis is almost impossible to exteriorize without trauma (Swindle et al., 1988; Swindle and Bobbie, 1987).

Castration (Orchiectomy)/Vasectomy

Swine may be castrated either by scrotal, prescrotal, or ventral midline approaches. The most common approach in small swine is prescrotal, while the scrotal approach predominates in adult males. For either the prescrotal or ventral midline approaches, the testicle is manually manipulated cranially and either a paramedian or midline incision is made over the testicle (Becker, 1992; Bollwahn, 1992; Mayo and Becker 1982; McGlone and Hellman, 1988; Swindle, 1983).

The skin and subcutaneous tissue are incised in the initial incision. The tunica vaginalis is incised without incising the testicular tissue. The testicle is exteriorized and the spermatic cord is dissected away from the mesorchium. Clamps are placed across the scrotal ligament and the spermatic cord and the testis is removed. The spermatic cord and the scrotal ligament are ligated with synthetic absorbable suture material. The incision is closed with continuous suture patterns in the tunical vaginalis and subcutaneous tissues. The skin is closed in a subcuticular pattern. It is unnecessary and undesirable to leave the castration incision open and draining as is performed in the agricultural setting. If adequate hemostasis is achieved, seromas or hematomas will not be a problem.

If a vasectomy is to be performed, the spermatic cord is identified as it passes from the scrotum to the inguinal canal at approximately a 45-degree angle to the midline from the scrotum to the brim of the pubis. At approximately one-half the distance between the scrotum and the inguinal canal, the spermatic cord can be palpated as a firm tubular structure. A skin incision is made over the spermatic cord and the tunic is incised. The vas deferens can be identified as a firm whitish structure approximately 2–3 mm in diameter. The vas deferens is isolated, doubly ligated and a segment removed. The tunic is closed with simple interrupted sutures, and the skin and subcutaneous tissues are closed in a routine manner (Fig. 8.2).

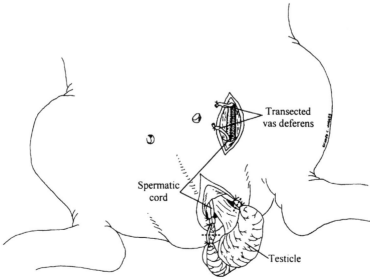

Transected vas deferens

Spermatic cord

Testicle

FIGURE 8.2   Castration and vasectomy site.

Ovariohysterectomy/Hysterectomy/Ovariectomy/Tubal Ligation

The female reproductive tract is usually approached through a ventral midline incision except in the case of a cesarian section (see below). The incision extends from the brim of the pubis to approximately two-thirds of the distance cranially to the umbilicus. Upon entering the abdomen, the fallopian tubes are likely to be the initial structures encountered in the nongravid system. They may be used to trace the origin of the ovaries and the horns of the uterus (Bollwahn, 1992; Christenson et al., 1987; Swindle, 1983).

The ovarian vessels are clamped, incised, and ligated proximally and distally. If only an ovariectomy is to be performed, then the fallopian tubes are divided surgically in the same manner, and the ovaries are removed. A tubal ligation may be performed by doubly ligating and dividing the structures or by placing occlusal devices on the structure for reversible sterilization (Rock et al., 1979).

If an ovariohysterectomy is to be performed, then it is necessary to dissect the horns of the uterus from the broad ligament of the uterus (Fig. 8.3A). This is performed by bluntly dissecting along the uterine vessels following the curvature of the uterine horns. The middle uterine vessels will have to be divided and ligated separately. The dissection is continued bilaterally to the level of the cervix.

At this point, the ovaries and uterine horns are retracted caudally, and the cervix is exteriorized. The blood vessels on the lateral sides of the vagina are individually ligated in place. The vagina proximal to the cervix is cross clamped and divided. The vaginal stump is sutured with transfixing ligatures in the case of nulliparous animals. In sows, the stump may have to be divided using an inverting technique such as a Cushing oversewn with a Lembert pattern. In the case of a hysterectomy, the instructions for the ovariohysterectomy are followed except that the ovaries are left intact, and the initial surgical transection starts with the fallopian tubes (Fig. 8.3B).

The middle uterine artery may be surgically constricted to reduce blood flow to the fetuses dependent upon the blood supply to the uterus. If performed in the second trimester of pregnancy it retards fetal and placental growth and development. It also reduces maternal estrogen blood levels (Molina et al., 1985).

Unlike many species of domestic animals, such as the dog and cat, swine rarely develop pyometritis, and the indications for these procedures are rarely clinical. Consequently, there are rarely problems associated with removal of the gonads and retention of the uterus. Rather, these procedures tend to either be research techniques or be surgical sterilization procedures for the pet pig. In the case of pet pigs, the ovaries should be removed in order to avoid the behavioral problems associated with estrus.

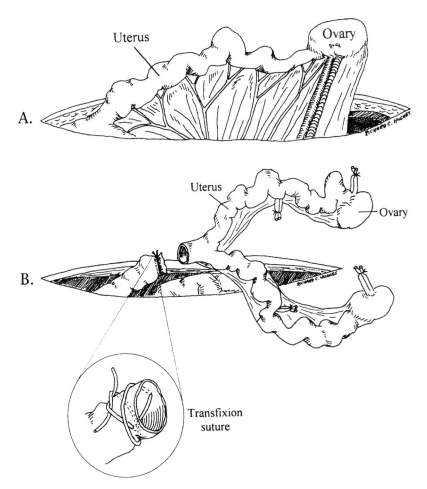

FIGURE 8.3A,B   Ovariohysterectomy.

Cesarian Section (C-Section)

A C-section may be performed using a midline, paramedian or flank surgical approach. (Bollwahn, 1992; Swindle et al., 1996) The midline and paramedian incisions are made as described above for ovariohysterectomy. If it is to be performed as a survival procedure with the pigs being allowed to nurse the sow, then it is best to avoid the midline approach. The midline will be constantly irritated by the pigs, and infection and refusal to nurse will be encountered as complications.

The paramedian incision is made along the dorsolateral margin of the mammary glands with the pig in lateral recumbency. The incision is made from the cranial margin of the retracted rear leg (approximately the brim of the pubis) to approximately the level of the umbilicus. In the pregnant sow, the muscle in this region will be thin and relatively avascular when cut; however, several branches of the caudal abdominal artery will have to be ligated or cauterized.

The flank approach is the most commonly employed approach for a C-section when the pigs are going to be allowed to nurse. A vertical incision is made from the level of the wings of the lumbar vertebrae ventrally to a point halfway to the mammary glands. The incision is located approximately one-half of the distance between the cranial surface of the thigh to the last rib. After making the skin incision, the muscles may either be bluntly dissected or transected in layers until the abdominal cavity is exposed.

Depending upon the number of fetuses and the experimental purpose of the surgery, multiple incisions will probably have to be made along the uterine horn, rather than making a single incision in the body of the uterus and removing all of them through a single incision. If the uterus and fetuses are large, it may be possible to remove all of the fetuses and membranes through an incision in the uterine horn. If fetuses have been manipulated experimentally, however, then an incision either over each fetus or between two fetuses may be required.

When the decision has been made to incise the uterus, the surgical site is packed off with warm saline-wetted laparotomy sponges. The uterotomy incision may be made using a scalpel; however, better hemostasis is achieved using absorbable GIA-60 3.8-mm staples. The device is inserted and fired after making a stab incision into the amniotic cavity. The fetus and membranes are extracted and handed to an assistant who cleans and resuscitates the piglet after ligation of the umbilical vessels. The uterus will contract relatively rapidly following removal of a fetus, which hampers the effort to remove multiple fetuses from the same incision. Hemorrhage from removal of the fetal membranes is usually minimal, providing that the C-section is performed at full-term gestation.

If a fetus is being removed prior to full-term gestation, then it is necessary to ligate and transect the umbilical vessels first. After this procedure, the membranes are bluntly separated from the uterine wall and extirpated. Gauze sponges may have to be used to provide hemostasis of the uterine wall following this procedure.

The uterotomy may be closed with a two-layer suture pattern of Cushing or Connell sutures oversewn with a Lembert suture pattern. It may also be closed with a staple surgical device, such as a TA-90 3.8 mm with absorbable staples, if staples were used to perform the uterotomy. In this case, the initial lines of staples are lifted together using Babcock forceps, and the TA device is closed distal to the suture line. After firing the device, a scalpel is used to trim the uterus between the device and the GIA staples. The line of TA staples is oversewn with a continuous Lembert pattern using absorbable sutures. The celiotomy incision is closed in a routine manner.

Fertility may be impaired following a C-section and this must be considered when making a clinical decision concerning performing the surgery as a survival procedure in the sow. Oxytocin may be given postoperatively if there is reason to believe that intrauterine hemorrhage may occur or that membranes remain in the uterus.

Fetal Surgery/Fetal Catheterization

The use of the pig as a fetal surgical model has been described and its usage is increasing because of the metabolic and anatomic similarities to humans and the availability of miniature breeds. Miniature breeds should be used whenever possible, because of the ease of handling smaller animals, which make them significantly more safe for personnel. For instance, a pregnant Yucatan sow may weigh 45–60 kg in contrast to a pregnant domestic farm pig that will probably weigh in excess of 135 kg. In this section, only the general surgical principles and the fetal catheterization techniques will be described. Other models will be described with the systemic sections of this text (Care et al., 1986; Dungan et al., 1995; Jackson and Egdahl, 1960; Jones and Hudak, 1988; Kraeling et al., 1986; Randall, 1986; Rosenkrantz et al., 1968; Sims et al., 1997; Swindle et al., 1996; Wiest et al., 1996).

Timing of the surgery may make a difference in the selection of the breed because of size of the fetus. Each trimester of pregnancy is 38 days in a species with a 114-day gestation period. The last trimester of pregnancy (>78 days) is used for many procedures, because the size of the fetus makes it amenable to catheterization and device implantation. The consistency and volume of the amniotic fluid changes as gestation progresses. For the first two trimesters the amniotic fluid has a watery consistency and occupies a relatively large volume of the amniotic sac. As parturition approaches, the amniotic fluid becomes relatively thick and yellowish in color from the passage of meconium. In the last few days of pregnancy, the fluid volume is substantially decreased.

Some relative sizes of the fetus at different stages of pregnancy for various breeds are in Table 8.1.

Maintenance of normothermia and homeostasis of the sow is imperative in order to be successful with these procedures. This can be achieved by a combination of keeping the room temperature greater than 29°C, use of circulating water blankets both below and above the sow's thorax, use of heat lamps suspended near the surgical site and/or dripping 37°C saline into the amniotic

Table 8.1.   Relative fetal sizes for various breeds at different stages of pregnancy

Breed	Gestation day	Crown/rump length (cm)	Weight (g)
Yucatan	100	15.7–16.9	350–391.3
	90–92	15.8–17.5	318–403.5
Göttingen	111–112	13–16	305.3–370.4
Landrace	80	16.5–17.5	332.5–377

cavity during surgery. Use of the warmed saline drip allows lowering the room temperature and discontinuance of the heat lamps that can be desiccating to delicate fetal tissues.

Other perioperative procedures that contribute to the success of these procedures include restricting the fetus from breathing by keeping the head submerged in amniotic fluid; meticulous attention to asepsis; and the prophylactic use of systemic antibiotics, such as the cephalosporins; delicate handling of tissues; and an anesthetic protocol that does not significantly depress the sow or fetus. Anesthesia is discussed in a separate chapter; however, analgesics and muscle relaxants may be delivered directly to the fetus if necessary. For example, pancuronium may be administered to restrict fetal breathing if the fetal head has to be removed from the uterus during surgery. Hemostasis is essential in any of the procedures performed because of the small blood volume of the fetus. Vessels should be ligated in advance of transection, if possible, and electrocautery on a low setting should be used. Use of microsurgical instruments and microsurgical cannonball and spear-shaped swabs are helpful in some procedures. All fetal tissue is extremely friable and can be readily traumatized by use of adult-sized surgical instruments. Ophthalmic and pediatric instruments are useful in cases in which the smaller microsurgical instruments are not required. All gauze should be wetted, and the fetus and membranes should be bathed regularly in saline warmed to 37°–38°C. Monitoring the fetal heart rate is a very helpful indicator of fetal distress and hypothermia. In an 80- to 90-day-old fetus, the heart rate is approximately 180 beats per minute.

The paramedian surgical approach, as described for C-section, is preferred to avoid having undue pressure placed on the aorta when the sow is restrained in dorsal recumbency. This may lead to cardiovascular compromise and/or utero-placental ischemia. The line of incision is made in an avascular section along the antimesometrial border of the uterus. The uterotomy is best performed using staple surgical devices as described for C-sections (Fig. 8.4). If the uterotomy is done using conventional surgical techniques, hemostasis becomes problematic for the fetal membranes. They are too friable for most hemostatic techniques, and electrocautery does not function well. Babcock forceps can be placed on the edges of the incision in such a manner as to provide occlusion of the hemorrhaging vessel. Use of surgical staples seems to help prevent the edematous reaction that occurs in the fetal membranes if conventional surgical methods are used.

The position of the fetus in the uterus can be determined prior to performing the uterotomy by careful palpation. The snout tends to be readily identifiable after the middle of the second trimester of pregnancy. Care should be taken to avoid damaging the membranes or the umbilical cord during the palpation and the surgical procedure. Hemorrhage in the membranes can lead to abortion, fetal mummification, or resorption. In the first trimester of pregnancy, pinching the membranes and the fetal head can be used as a technique to reduce the number of fetuses in utero.

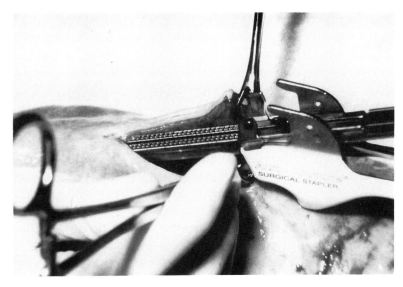

FIGURE 8.4   Uterotomy using a staple device. *Reprinted with permission from Swindle et al., 1996, Fetal surgical protocols in Yucatan miniature swine, Lab. Anim. Sci. 46(1): 90-95.*

The smallest incision possible should be used to expose the area of interest in the fetus. Following uterotomy the fetal surgical site should be gently rotated into the incision taking care to avoid torsion of the umbilical vessels. An assistant can retain the fetal surgical site in the uterotomy exposure by applying gentle pressure beneath the fetus. The fetus can also be positioned by exposing a fetal leg and manually restraining it using a wetted gauze sponge. Loss of amniotic fluid is not harmful provided it is replaced with a similar volume of sterile saline. By using the continuous drip of warmed saline method of providing heat to the fetus, this volume is continuously replaced.

Once the fetal incision is made, the edges can be retained by clamping them to the edges of the uterotomy incision with Babcock forceps. Microsurgical or ophthalmic self-retaining retractors can also be applied into the incision and held by an assistant.

The site of the fetal surgical incision will depend upon the technique being performed; however, some general guidelines are useful. The area of the umbilicus and the cranial abdominal midline are problematic for incisions because of the possibility of damaging the umbilical vessels or causing vasospasm. It is best to use either lateral thoracotomies and paramedian or flank incisions to enter the thorax and abdomen rather than median sternotomies or midline celiotomy incisions. The flank region offers the most easily dissected subcutaneous tissue for implantation of devices. Catheterization of the neck vessels can be done from either a ventral midline or preferably a paramedian incision made over the external jugular vein as described for the adult (Fig. 8.5). The femoral vessels can be catheterized by externalizing the rear leg and performing the cutdown in the same manner as for adults. The axillary vessels are potentially useful, however, they are difficult to access and catheterize because of the acute angles involved in catheter insertion. The umbilical vessels can be catheterized, however, their tortuous course and friability frequently lead to extravasation especially after they enter the abdomen and turn cranially. When manipulating the fetus without observing the umbilical vessels, as for these procedures, care must be taken to avoid torsion of them.

A variety of catheterization techniques have been described for fetal swine. The system of using vascular access ports has proved to be reliable and minimizes the opportunity for infection. The catheter system designed for use in our lab (Access Technologies, Inc., Skokie, IL) is a 4-Fr catheter for the carotid artery and a 2-Fr catheter for the external and internal jugular veins and femoral vessels in a third-trimester fetus. These silicone catheters must be manufactured inside a larger 6-Fr catheter sheath to avoid kinking in the abdomen. The catheters are passed into the abdominal cavity using a trochar from the lateral wings of the lumbar vertebrae. The ports are either sutured to the dorsum of the pig or implanted subcutaneously. If externalized, they should be covered with a pouch or an adhesive plastic sheet (Fig. 8.6). When threading the catheters into the blood vessels, it is essential to have a beveled tip and to preplace a 2-Fr wire catheter insertion aid into the lumen of the catheter. Polydiaxonone or other monofilament sutures are used to avoid vasospasm caused by braided sutures when tying the catheters in place. Catheter care should be the same as described for adults.

The closure of fetal incisions should be performed using atraumatic technique and noninflammatory sutures. Continuous suture patterns are accept-

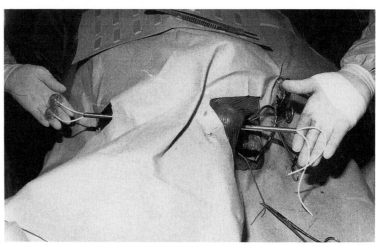

FIGURE 8.5   Trocar placement for catheterization of the neck vessels with the sow in lateral recumbency. *Reprinted with permission from Swindle et al., 1996, Fetal surgical protocols in Yucatan miniature swine, Lab. Anim. Sci. 46(1): 90-95.*

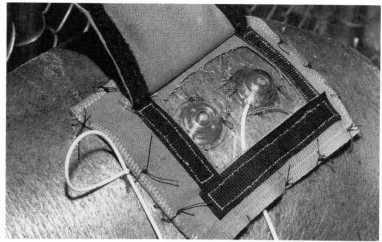

FIGURE 8.6   Canvas pouch sewn to skin of the dorsum to protect externalized
catheters. *Reprinted with permission from Swindle et al., 1996, Fetal surgical
protocols in Yucatan miniature swine, Lab. Anim. Sci. 46(1): 90-95.*

able, and multiple muscle layers can be closed together depending upon the
thickness of the layer. If subcuticular sutures are not used, then care should be
taken to cut the suture ends close to the knot to avoid irritation of the fetal
membranes.

Closure of the uterotomy and fetal membranes may be performed with staples as described for the C-section above. A technique described by Randall
(1986) for suturing the fetal and maternal membranes to reduce the possibility
of conjoining the circulations should be used if staples are not available (Fig.
8.7). The suture pattern consists of a continuous pattern in which the suture
passes from the outside throughout the myometrium, endometrium, and allantochorion into the amniotic cavity. The suture then continues through
both sides of the allantochorion passing across the incision in such a manner
as to invert the edges of the membranes. The suture then passes completely
through all three layers to the outside. The same suture is then reinserted
through the myometrium and endometrium close to the edge of the incision,
passed across the incision and passed out through the endometrium and myometrium. After tying the suture, the effect from the outside is to have a vertical mattress type pattern with inverted edges. This pattern is continuous along
the entire edge of the incision. It is then oversewn with continuous or interrupted Lembert sutures. The suture used for these patterns should be a 2/0 or
3/0 synthetic absorbable material. If the goal of the project involves the necessity of preventing conjoinment of the maternal and fetal circulations, then the
absence of gamma-globulins in the fetal plasma can be used as confirmation.
Staple closures provide better hemostasis and a tighter seal and are more likely
to prevent this phenomenon (Fig. 8.8). They also greatly reduce operative time.

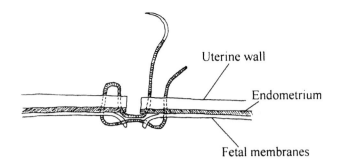

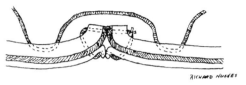

FIGURE 8.7   Manual suturing technique for fetal membranes.

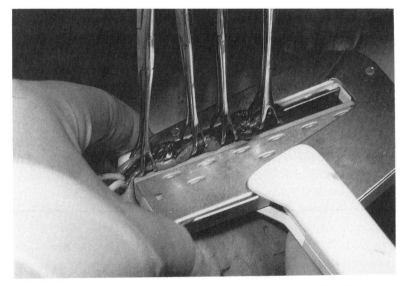

FIGURE 8.8   Closure of the uterus with staples. *Reprinted with permission from Swindle et al., 1996, Fetal surgical protocols in Yucatan miniature swine, Lab. Anim. Sci. 46(1): 90-95.*

Regardless of which uterine closure method is used, the final suture pattern is a Lembert to oversew the other layers, and catheter flanges are sutured to the uterine wall (Fig. 8.9).

Complications of the surgery include sepsis, fetal death, and mummifica-

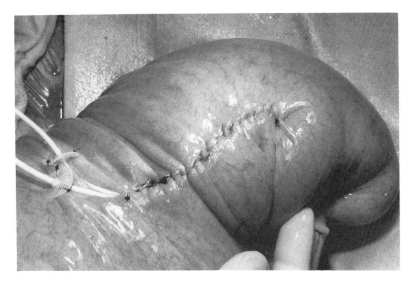

FIGURE 8.9   Lembert sutures oversewing the staple line and catheter flanges sewn to
the uterine wall. *Reprinted with permission from Swindle et al., 1996, Fetal
surgical protocols in Yucatan miniature swine, Lab. Anim. Sci. 46(1): 90-95.*

tion, which may be followed by abortion. In our experience, the presence of a
bloody vaginal discharge within 5 days postoperatively always leads to abortion. If this sign is noted, then an acute physiologic experiment should be performed. Fetal death may lead to mummification without abortion. Fetal sepsis
may lead to pyometritis and systemic sepsis; however, it is more likely to lead
to abortion. Factors that appear to lead to the complication of abortion include
animals from herds susceptible to abortion, invasive procedures likely to be life
threatening to the fetus, the presence of fetal distress at the time of surgery,
and the presence of uterine contractions and other signs of uterine irritation.
If abortion occurs as a complication, then the protocol should be reviewed for
refinement, and progestins and agents that relax smooth-muscle contractions
may be used for prophylaxis.

The progesterone agents include medroxyprogesterone (Depo-Provera, Up-
john Co., Kalamazoo, MI), 15–50 mg im, 2 days before surgery, the day of
surgery, and 2 days after surgery, or an oral progestin (ReguMate, Hoecst Rous-
sel, Philadelphia, PA), 0.1 mg/kg/d po, for the same time period. Nitroglycerine
infusions or infusions with terbutalin may be used intraoperatively to prevent
uterine contractions. Indomethacin may be given postoperatively for uterine
relaxation as well. Pancuronium, 0.02–0.15 mg/kg, is used as a muscle relaxant
during surgery to increase exposure of the uterus, however, it is not effective in
relaxing smooth muscle. Postoperative and intraoperative analgesia with
buprenorphine, 0.05–0.1 mg/kg im, prevents anxiety and straining by the sow.
Third-generation cephalosporins are useful as prophylaxis against infection
starting the day prior to surgery in order to allow the antibiotic to cross the fetal membranes. They may also be used as a dilute flush in the amniotic sac

prior to closing the incision. Tether and harness systems for providing chronic infusions have been developed (Fig. 8.10).

Most fetal surgical models that have been applied in other species, notably the lamb, could be modified to be performed in swine. Other than fetal vascular catheterization, models that have been created include craniofacial defects, thoracotomy with pacemaker implantation, hydronephrosis, and endocrine gland ablation.

Prolapse of the Reproductive Tract

Prolapse of the vagina and/or uterus may occur during parturition or in the immediate peripartum period. Modifications of the techniques of Bollwahn (1992), Ladwig (1975), and Markham (1968) are described here. The prolapsed tissue should be examined to determine if it contains the urinary bladder, and a determination made whether fetuses are retained in the uterus. Prolapse of

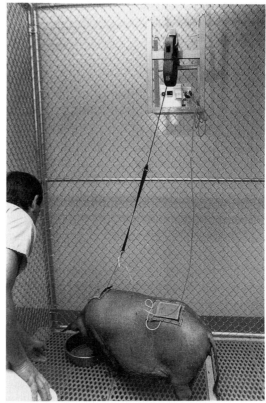

FIGURE 8.10   Harness and tether device for chronic infusion of vascular catheters in the sow and fetus. *Reprinted with permission from Swindle et al., 1996, Fetal surgical protocols in Yucatan miniature swine, Lab. Anim. Sci. 46(1): 90-95.*

the uterus and bladder or retention of additional fetuses requires a celiotomy. Any prolapsed tissue should be examined for necrosis and cleaned carefully with mild surgical soap solutions. Flushing the tissue with antibiotic solutions prior to reduction is also indicated.

If the vagina is prolapsed, it may be reduced by manual manipulation. The vagina is gently manipulated through the vulva after cleaning. This should not be done with sharp instruments or the extended fingers because the tissue will be friable and easily ruptured. If the prolapsed material can be manipulated into the vulva, it should be extended into the pelvic cavity. A deep subcutaneous purse-string suture should be placed to prevent recurrence, and the bladder should be catheterized.

If the uterus or bladder are involved, then a paramedian flank or midline abdominal incision is performed as previously described. The prolapsed structures are gently reduced, and any remaining fetuses are removed by C-section as described above. Oxytocin should be administered to promote uterine contraction. Use of the purse-string suture described above for the vagina may help prevent recurrence. Use of a modified technique for primates may be useful, however, if the animal is to be retained for the long term (Adams et al., 1985). The technique involves suturing a loop of the ovarian ligament on both horns of the uterus to the abdominal wall on its corresponding side. This provides security against future prolapses by surgical fixation of the cranial poles of the uterus to the abdominal wall. The celiotomy incision is closed in a routine fashion, as previously described.

If the tissue is necrotic, an amputation of the prolapsed stump may have to be performed. As described above, a determination should be made to ensure that additional fetuses or the bladder are not involved in the prolapse and a laparotomy performed if they are. The vaginal stump is best amputated using staple surgical techniques. If it is performed manually, then a V-shaped incision is made from the perineum to the tip of the viable tissue in the stump. The vessels are ligated, and the edges of the stump are oversewn with a continuous interlocking suture to ensure hemostasis and to provide a patent opening in the reproductive tract. Alternatively, an ovariohysterectomy may be indicated and performed as described above.

If any of these conditions occur, then consideration should be given to restriction of future breeding and the use of C-section delivery of fetuses if breeding is necessary for research purposes.

Mammectomy

Most sows have seven pairs of mammary glands on the abdomen; however, the number can have substantial variability depending upon the breed. Surgical removal of a mammary gland may be indicated in the case of chronic infection or trauma. Modifications of the techniques of Bollwahn (1992) and Mbiuki

(1982) are described here. The vascular supply to the mammary glands is derived from branches of the external thoracic and cranial and caudal epigastric arteries and veins.

A paramedian skin incision is made over the center of the glandular structure to be excised. The skin is bluntly dissected to both edges of the gland. The vascular supply is identified, ligated, and transected prior to removal of the gland. The subcutaneous dissection is easily performed using Metzenbaum scissors. The vascularity of the gland increases substantially with lactation, and leakage of milk from adjacent glands should be prevented by taking care not to damage them during the dissection. After removal of the gland, the skin is trimmed and the nipple excised with the excised tissue. The subcutaneous pocket must be closed carefully to avoid a seroma. The skin is closed with subcuticular sutures. A circumferential bandage of the torso including the surgical site is indicated for the first 24 hours to prevent seroma formation.

References

Becker, H.N. 1992. Castration, vasectomy, hernia repair, and baby pig processing. In Leman, A.D., Straw, B.E., Mengeling, W.L., D'Allaire S., and Taylor D.J. Diseases of Swine, 7th ed. Ames: Iowa State University Press, pp. 943–956.

Bollwahn, W. 1992. Surgical procedures in boars and sows. In Leman, A.D., Straw, B.E., Mengeling, W.L., D'Allaire, S., and Taylor, D.J. (eds), Diseases of Swine, 7th ed. Ames: Iowa State University Press, pp. 782–793.

Care, A.D., I.W. Caple, R. Singh R, and M. Peddie. 1986. Studies on calcium homeostasis in the fetal Yucatan miniature pig. Lab. Anim. Sci. 36(4): 389–392.

Christenson, R.K., K.A. Leymaster, and L.D. Young. 1987. Justification of unilateral hysterectomy-ovariectomy as a model to evaluate uterine capacity in swine. J. Anim. Sci. 65(3): 738–744.

Dungan, L.J., D.B. Wiest, D.A. Fyfe, A.C. Smith, and M.M. Swindle. 1995. Hematology, serology and serum protein electrophoresis in fetal miniature Yucatan swine: Normal data. Lab. Anim. Sci. 45(3): 285–289.

Jackson, B.T., and H. Egdahl. 1960. The performance of complex fetal operations in utero without amniotic fluid loss or other disturbances of fetal–maternal relationships. Surgery 48: 564–570.

Jones, M.D., and B.B. Hudak. 1988. Fetal and neonatal surgery. In Swindle, M.M., and Adams, R.J. (eds), Experimental Surgery and Physiology: Induced Animal Models of Human Disease. Baltimore: Williams and Wilkins, pp. 300–308.

Kraeling, R.R., C.R. Barb, and G.B. Rampacek. 1986. Hypophysectomy and hypophysial stalk transection in the pig: Technique and application to studies of ovarian follicular development. In Tumbleson, M.E. (ed), Swine in Biomedical Research, Vol. 1. New York: Plenum Press, pp. 425–436.

Ladwig, V.D. 1975. Surgical procedure to control hemorrhage of porcine vulva. J. Am. Vet. Med. Assoc. 166(6): 598–599.

Markham, L. 1968. Replacement of prolapsed uterus in a sow. Vet. Rec. 82: 605–606.

Mayo, M.B., and H.N. Becker. 1982. Unilateral castration to correct a peritesticular hematoma in a boar. Vet. Med. Sm. Anim. Clin. 77(3): 449–451.

Mbiuki, S.M. 1982. Mammectomy for treatment of chronic mastitis in sows. Vet. Med. Sm. Anim. Clin. 77(10): 1516–1517.

McGlone, J.J., and J.M. Hellman. 1988. Local and general anesthetic effects on behavior and performance of two and seven week old castrated and uncastrated piglets. J. Anim. Sci. 66(12): 3049–3058.

Molina, J.R., A.I. Musah, D.L. Hard, and L.L. Anderson. 1985. Conceptus development after vascular occlusion of the middle uterine artery in the pig. J. Reprod. Fert. 75(5): 501–506.

Randall, G.C.B. 1986. Chronic implantations of catheters and other surgical techniques in fetal pigs. In Tumbleson, M.E. (ed), Swine in Biomedical Research, Vol. 2. New York: Plenum Press, pp. 1179–1186.

Rock, J.A., Z. Rosewaks, and E.Y. Adashi. 1979. Microsurgery for tubal reconstruction following Falope-Ring* sterilization in swine. J. Microsurg. 1:61–64.

Rosenkrantz, J.G., R.C. Simon, and J.H. Carlisle. 1968. Fetal surgery in the pig with a review of other mammalian fetal techniques. J. Pediatr. Surg. 3(3):392–397.

Scambler, J.D. 1968. Replacement of prolapsed uterus in a sow. Vet. Rec. 82:712–715.

Sims, C.D., P.E.M. Butler, R. Casanova, M.A. Randolph, and M.J. Yaremchuk. 1997. Prolonged general anesthesia for experimental craniofacial surgery in fetal swine. J. Invest. Surg. 10(1): 53–57.

Swindle, M.M. 1983. Basic Surgical Exercises Using Swine. Philadelphia: Praeger Press.

Swindle, M.M., and D.L. Bobbie. 1987. Comparative anatomy of the pig. Charles River Technical Bulletin, Charles River Laboratories 4(1): 1–4.

Swindle, M.M., A.C. Smith, and B.J.S. Hepburn. 1988. Swine as models in experimental surgery. J. Invest. Surg. 1(1): 65–79.

Swindle, M.M., D.B. Wiest, A.C. Smith, S.S. Garner, C.C. Case, R.P. Thompson, D.A. Fyfe, and P.C. Gillette. 1996. Fetal surgical protocols in Yucatan miniature swine. Lab. Anim. Sci. 46(1): 90–95.

Wiest, D.B., M.M. Swindle, S.S. Garner, A.C. Smith, P.C. Gillette. 1996. Pregnant Yucatan miniature swine as a model for investigating fetal drug therapy. In Tumbleson, M.E., and Schook, L.B. (eds.), Advances in Swine in Biomedical Research, Vol. 2. New York: Plenum Press, pp. 629–636.

9 CARDIOTHORACIC AND VASCULAR SURGERY

General Principles of Cardiothoracic Surgery

Swine share important characteristics with humans in anatomy and physiology of the cardiovascular and pulmonary systems, making them useful models in the study of human diseases (Corin et al., 1988; Gardner and Johnson, 1988; Horneffer et al., 1986; Hughes, 1986; Lee, 1986; McKenzie, 1996; Smith et al., 1990; Smith et al., 1994; Stanton and Mersmann, 1986; Swindle, 1983; Swindle, 1986; Swindle, 1992; Swindle and Adams, 1988; Swindle and Bobbie, 1987; Swindle et al., 1986; Swindle et al., 1988). Besides the size and morphologic characteristics, there are physiologic similarities in the areas of coronary blood flow, growth of the cardiovascular system, and neonatal pulmonary development. The coronary circulation of the pig has few subepicardial collateral anastomoses, like 90% of the human population. The circulation to the conduction system is predominantly right-side dominant from the posterior septal artery, in contrast to the dog. Consequently, the pig responds in a similar manner to humans with acute myocardial infarction (Bloor et al., 1986; Bloor et al., 1992; Gardner and Johnson, 1988; White et al., 1986). There are some differences from humans in physiologic composition of the conduction system. The pig endocardium and epicardium are activated simultaneously because of differences in distribution of the specialized conduction system in the ventricles (Brownlee et al., 1997; Gillette et al., 1991; Hughes and Bowman, 1986; Schumann et al., 1994; Smith et al., in press; Tong et al., 1995; Verdouw and Hartog, 1986). Atherosclerotic and coronary occlusion models are readily induced in swine and are discussed in this section; there is also additional information in Chapter 12 (Gal and Isner, 1992; Mitchell et al., 1994; Murphy et al., 1992; Rogers et al., 1988; Rysavy et al., 1986; White et al., 1992). The aorta has a true vaso vasorum unlike many species of animals but similar to humans; this structure leads to a difference in reaction to aortic banding techniques. The growth of the cardiovascular system from fetus to sexually mature adult in swine parallels the growth and development of the cardiovascular system of humans into early sexual maturity (Brutel de la Riviere et al., 1983; Pae et al., 1981).

The pulmonary tissues and pulmonary circulation have been studied from fetal life to 6 months of age and show similarities morphologically and functionally (Greenberg et al., 1981; Haworth and Hislop, 1981; Sparrow, 1996). Pulmonary function matures by 2 weeks of age, but growth and remodeling continue into adult life. It is beyond the scope of this text to review all of the data relating to the use of swine in cardiovascular research, and readers are referred to the general references found in the appendix as well as literature on particular models.

Lateral thoracotomies (Fig. 9.1) in the pig can be a challenge because of the width of the ribs and the narrowness of the intercostal spaces, which can result in minimal exposure of the structures of interest. Placing a rolled up towel or sandbag under the thorax to make the operative side more convex will increase surgical exposure. Also, the incisions should be performed within the intercostal spaces parallel to the ribs. This means that lateral thoracotomy incisions will be oblique rather than vertical because of the anatomy of the ribs in swine. The pig usually has 15 pairs of ribs including the floating rib, and they can be counted to locate the appropriate intercostal space (Swindle, 1983; Swindle et al., 1986).

Median sternotomy (Fig. 9.2) incisions can be performed successfully in swine as a survival procedure, unlike in many other animals. Pigs experience relatively little discomfort with the procedure, especially if the manubrium sterni is left intact, as it can be for many cardiac procedures. Care must be taken

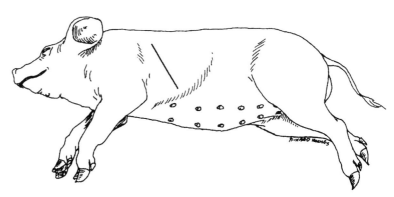

FIGURE 9.1   Lateral thoracotomy.

when performing this procedure, because the heart is in sternal contact between the fourth and seventh costal cartilages in most pigs. The sternum may be bisected using a Stricker saw if a scalpel handle or straight ribbon retractor is held along the interior surface of the sternum to prevent cardiac trauma. It may also be bisected using sternal cutters of all the various configurations used for humans. The apex of the heart is in close apposition to the diaphragm at its most cranial attachment to the sternum at the level of the seventh costal cartilage. The heart will remain in a pericardial cradle after this procedure is performed because of the close attachment of the pericardium to the sternum (Swindle et al., 1986; Swindle et al., 1988).

Cardiac and pulmonary tissue is very friable in swine, especially in the smaller farm pigs commonly used in research. This tissue friability decreases with maturity and, consequently, miniature pigs tend to be easier to manipulate surgically at the same weight as farm breeds because of their greater age at the same weight. Gentle handling of tissues using appropriate instrumentation is imperative to prevent complications, such as tearing of atrial tissue and

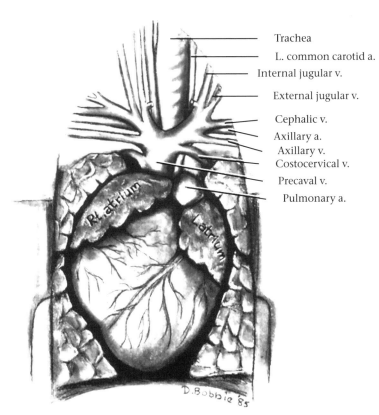

FIGURE 9.2   Median sternotomy. *Reprinted with permission from Swindle, et al., 1986, Anatomic and anesthetic considerations in experimental cardiopulmonary surgery in swine, Lab. Anim. Sci. 36(4): 357–361.*

rupture of pulmonary tissue, which may cause emphysematous bullae. Vessels are similar to those in humans except for the presence of the left azygous (hemiazygous) vein (Fig. 9.3) that crosses from the intercostal vessels ventral to the left hilum of the lung to drain into the coronary sinus (Swindle, 1983; Swindle and Bobbie, 1987; Swindle et al., 1986).

The edges of thoracotomy incisions should by protected with wetted gauze laparotomy sponges when using retractors. The self-retaining retractors indicated for most swine will need to be pediatric instruments with blunt blades in order to avoid injuring the underlying pulmonary tissue with retraction blades that extend too deep into the thoracic cavity. The mediastinum is thin and easily ruptured in swine. Chest tubes or instruments will readily injure the structure and, as a practicality, the mediastinum should be considered incomplete, because it is likely that fluids or surgical hemorrhage from one side of the thoracic cavity will extend into the other side through inadvertent rents.

Closure of thoracic surgical incisions is comparable to other species. Lateral thoracotomies are closed with heavy gauge (0–1) circumferential sutures that

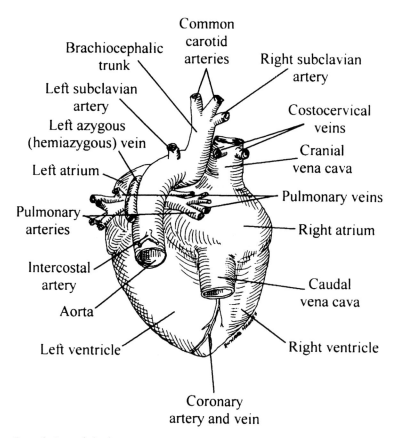

FIGURE 9.3   Dorsal view of the heart.

have been preplaced around the cranial and caudal ribs adjacent to the incision. Three to five sutures are usually required to close the incision adequately. Sutures may either be absorbable polydiaxonone or nonabsorbable materials. After preplacing all of the sutures, the central one in the incision is tied first, followed by the peripheral ones, with alternated tying of sutures in both directions. Rib-approximating forceps are helpful for tying the first suture. The latissimus dorsi always requires closure as a separate layer, even in the smallest pig. However, the decision whether or not to close the rest of the muscles in layers varies with the size of the pig. Muscle layers can be closed either with interrupted or continuous sutures of any of the synthetic absorbable materials. The subcutaneous tissues are also variable in thickness depending upon the size of the pig, but this layer is closed, if necessary, using synthetic absorbable materials. The skin layer is best closed with a subcuticular layer of 2/0 or 3/0 synthetic absorbable suture. Other types of closure may be used if preferred.

A median sternotomy is closed in a similar fashion to the lateral thoracotomy. Nonabsorbable heavy gauge (0–2) sutures are preplaced in the intercostal spaces from cranial to caudal. Care should be taken not to occlude unnecessarily the interior mammary artery with these sutures; however, it may be sacrificed if necessary. If the manubrium sterni was not transected, then the pig will have an easier recovery with less postoperative discomfort, and the surgical incision will be easier to close in proper alignment. If it was transected, then great care should be taken to ensure that closure of the sternotomy is performed in an anatomically correct fashion. The sutures are tied sequentially from cranial to caudal. The pericardium does not need to be sutured as a separate layer. A single-layer closure of muscle and subcutaneous suture using 2/0–3/0 synthetic absorbable suture should be placed next. The skin is closed in the same fashion as for the lateral thoracotomy.

Evacuation of air from the chest can be performed by a variety of methods. The lungs should be expanded to their maximum capacity to reduce the air volume of the thorax while closing the initial layer of the thoracotomy, whether it is a lateral or median incision. For simple procedures in which postoperative bleeding and leakage of air are not expected, the chest may be evacuated with a needle or preferably a small-gauge catheter and syringe with an attached three-way valve. The insertion is in the dorsocaudal area of the thoracic cavity, taking care to avoid damage of the lung with the needle or catheter. This evacuation may be performed after closing the internal muscle layers so that a watertight seal exists. If a chest tube is to be placed, it is inserted while the incision is still open. It is placed in a dorsocaudal position at least two intercostal spaces caudal to the lateral thoracotomy. The tube is passed through the skin after making a stab incision, and then advanced into the thoracic cavity. For a median sternotomy, single or double chest tubes are placed on the ventrolateral aspects of the midthorax cranial to the attachment of the diaphragm. Tubes may either be the one-way valve Heimlich type for short- or mid-term usage, or the use of water-sealed systems may be required for more involved procedures that have the possibility of increased complications. Chest tubes are placed with purse-string sutures around them in the skin, and the chest tubes are removed and the purse-string sutures are tightened after it has been determined that pneumothorax or hemorrhage are no longer likely.

The major difficulties encountered in thoracic surgical procedures are likely to be cardiac arrhythmias and cardiodepression. Methods of preventing these common complications are detailed in the chapter on anesthesia. Inherent in the design of these surgical protocols is the necessity of designing an appropriate anesthetic and analgesic protocol for the procedure being performed. Good surgical technique alone is not sufficient to have a successful outcome for a thoracic surgery. Intraoperative and postoperative monitoring of heart rate, electrocardiogram, blood pressures, and blood gases is essential in these cases if survival is expected.

General principles of vascular surgery are discussed within the text in the sections on vascular cannulation and anastomosis below.

Pulmonary System

Tracheostomy/Tracheotomy

Tracheostomy can be performed in the pig as a survival procedure either following an emergency or as part of a planned experiment. With the pig in dorsal recumbency, the cricothyroid cartilage can be palpated easily, even in large swine. The caudal end of the cartilage has a blunted tip like a bird's beak. The cricothyroid membrane is immediately caudal to this structure and is the preferred location for a tracheostomy (Swindle, 1983).

A 1- to 2-cm incision is made over the membrane on the ventral midline. The cutaneous coli and sternohyoideus muscles are separated longitudinally, and the membrane is identified. This procedure can be performed bloodlessly in seconds in an emergency. The cricothyroid membrane is incised, and either a tracheostomy tube or an endotracheal tube of the appropriate size can be inserted (Fig. 9.4). The larynx may be held between the thumb and forefinger of the surgeons hand for countertraction to aid this procedure. As an option, the membrane between the first and second tracheal rings can be incised and used for this procedure. For a survival procedure, however, this transection does not heal as readily as an incision in the cricothyroid membrane. The larynx of swine is large, and the tracheal rings will be somewhat obscured by this structure, necessitating a longer incision.

The cricothyroid membrane can be sutured with continuous pattern using synthetic absorbable sutures. Problems have not been noted with the suture material entering the lumen of the larynx; however, some surgeons may wish to use a continuous Lembert pattern instead. The sternohyoideus muscle is

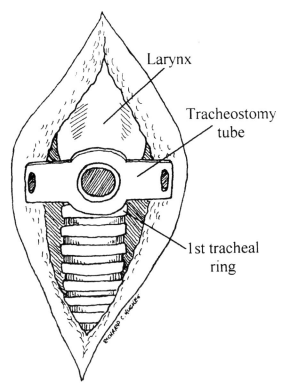

FIGURE 9.4   Tracheostomy tube surgically implanted into the cricothyroid
                    membrane.

closed with a continuous suture pattern and the skin, with a subcuticular pattern using synthetic absorbable material.

Chronic ostomies can also be maintained by suturing a standard tracheostomy tube to the skin after closing the muscular and subcutaneous tissues around the device. By making the incision in the cricothyroid membrane, complications associated with the vocal cords can be avoided as long as the surgeon passes the tracheostomy device caudally. An ostomy can also be formed by suturing the edges of a tracheal window to the skin. A tracheal window can be formed by resecting a rectangular section from the first few tracheal rings on the ventral surface. The trachea is too deep in the musculature of the neck to use this procedure beyond the area immediately caudal to the larynx.

Pneumonectomy/Lobectomy

The hilum of either lung is surgically approached through the fourth intercostal space. A total pneumonectomy is more easily performed on the left side and is described here (Swindle, 1983; Swindle et al., 1986). With the pig in right lateral recumbency, the left foreleg is drawn cranially, and a sandbag is positioned under the thorax. The incision is made obliquely from the dorsal caudal border of the scapula ventrocaudally toward the first nipple. After making the skin incision, the ribs may be palpated; the fourth intercostal space is the most cranial one approachable with this skin incision. The muscle layers are successively divided, and the thoracodorsal artery and vein within the body of the latissimus dorsi muscle will be the only major blood vessels encountered. The muscles are easily divided, and the intercostal muscles may be divided along the cranial border of the fifth rib using Metzenbaum scissors. At the dorsal edge of the incision the superior intercostal vessels may be encountered and at the distal margin of the incision, the internal thoracic vessels should be avoided. Care should be taken to enter the thorax without damaging the lungs. This can be facilitated by underinflating the lungs and cutting the last muscle layer with Metzenbaum scissors.

After placing self-retaining retractors, the pulmonary ligament is identified at the dorsocaudal aspect of the caudal lobe of the lung. This fibrous structure cannot be seen through the thoracotomy and must be cut blindly with Metzenbaum scissors while retracting the tip of the caudal lobe proximally with the fingers. The caudal and apical lobes of the lung can now be exteriorized to expose the hilum of the lung. The lobes of the lung are retracted dorsally using wetted gauze pads.

The hilum of the lung (Fig. 9.5) is dissected, and the blood vessels are identified and surgically transected in this order: cranial ventral branch of the pulmonary vein, left pulmonary artery, apical branch of the pulmonary vein, and caudal diaphragmatic branch of the pulmonary vein. The first branch of the pulmonary vein has to be transected in order to expose adequately the pulmonary artery branch. If these transections are being performed manually, then it is best to use transfixion sutures in the pulmonary artery. During this dissection, the left azygous (hemiazygous) vein that crosses ventrally to these vessels should not be damaged. However, it may be sacrificed, if necessary. The lung is then retracted ventrally to expose the bronchial artery on the dorsal aspect of the bronchus in order to transect it. If vagal stimulation resulting in bradycardia and/or cardiac standstill is problematic during the deep dissection of the hilum, atropine should be administered.

After all the vessels have been ligated, then the bronchus is cleared of fascial tissue and transected. This transection is best performed with staples. However, if it must be performed manually, the bronchus is cross clamped distally, and the bronchus is cut on the proximal end of the clamp a few millimeters at a time, while placing simple interrupted sutures using nonabsorbable suture material. As an alternative, a continuous horizontal mattress pattern can be used. This cut-and-suture technique is performed from the caudal end to the cranial end of the bronchus. The bronchus is checked for leaks with saline, and any leak noted is repaired with additional sutures. Leaks are most likely to occur at

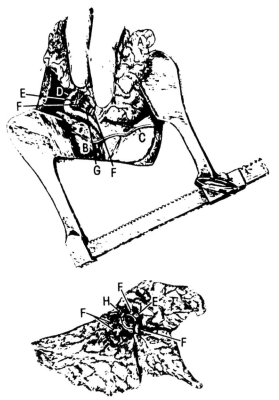

FIGURE 9.5   The hilum of the lung to be dissected with a left total pneumonectomy.
Note the oblique incision. *Top*-Lateral thoracotomy approach to the left
lung hilum, *Bottom*-Medial aspect of left lung following pneumonectomy, *A*-Left lung, *B*-Heart, *C*-Phrenic nerves crossing the diaphragm,
D-Left azygous vein, *E*-Pulmonary artery, *F*-Pulmonary veins,
G-Bronchus, *H*-Bronchial artery. *Reprinted with permission from Swindle et
al., 1986, Anatomic and anesthetic considerations in experimental
cardiopulmonary surgery in swine, Lab. Anim. Sci. 36(4): 357–361.*

the middle of the bronchus where there is an indentation in the dorsal border.
The leak can usually be repaired by placing a horizontal mattress suture in this
area.

The right lung can be removed in a similar manner. However, the right cranial lobe bronchus branches directly from the trachea separate from the
bronchus, which branches to supply the caudal and accessory lobes. Consequently, both bronchi have to be divided surgically. Access to the accessory
lobe is difficult because of the location of the vena cava, which makes dissection of the pulmonary veins difficult.

Lobectomies and partial lobectomies of the lung in swine are technically
feasible but difficult. Division of the friable lung tissue always leads to leakage

of air and frequently the formation of emphysematous bullae. The two best locations for attempting the procedure are the right cranial lobe followed by the left cranial lobe at the caudal interlobular fissure. These two locations provide the deepest fissure between lung tissue and have a single branch of the bronchus to transect.

The lung is divided using staples at the identified location. If staples are not available, manual suturing using a horizontal mattress suture pattern can be used; however, the pulmonary tissue frequently ruptures with this technique. The branches of the pulmonary artery and veins supplying the resected section are identified and surgically transected. The branch of the bronchus is then dissected free and transected with staples. The transected edge of the lung remaining in the animal will have to have the leaks sealed in the tissue following removal of the resected lobe. Various tissue glues and oxycellulose patches have been used to seal these leaks in the past with variable success. The complication rate is high with this procedure because of the friability of the pulmonary tissue and the high potential for air leaks. Development of better methods of sealing the cut edges of the lung would help in this species.

The lateral thoracotomy is closed as described above.

Pulmonary Transplant

Swine have been used for single-lung transplantation and heart-and-lung transplantation (Baumgartner et al., 1988; Calne et al., 1976; Calne et al., 1978; Hall et al., 1986; Harjula and Baldwin, 1987; Qayumi et al., 1990; Qayumi et al., 1991; Qayumi et al., 1993; Saito and Waters, 1994; Swindle et al., 1986). A left single-lung transplant is more applicable than a right-lung transplant because of the presence of the right cranial bronchus, which makes it substantially different from humans. Consequently, a left single-lung transplant is described here. Pulmonary denervation can lead to respiratory insufficiency, which can be a problem for long-term studies.

The donor is prepared for a complete median sternotomy. The left lung is removed following heparinization and subsequent transection of the following structures: left main bronchus, pulmonary artery, and atrial cuff containing the pulmonary veins. All of the structures should be transected so that the longest possible segment remains attached to the donor lung. It is perfused with cold preservation solution through the pulmonary artery while awaiting transplantation.

The recipient is prepared in a similar manner. The donor lung is sutured in place in the following order: atrial cuff with pulmonary veins, pulmonary artery, and bronchus. Suture selection depends upon the size of the animal and the experience of the surgeon. However, continuous suture pattern with nonabsorbable suture is the most common technique.

Heart and heart–lung transplantations are discussed and illustrated below.

Cardiovascular System

Peripheral Vascular Cannulation and Chronic Catheterization Techniques

Many of the vascular access sites in swine are relatively deep in the tissues. Venipuncture techniques have previously been described in Chapter 1 (Bobbie and Swindle, 1986; Swindle, 1983). The Seldinger technique for vascular access for cardiac catheterization studies is discussed in Chapter 12 (Gaymes et al., 1995; Smith et al., 1989). In this section, the surgical principles of vascular access to the main blood vessels will be described (Hand et al., 1981; Nicolau et al., 1996; Purohit et al., 1993; Smith et al., 1989; Swindle, 1983; Swindle et al., 1986; Swindle et al., 1996; Swindle et al., 1998).

Peripheral blood vessels of swine are prone to vasospasm and are relatively easy to rupture during catheterization techniques. Good surgical technique and gentle handling of tissues cannot be replaced by use of topical antispasmodic agents such as lidocaine or papaverine. When performing vascular access surgery, the division of muscular tissues should be performed in fascial planes between muscle bodies and not by dividing musculature. Blood vessels should be handled gently and suture material used around the blood vessels should not be abrasive; for example, silk should not be used. The use of elastic vessel loops, especially the rounded types, is the preferred method of isolating and occluding blood vessels during catheterizations. Experience has shown that they do not have the sawing action that braided suture materials have on vessels, which frequently leads to vasospasm. When using gauze, it should be wetted with warm saline to prevent hypothermic vasoconstriction. Gauze should be pressed and held on a bleeding site, never rubbed. The use of electrocautery for hemostasis and ablation of collateral branches works well, as long as the power settings are not high enough to cause collateral cauterization and vasoconstriction.

Catheter selection is based upon the technique and purpose of the experiment and the surgeon's preference and experience. Many laboratories manufacture their own catheters for cost savings; however, inappropriate designs and flaws can lead to problems more readily than if commercial catheters are used. Consequently, it is not recommended that investigators manufacture their own catheters for cost savings alone. There either should be an experimental reason or the laboratory should be experienced in design and manufacture of catheters without sharp edges, surface flaws, or contaminants (Dougherty, 1981; Hand et al., 1981; Harvey and Jones, 1982; Swindle et al., 1988; Swindle et al. 1998).

Hickman (Fig. 9.6) and Broviac catheters are excellent catheters if large-bore or multiple-channel cannulae are required. Subcutaneously implantable catheters, referred to as vascular access ports (Figs. 9.7–9.9), are manufactured by several companies including Access Technologies, Inc, (Skokie, IL) or Pharmacia Deltec (Madison, WI). These catheters may be modified or designed by the manufacturers to specifications for particular experimental purposes (Bailie et al., 1986; Swindle et al., 1986). The subcutaneous implantable catheters may be sutured to the skin instead of being implanted subcutaneously. They offer an advantage of improved asepsis because of the closed nature of the design system. These catheters can also be procured with a tapered edge on the tip to help prevent vascular damage and thrombosis. Small catheters for short-term catheterization include the use of iv catheters available from any hospital supply.

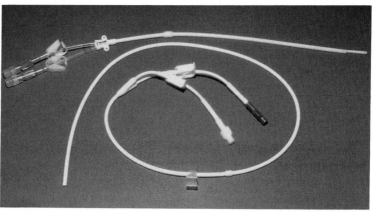

FIGURE 9.6   Hickman catheters.

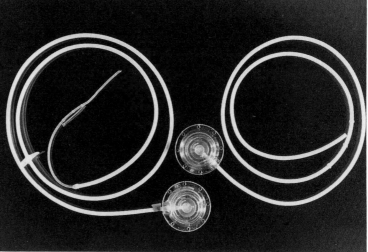

FIGURE 9.7   Intravascular vascular access ports and catheters. The catheter on the left has a retention flange for anchoring in the soft tissues and an introducer inserted in the tip. Both catheters have intravascular retention beads. *Photo courtesy of Access Technologies, Inc., Skokie, IL.*

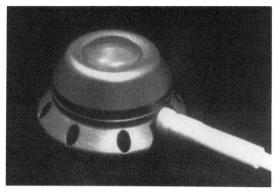

FIGURE 9.8   Titanium vascular access port. *Photo courtesy of Access Technologies, Inc.,*
                    Skokie, IL.

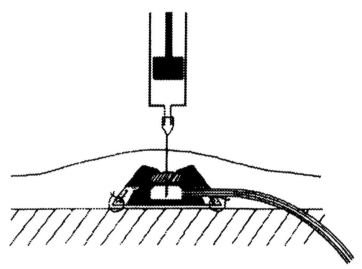

FIGURE 9.9   Schematic of the insertion of a Huber point needle into a sub-
                    cutaneously implanted vascular access port. *Photo courtesy of Access*
                    Technologies, Inc., Skokie, IL.

More-rigid catheters, such as those made from polypropylene, polytetrafluoroethylene, or polyethylene, are easier to insert into small blood vessels; however, their stiffness may lead to erosion or perforation of the vessel. Silicone (Silastic) catheters offer the advantage of being more flexible; however, small bores may easily kink in locations such as the abdomen, and silicone is porous and subject to contamination. Kinking can be prevented by placing a small-bore catheter of rigid material inside the bore of a larger silicone catheter, leaving only the length of rigid material inserted in the vessel exposed.

The technique of incising the vessel for insertion of the catheter depends upon the catheter design and the experience of the surgeon. Systems with needles and guidewires are reliable in swine (see Chapter 12). The vessel should be occluded with elastic vessel loops cranial and caudal to the site of entry and the vessel allowed to fill with blood. The vessel may be entered with either a no. 11 surgical blade or iris scissors or a needle tip. The author prefers to use iris scissors, because they tend to be less traumatic in small vessels and serve to prevent vasospasm. Suture material for tying the catheters in place for chronic cannulation depends upon the length of time that the animal will survive. Polydiaxonone is a good first choice if 3–6 months of suture retention is sufficient. Other synthetic absorbable or nonabsorbable materials may be more appropriate for some projects. Silk and surgical gut should not be used because of their inflammatory characteristics in swine. Both arteries and veins may be repaired surgically following catheterization using 5/0–6/0 cardiovascular suture material in a simple interrupted pattern.

Catheters for chronic implantation should have retention beads permanently fixed to the catheter at the site of vascular insertion (Fig. 9.10). These can be simply beads of silicone glue instead of manufactured structures. When sutures are placed in between the beads, it provides some security that the catheter will not move after implantation. A loop of the catheter should also be coiled in the area of venous access to prevent tension on the catheter as a result of movement or growth. Retention beads or Velcro cuffs may be necessary in the subcutaneous tissue to prevent the catheter from moving into and out of the skin causing contamination. Nylon velour cuffs or cuffs of other porous material allow tissue ingrowth to form a barrier against contamination. When closing the skin around a catheter exit site, synthetic absorbable materials should be used in subcuticular purse-string fashion. Catheters for vascular access should never be exited through the surgical site, because of the stress on the suture line and the high probability of contamination. Monofilament sutures may be used on the surface of the skin for a tight closure. Tissue glues may be helpful for the purpose of sealing the exit site.

Catheters should be exteriorized on the dorsal surface of swine. Pigs do not scratch or bite at catheters because of their body conformation. Rather, they rub sites that irritate them. The cage design should be free of materials that a pig could reach by rubbing. Exteriorized catheters can be protected by pouches or covers sutured to the skin or secured with adhesives. Use of nylon jackets and vests designed for research purposes can also be used as well as tether and harness systems.

For continuous infusion catheters, such as those attached to portable infusion pumps, flow rates of 3–5 ml/h are generally high enough to prevent occlusion. Catheters should be filled with full-strength heparin (1:1000 solution) if they are static. Some prefer to add hypertonic solutions, such as 50% glucose, to the heparin solution to aid in prevention of thrombosis or antibiotic solutions to aid in the prevention of infection. These are unnecessary if meticulous attention is paid to aseptic handling of the catheters during sampling and if

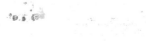

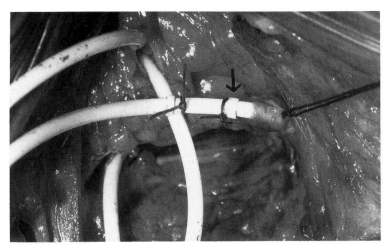

FIGURE 9.10   Surgical cutdown on the external jugular vein. Note the retention beads
                     (*arrow*) on the implanted catheter. *Reprinted with permission from Swindle
                     et al., 1996, Fetal surgical protocols in Yucatan miniature swine, Lab. Anim.
                     Sci. 46(1): 90–95.*

the catheter solutions are withdrawn, flushed with sterile saline, and refilled
with heparin two to three times a week. Closed systems, such as the vascular
access ports, are more reliable in the prevention of complications than systems
using three-way valves attached to the ends of open catheters.

     Catheter sites that are commonly approached surgically include the follow-
ing: external jugular vein, internal jugular vein, carotid artery, cephalic vein,
femoral vein, femoral artery, and medial saphenous artery. Except for the
carotid artery, these vessels may be ligated and sacrificed bilaterally instead of
being surgically repaired, without significant postoperative complications.
Collateral circulation is sufficient with one intact carotid artery. One of either
the external or internal jugular veins on each side of the neck should also be
left intact, but this is not essential. Other vessels that are chronically cannulated for specific research purposes include: portal vein, pulmonary artery, and
aorta. These vessel approaches will be discussed in this section. Using these
vessels as an example, many other blood vessels can be cannulated if indicated
by the research protocol. Superficial access to some veins makes it possible to
cannulate the central venous system either percutaneously or with minor skin
incisions. These veins include the auricular vein, the cephalic vein at the level
of the thoracic inlet, and the cranial epigastric vein on the ventral abdomen.

     The neck vessels can all be approached from an incision in the jugular fur-
row (Fig. 9.11). By retracting one leg caudally with the pig in dorsal recumbency, the jugular furrow can be seen along a line drawn slightly medial from
the point of the jaw to the point of the shoulder. An incision made in this
plane will provide access to the external jugular vein, which is deep in the in-

termuscular plane between the brachiocephalic and sternocephalic muscles at the same level as the trachea. After incising the skin, subcutaneous tissue, and cutaneous coli muscle, the external jugular vein can be isolated by blunt dissection. From this incision, the two mandibular branches of the vein and the main trunk can be easily isolated.

The internal jugular vein, carotid artery, and vagus nerve can be isolated from this same incision or they can be approached by a ventral midline incision followed by dissection of the fascial plane parallel to the trachea. They are located at the same depth as the external jugular but are medial and lie along the ventral surface of the cervical vertebrae parallel to the trachea. They are exposed from the jugular furrow incision by dissecting the fascial plane on the dorsal surface of the sternocephalic muscle. After dissecting this fascia, the floor of the vertebrae and the carotid pulse can be palpated easily. The blood vessels can be retracted into the area of the external jugular vein with a right angle forceps and isolated with vessel loops for cannulation.

From this location, all three vessels can be cannulated and the catheters ex-

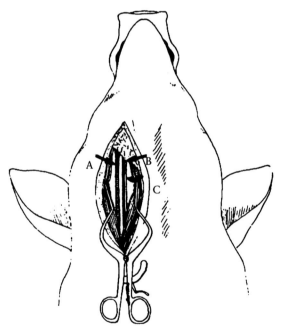

FIGURE 9.11   Surgical cutdown on the neck vessels from a paramedian incision over the jugular furrow. *A*-External jugular vein located between the sternohyoideus muscle laterally and the sternomastoideus muscle medially, *B*-Common carotid artery located medially to the external jugular vein, in the same muscle plane; note the parotid salivary gland at the rostral portion of the incision, *C*-Internal jugular vein medial to common carotid artery. *Reprinted with permission from Smith et al., 1989, Technical aspects of cardiac catheterization of swine, J. Invest. Surg. 2(2): 187–194.*

teriorized if desired. Placement of the tip of the catheter in the correct location is important, and premeasurements in similar-sized pigs can be made to determine the length and to premark the catheter with retention beads. Alternately, the catheter placement can be checked radiographically or pressure wave tracings can be used for confirmation. Generally, catheters in the jugular veins are meant for chronic infusion and sample withdrawal. Placement of the tip at the entrance of the precava to the right atrium (approximately at the second intercostal space) is optimal, because the turbulence and velocity of venous blood in this location helps prevent thrombosis. Placement into the atrium or ventricle can lead to cardiac arrhythmias, valvular damage, or atrial appendage thrombosis and/or rupture.

Exteriorization of the catheters is best done on the dorsal surface of the caudal neck between the scapulas. In order to perform this surgery without repositioning the pig during surgery, the pig should be in lateral recumbency. The major neck vessels can all be isolated from the same incision, and the catheters passed through a rod tunneled through the subcutaneous tissues exiting the skin on the dorsum of the neck (see Chapter 8, Fig. 8.5). If a subcutaneously implanted vascular access port is used, the tunneling rod is passed caudoventral to the axillary space to the lateral aspect of the thoracic wall. The port is implanted subcutaneously in the dorsal region of the chest wall. The subcutaneous pocket incision should be made either cranial or caudal to the site of the device implantation. The subcutaneous tissues are carefully dissected, and complete hemostasis must be ensured to prevent hematomas and seromas. The device should be anchored to the muscle fascia and the dead space closed adequately with subcutaneous and subcuticular sutures. The suture line should not be under tension and should not overlap the device; this prevents the complications of suture line dehiscence and necrosis. Skin sutures are placed as required.

The neck incision is closed in three layers in most swine: muscles, subcutaneous tissues, and skin. In larger swine, dead space in the deep fascial plane of the incision may also have to be closed.

The cephalic vein can be percutaneously catheterized on the cranial aspect of the foreleg as well as the ventral surface of the neck at the thoracic inlet, as described in Chapter 1. The vein can be identified by applying digital pressure at the thoracic inlet and watching it fill with blood along its course from the leg through the neck. An incision over the vessel is made, and the dissection is continued through the skin, subcutaneous tissue, and thin body of the cutaneous coli muscle. The vein may be cannulated and the catheter tunneled subcutaneously as described for the other neck vessels. For short-term catheterization, the exteriorization may be done on the ventrolateral aspect of the neck. The pig is likely to traumatize this site, however, unless it is protected with a bandage.

The femoral vessels and the medial saphenous vessel are all approached (Fig.

9.12) with the pig in dorsal recumbency and the rear leg retracted caudally. The pulse of the medial saphenous artery may be consistently palpated over the medial aspect of the stifle joint. This pulsation may be followed cranially to the level of the thigh, where the artery courses deeply into the musculature of the medial aspect of the leg. The division of the musculature where the arterial pulse disappears is the fascial division of the sartorius and gracilis muscles. The femoral artery, vein, and nerve are located below the edge of the body of the gracilis muscle.

The surgical incision for the medial saphenous artery may be made directly adjacent to the arterial pulse along the medial aspect of the stifle joint or tibia. The artery is superficial and may be isolated after dissection of the subcutaneous tissue. The vein is usually a plexus in this region and not useful for cannulation. The artery may be cannulated as a superficial site for measuring arterial pressures and taking samples, or catheters may be passed into the femoral artery from the access site. Most small swine can accommodate 18- to 20-ga catheters in this vessel.

The femoral vessels may be approached by making either a longitudinal or a transverse incision over the fascial muscular division described above on the medial aspect of the rear leg. There are lateral and deep branches of both the artery and vein that should be ligated or cauterized during the isolation of the vessels. Rupture of these branches usually leads to bleeding in the sheath of the vessels and vasoconstriction.

If the vessels are to be chronically cannulated, the catheters are tunneled subcutaneously to the flank of the pig on the same side for exteriorization (see Chapter 8, Fig. 8.6). The more dorsal the cannulae can be exteriorized, the less

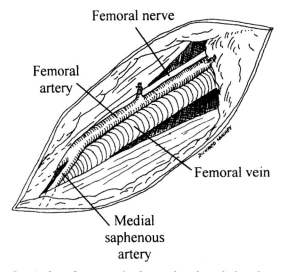

FIGURE 9.12   Surgical cutdown on the femoral and medial saphenous vessels.

likely that they will be traumatized by the pig. In large swine, this may require that the position of the pig be rotated to an oblique or ventral recumbency for the exteriorization process. The femoral incision is usually closed in three layers; muscle, subcutaneous, and subcuticular. Dead space in the subcutaneous region of the thigh should be closed to prevent seromas.

The portal vein may be catheterized through a ventral midline incision from the xiphoid process to the umbilicus. Access to the region is difficult, especially in large swine, and all of the principles of abdominal surgery previously described should be followed. The liver needs to be retracted cranially and the stomach and duodenum, caudally. The intestinal mass will have to be excluded from the surgical area by packing them off with wetted laparotomy sponges. The portal vein can be identified at the hilum of the liver as it passes through the pancreas and dorsal to the duodenum. The common bile duct runs on its ventral surface (Hand et al., 1981).

The portal vein may be carefully dissected around its dorsal surface above and below the area where the cannula is to be inserted. Elastic vessel loops are placed around the vessel to provide occlusion during the venotomy. The portal vein is thin walled, and extensive hemorrhage can occur if it is damaged. A preplaced purse-string suture is placed around the venotomy site. The best location for access is usually in the ventrocaudal portion close to the duodenum.

The portal vein is incised with either a no. 11 scalpel blade or iris scissors after cranial and caudal occlusion of the vessel with the vessel loops. A catheter with a retention bead is fed into the venotomy toward the liver. If the catheter actually passes into the liver, it is more likely to occlude. After placing the tip in the desired location, the purse-string suture is tightened so that a retention bead remains within the vessel. The cranial and then the caudal occlusion loops are loosened. The catheter should either be sutured to the side of the portal vein wall between two retention beads or to some other structure in the region to prevent kinking. The catheter should be checked for patency at this stage. Experience from liver transplantation experiments has shown that greater than 15 minutes of occlusion of the portal vein leads to irreversible portal hypertension. The catheter may be exteriorized through the abdominal wall caudal to the ribs. If a vascular access port is used, it is placed on the lateral surface of the ribs. Experience from many laboratories does not give a consensus on the best type of catheter or technique to use for catheterization of this vessel. Most would consider 6 weeks of patency to be exceptional. Postoperative problems include thrombosis and erosion of the portal vein because of the low velocity in a thin-walled vessel. The portal vein can also be cannulated retrogradely from the splenic vein (Drougas et al., 1996).

Other blood vessels may be cannulated by following the surgical approach for exposure of the organ or structure of interest. For instance, the left hemiazygous vein can be cannulated and the cannula threaded to the coronary sinus to measure venous coronary blood flow by following the applicable surgical instructions for the left total pneumonectomy described above. Using these principles of catheter placement, reasonable success rates can be expected.

For survival procedures, meticulous aseptic technique is obligatory not only intraoperatively, but also postoperatively. Every aspect of the use of chronic catheters must include attention to aseptic technique. The outside of the catheter should be prepped with iodine solution, and personnel should wear gloves when injecting or withdrawing samples. Therapeutic levels of antibiotics at the time of the surgery for device implantation have been shown to be useful, but chronic administration of antibiotics is not a reliable replacement for aseptic technique. Infected implants will have to be surgically removed in order to resolve a chronic infection (Swindle et al., 1998).

Vascular Anastomosis

Anastomosis of blood vessels (Fig. 9.13) is a routine procedure required for experimental procedures, such as organ transplantation or implantation of vascular grafts. It may also be required clinically for trauma. The basic techniques of suturing are the same as for other species. Two characteristics of the porcine vascular system are important considerations. These are the tendency to vasospasm and the pig's rapid clotting time, which necessitates frequent administration of heparin for some procedures. The iv dosage of heparin is 100–300 units/kg as a priming dose with maintenance doses of 100–200 units/kg given approximately every 45 minutes (Gaymes et al., 1995; Smith et al., 1989; Swindle, 1983). Porcine graft implants have been shown to have a smooth fibrin surface and be relatively resistant to experimental infection; these characteristics may make them useful for some preclinical studies (Mehran et al., 1991; Ricci et al., 1991a; Ricci et al., 1991b).

The surgical approach to the blood vessels will be dictated by the procedure being performed. For instance, the abdominal aorta can be approached from

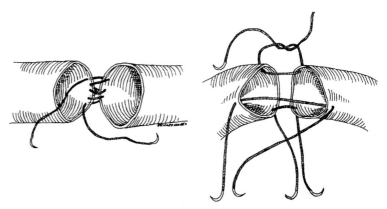

FIGURE 9.13   Anastomosis of the aorta using triangular and continuous closure techniques.

either a retroperitoneal flank incision or a midline incision. If the procedure being performed is a simple anastomosis or implantation of a short graft segment, then the retroperitoneal approach should be considered because of the better exposure without the intestinal mass having to be retracted. On the other hand, if the aortic anastomosis is to be performed in conjunction with another procedure on the vena cava, then the midline incision may be more appropriate. Other vessels, such as the femoral or neck vessels, may be approached from the standard incisions described under vascular cannulation.

Isolation of the vessel and ligation of branches in the proximity of the anastomotic site should be performed gently to avoid vasospasm. The blood vessels to be anastomosed are cross clamped with atraumatic vascular forceps, such as bulldog clamps for small vessels and Satinsky or DeBakey clamps for larger vessels. Cross clamping resulting in total occlusion of blood flow is problematic in some regions, notably the aorta. When cross clamping the aorta or other major vessel without substantial collateral circulation, heparin should always be administered. The total cross-clamp time of the prerenal descending aorta that is tolerated without ischemic damage to the spinal cord is approximately 15 minutes. The number of branches to the psoas musculature that are ligated during isolation of the aorta should be limited to the minimal number required for the procedure. Ligation of substantial numbers of these branches, i.e., four to six continuous pairs in most regions, can also result in spinal cord ischemia. Lymphatic vessels in the region of the aorta should either be avoided or ligated to avoid leakage of chyle. Consequently, it is preferential to perform vascular surgery using tangential clamps that only partially occlude the aorta. Bypass procedures can also be used as for some types of organ transplantation. Peripheral vessels are less of a problem when cross clamped, but heparinization should be used if the goal of the procedure is to provide a patent vessel (Swindle, 1983; Qayumi et al., 1993).

Synthetic nonabsorbable 5/0–6/0 cardiovascular suture is indicated for most vascular anastomoses in swine. Larger vessels, such as the aorta, are sutured in a continuous pattern and smaller vessels are sutured using simple interrupted sutures. For large vessels, the wall of the aorta most distal from the surgeon is the starting point. A double-armed cardiovascular suture is passed from inside the lumen to outside, and a knot is tied at the middle of the suture length to ensure that the knot is outside the lumen. Suture bites of approximately 2–3 mm are necessary to avoid tearing the vessel. The strands are tied in a continuous pattern to a position opposite the first knot one at a time toward the surgeon. The distal clamp may be partially released at this point to allow the vessel to fill and to remove air bubbles. The knot is tied and the distal clamp is released slowly to check for leaks. This is followed by gradual release of the proximal clamp one notch at a time. If substantial leakage occurs, then the leaks can be repaired with simple interrupted sutures. If leakage is minor, then the anastomotic incision may be packed with gauze for 3–5 minutes. This is usually sufficient for clotting to occur at the needle puncture sites. Longitudinal incisions in blood vessels, such as the aorta, may also be utilized. They may be closed in a similar fashion or, if extra security is required, a continuous mattress suture with buffering tags at the knots may be used. This suture pattern is oversewn with simple continuous or continuous Lembert sutures.

When smaller vessels are repaired with simple interrupted patterns, the basic procedure is the same. The wall of the vessel distal from the surgeon is sutured first and the sides are sutured alternatively until the portion of the wall most proximal to the surgeon is closed last. A triangular pattern may also be used for appropriately sized vessels with the first sutures placed distal to the surgeon as for the other patterns. Vascular picks are helpful in positioning the walls of the smaller vessels for proper alignment during suturing.

Veins may be sutured in the same manner as arteries; however, they are much more friable and easily torn with sutures. Closure of the surgical incision is routine for the area in which the vessel is located.

Postoperative anticoagulant and antimicrobial therapy may be required for some procedures, such as the implantation of synthetic grafts. Oral coumarin and aspirin, 25 mg/kg once daily, are readily administered to swine in their food. Antibiotics are given intraoperatively for graft implantation and postoperatively if contamination is suspected (Rogers et al., 1988).

Arteriovenous and Venovenous Fistulas/Vascular Shunts

Arteriovenous fistulas (Fig. 9.14) and shunts are usually created in swine to produce a model of volume overload heart failure (Randsbaek et al., 1996; Wittnich et al., 1991) that leads to cardiac dilatation and subsequent eccentric cardiac hypertrophy (Carroll et al., 1995; Gardner and Johnson, 1988). They have been used in other species to create a dilated vascular space for enhanced vascular access as for human dialysis patients.

The technique involves performing a side-to-side anastomosis between an artery and a vein or the suturing of a vascular prosthesis in an end-to-side vascular window technique between an artery and a vein to produce a left-to-right shunt. The more peripheral the location, i.e., femoral vessels, the longer the time course for production of volume overload. Fistulation between the aorta and pulmonary trunk will have significant immediate effects. This is in contrast to a period of months for clinical effects if peripheral vasculature is used. A fistulation between the carotid artery and the internal jugular vein would be intermediate in time for development of clinical effects. The size of the shunt required differs with the age and breed of the pig and location of the shunt. As a generality, the fistulation needs to be 2.5 times the outside diameter of the blood vessels in length for peripheral vessels. If this size fistula were used in a neonatal pig aorta–pulmonary shunt, it would die acutely. Miniature pigs are less susceptible to the effects of arteriovenous fistulas and shunts, at least in the acute and short-term phases. Because there are relatively few references in the

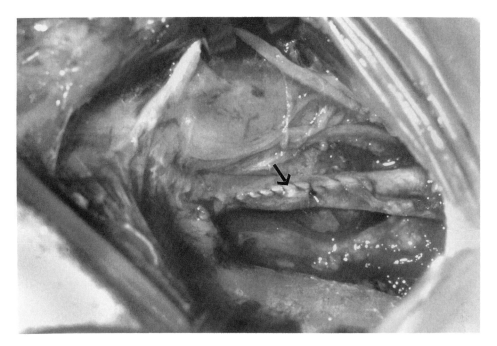

FIGURE 9.14   Femoral arteriovenous fistula (*arrow*).

literature to creation of this model in swine, no consensus on the best surgical technique or breed and age of pig has been reached.

A portocaval shunt may be created by side-to-side or end-to-side anastomosis of the portal vein and the posthepatic caudal vena cava. This model has been used to study the effects of the portocaval shunt on the metabolism of lipids and lipoproteins. Attempts to produce a model of portal hypertension with gastric ulcers and esophageal varices have been made in swine. This involves creation of an end-to-side anastomosis of the vena cava to the portal vein and gradual constriction of the portal vein with devices such as an ameroid constrictor. Collateral circulation in the region helps lower the portal pressure in swine. Irreversible hypotension has also been reported as a complication in hepatic transplantation with prolonged portal vein occlusion, and this should be avoided during portal vein surgery (Carew et al., 1976; Dupont et al., 1985; Gadacz, 1988; Jensen et al., 1983; Kahn et al., 1994; Nestruck et al., 1977).

An arteriovenous malformation model has been created in swine by using a transorbital puncture into the cavernous sinus to create an arteriovenous communication between the rostral rete and the cavernous sinus. The model is possible because of the presence of a rete mirabile in the cavernous sinuses of the skull base (Chaloupka et al., 1994).

The surgical approaches to the vessels will be the routine approaches described for isolation of the vessels in the other sections, i.e., vascular cannulation for femorals or caudal celiotomy for the iliacs. The techniques for suturing the vessels are described in the section on vascular anastomosis.

Atriotomy/Ventriculotomy

The atria on either side can be approached through the fourth or fifth intercostal space or a median sternotomy using the standard thoracotomy incisions described above. Indications would include cannulation procedures and surgical approaches to the foramen ovale, atrioventricular valves, and high membranous ventricular septal defects. Cannulation and other procedures should be performed in the atrial appendage if possible (Fig. 9.15). However, this approach would not be useful for the valvular rings. Cardiopulmonary bypass (Chapter 2) would be required for most procedures except simple cannulations. The atria are extremely friable in swine and should be handled gently with appropriate instruments (Ehler et al., 1990; Hall et al., 1986; Horneffer et al., 1986; Swindle et al., 1986).

The appropriate portion of the atrium is incised with a scalpel or punctured with a scalpel and the incision extended with scissors. Gentle handling of the tissues using cardiovascular instruments is essential to prevent tearing of the atrial incision. Care should be taken to avoid traumatizing the conduction system especially in the region of the sinoatrial (SA) node, atrioventricular (AV) node and bundle of His in the right atrium.

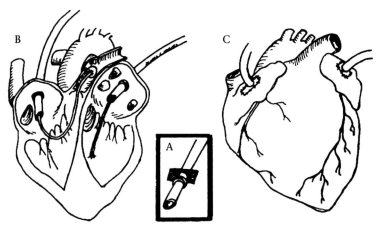

FIGURE 9.15   Atrial cannulation. **A.** Tip of silastic catheter showing placement of silastic ridge and sheeting. **B.** Cutaway view of heart showing a balloon-tipped catheter in the main pulmonary artery and a biopsy catheter in the left ventricle. **C.** External view of the heart with left and right atrial catheters sutured in place. *Reprinted with permission from Smith et al., 1989, Technical aspects of cardiac catheterization of swine. J. Invest. Surg. 2(2): 187–194.*

After the procedure is performed, closure of the incision should be undertaken with great care. Synthetic monofilament nonabsorbable cardiovascular suture material 5/0–6/0 is usually indicated. A purse-string suture may be sufficient for the implantation of a catheter into the atrial appendage. However, such simple suturing techniques for the atria will probably be insufficient, especially in immature animals. Continuous suture patterns can be used if care is taken with their placement and the tension on the suture line. The use of continuous horizontal mattress suture patterns with buttress pledgets at both ends of the suture line offer more security. This pattern may be oversewn with a simple continuous patten for control of leaks. Prior to tying the suture, the usual precautions for closure of cardiac incisions on bypass should be taken. This would include such procedures as the removal of air from the atrium and filling with blood. If leakage occurs from the atrium, it may be repaired by either packing with gauze sponges or the judicious placement of simple interrupted sutures. A small amount of leakage can be tolerated in a heparinized animal and controlled postoperatively with chest tube drainage. The use of protamine to counteract heparin is not recommended as a routine in swine; however, it can be administered slowly with monitoring of blood pressure if indicated.

Intracardiac surgery should be limited to atrial approaches if at all possible, because of the potential complications with ventricular incisions. The surgeon must take care to avoid compromising the coronary circulation and the conduction system. There is also the potential of developing a surgical scar causing arrhythmias. Consequently, most procedures are limited to small puncture wounds or windows with internal instrumentation except for outflow tract approaches and aneurysm repair. Examples would include cutting tendinous chordae or dilation of valves. When incising the ventricle without cardiopulmonary bypass, a purse-string suture should be preplaced around the entry site. Following the removal of the instrument, the purse-string suture is tightened.

Epicardial implantation of devices is easily performed if the same precautions concerning the blood supply and conduction system are taken. The ventricle is easily catheterized from peripheral vessels with or without the use of fluoroscopy, and that is the preferred method of placing internal catheters. Cardiac catheterization is discussed in Chapter 12.

Closure of the incision and postoperative care techniques are the routine ones described for thoracotomy.

Valvular Surgery

The AV valves, the pulmonary valve, and the aortic valve are approached for surgical replacement during cardiopulmonary bypass. The AV valves are usually approached using the appropriate atriotomy incision after a lateral thoracotomy at the fourth to fifth intercostal space on the appropriate side. A median sternotomy approach can also be used as it is in humans, particularly for the right atrium. The mitral valvular approach is problematic regardless of the incision site selected. The pulmonary and aortic valves are approached by longitudinal or transverse incisions over the site of the valve from a median sternotomy or, alternatively, a left lateral thoracotomy may be used for the pulmonary artery (Litzke and Berg, 1977; Shimokawa et al., 1996; Smith et al., 1994; Swindle et al., 1986).

For valvular replacement, the existing valve needs to be excised taking care to not damage the conduction system. The selected valve is sutured in place using the manufacturer's instructions. Most of the valves used will require sizing of the orifice and preplacement of a specified number of sutures using synthetic nonabsorbable suture material. The sutures are passed through the AV valvular tissue into the valve sleeve and then tied in turn. Experimentally, this procedure is usually performed to test new valves using a mitral valve implantation site. The porcine bioprosthesis valves prepared from glutaraldehyde fixed aortic valves collected at slaughterhouses are the preferred valvular implant if there is a choice. These valves offer the advantages of being of porcine origin and having minimal problems with thrombosis and emboli, thus eliminating the need for anticoagulant therapy. Sizing of the orifice for selecting a valve can be performed using two-dimensional echocardiography or may be performed intraoperatively. If mechanical valves of synthetic material are selected, lifetime anticoagulant therapy will be required.

Cutting of the valves to produce valvular regurgitation and creation of volume overload models of heart failure and eccentric ventricular hypertrophy can be performed from peripheral vessels without the use of thoracotomy or cardiopulmonary bypass. Using fluoroscopic guidance, an instrument, such as urologic grasping forceps, is advanced into the ventricle, tendinous chordae are grasped and then torn. Cardiac catheterization or echocardiography can be utilized to judge the degree of regurgitation.

Closures of the atriotomy and/or blood vessel and the thoracotomy are routine. Postoperative care should include antimicrobial therapy as well as the usual analgesic and cardiothoracic precautions.

Aortic and Pulmonary Artery Banding/Ligation of the Ductus Arteriosus/Chronic Instrumentation

The aorta and pulmonary artery are best approached through a left lateral thoracotomy in the third intercostal space. The pulmonary artery can also be approached throughout the fourth intercostal space in most animals. Both vessels can also be approached through a median sternotomy that does not bisect the manubrium. The ductus arteriosus also can be approached through the same lateral incision.

Indications for these surgical approaches to the aorta and pulmonary artery include cannulation for bypass procedures, implantation of devices or grafts and constriction banding to produce pressure overload of the ventricles

(Carroll et al., 1995; Dougherty, 1981; Gardner and Johnson, 1988; Harvey and Jones, 1982; Kaplan et al., 1995; Swindle et al., 1986). The ductus arteriosus can be ligated through the same approach if it is patent ductus arteriosus (PDA). Banding of the great vessels produces a model of concentric ventricular hypertrophy as compared to the models of eccentric hypertrophy produced by AV fistulas as described above. Banding of the aorta produces more severe postoperative consequences than banding of the pulmonary artery.

The surgical approach is routine, and the pericardium is incised, taking care to avoid damage to the phrenic nerve. The most difficult part of the surgery is dissection and isolation of the blood vessels, especially in immature animals. Most models require that the dissection be proximal to the ductus arteriosus close to the base of the heart. The tissue is dissected bluntly using either right-angle forceps or Metzenbaum scissors. In older animals, there may be a fat pad present in this location. In younger animals, the thymus gland may also extend to this region. The most common problems during the dissection are tearing of the right atrium, tearing the ligamentum arteriosus, or tearing of the great vessels. The pulmonary artery is more easily dissected than the aorta from the lateral incision; however, for complex instrumentation, the surgeon may prefer the sternotomy approach.

If the ductus arteriosus is to be ligated, the dissection is similar to the dissection to isolate the pulmonary artery. The vagus nerve crosses the region and should be retracted dorsally without damaging the structure. Atropine should be administered prior to this procedure. The ductus can be doubly ligated using nonabsorbable suture material. If a rupture occurs during this process, the aorta and/or pulmonary artery may have to be repaired by tangential clamping and suture closure of the tear. The method of reopening a closed ductus and using it as a model of PDA is discussed in Chapter 12.

Various methods have been utilized to band these blood vessels to produce a pressure gradient (Fig. 9.16). The method and type of banding material will be dictated by the research application. Generally, the bands are either placed with a pressure gradient in mature animals or they are placed loosely around the vessel in immature animals, which allows gradual constriction as the animal grows. When making bandings resulting in an acute pressure gradient, the constriction should produce a gradient of less than 20 torr. This varies with the age, weight, and breed of the animal, but may be used as a general guideline. Bradycardia will be readily detectable with a tight banding procedure. Making too tight a constriction acutely can result in heart failure. Procedures using angioplasty balloon implantation between the band and the blood vessel to produce a gradual constriction by periodic inflation of the balloon have been used in the dog and could possibly be applicable in this species (Keech et al. 1997).

Erosion of the blood vessel and resultant fatal hemorrhage occurs to some degree with virtually all banding techniques. Erosion tends to be less than in some species because of the presence of a true vaso vasorum in the aorta. However, the incidence may be minimized by the design of the band. The same

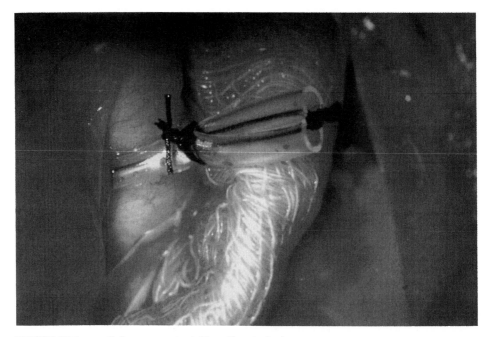

FIGURE 9.16   Pulmonary arterial banding technique.

principles of constriction banding are true for both the aorta and the pulmonary artery. The band should be wide and without sharp edges. Constricting the vessel with either suture material or umbilical tape tends to have a high incidence of erosions. Polytetrafluoroethylene (PTFE) or Teflon bands used clinically have fewer problems. Placing a piece of nonabsorbable suture material inside silicone tubing also has a low incidence of erosion. In this technique, the ends of the suture material can be tied after passing it through a piece of tubing that is long enough to encircle the blood vessel with some overlap. The ends of the tubing are then clamped together at a location to produce the appropriate amount of constriction. Enough overlap of the ends of the tubing to suture around the tubing twice is needed to provide security against slippage. With this technique, only curved pieces of silicone tubing are in contact with the blood vessel, and neither the cut ends of the tubing or the knots in the suture material are in contact with the vessel walls.

A band that can be ruptured with balloon angioplasty techniques to reverse the stenosis can be developed by use of absorbable suture material within the silicone tubing. Three (3/0) polydiaxonone will lose its tensile strength inside a silicone constriction band within 2 months. The period of time to produce a band that loses its tensile strength enough to be ruptured with balloon expansion can be varied with the type and size of absorbable suture material used. For instance, 3/0 polyglactin will lose its tensile strength in approximately one-half the time as polydiaxonone. If these bands are not ruptured mechanically, they will eventually rupture from the pressure of the blood vessel. These same principles can be used to develop a model of coarctation of the aorta or peripheral vascular constriction in addition to the pulmonic and aortic stenosis models described here.

Closure of the incision is routine for thoracotomies as described above. In addition to the usual analgesic and antimicrobial administration postoperatively, treatment for congestive heart failure may have to be administered. Furosemide should be the initial agent used in cases of congestive heart failure.

Myocardial Infarction and Associated Arrhythmias

Swine have been extensively used as animal models of myocardial infarction for the reasons discussed above. These models have included acute and gradual onset occlusion of all of the various coronary arteries and the study of arrhythmias associated with infarction (Bloor et al., 1986; Bloor et al., 1992; Gardner and Johnson, 1988; Lee, 1986; Roberts et al., 1987; Verdouw and Hartog, 1986; White et al., 1986).

The surgical approach depends upon the vessel being instrumented. The left anterior descending (LAD or anterior interventricular) artery is best approached through a median sternotomy. The left circumflex (LCX) is best seen using a left lateral thoracotomy in the fourth intercostal space after lifting the left auricle. The proximal region of the LAD can also be seen through this approach. The right coronary artery (RCA) and its posterior interventricular branch are best seen from a right thoracotomy in the fourth intercostal space. The proximal portion of the RCA is also observed using a median sternotomy. All of the coronary vessels can be observed using a median sternotomy, if the heart is gently lifted from the pericardial cradle. However, prolonged lifting of the heart to see its dorsal aspect leads to compromise of the systemic circulation secondary to compression of the major blood vessels.

Occlusive techniques may either be intravascular or extravascular. Extravascular techniques include the use of snares, clips, and suture ligations for acute occlusion (Fig. 9.17). Gradual occlusion with chronic models can be performed by encircling the vessel with an ameroid constrictor or inflatable cuffs. Intravascular techniques would include occlusion with angioplasty balloon catheters, injection of embolic substances, such as microspheres (Borrego et al., 1996), to block the vessel, or gradual occlusion by creating an atherosclerotic plaque. Atherogenic occlusion can be created after initiating endothelial damage with an inflated angioplasty balloon in conjunction with feeding an atherosclerotic diet. Global ischemia is produced by administering cardioplegic agents during cardiopulmonary bypass. The midsternal approach may be used for coronary artery bypass procedures between the internal thoracic artery and the LAD or using grafts between the aorta and LAD. Additional information on the intravascular procedures may be found in Chapter 12.

Because of the paucity of collateral circulation, swine develop a high inci-

Top

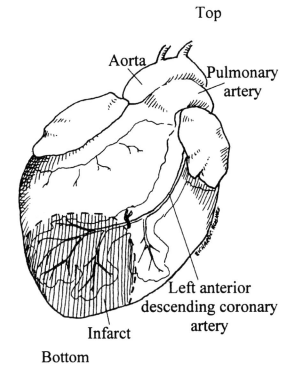

Bottom

FIGURE 9.17   Occlusion of the left anterior descending coronary artery.

dence of ventricular fibrillation following acute occlusion. This is especially true of the LAD, which has less collateral circulation than other vessels, such as the LCX. The incidence of arrhythmias can be decreased several ways. Using the gradual occlusion methods in miniature swine allows the collateral circulation to develop as it does in humans.

In acute infarctions, the incidence of fatal arrhythmias can be decreased by either limiting the time of occlusion, limiting the region of occlusion, or administering antiarrhythmics (Bloor et al., 1986; Horneffer et al., 1986; Swindle, 1994; Verdouw and Hartog, 1986; White et al., 1986). Generally, the incidence of arrhythmias increases substantially after 15 minutes and approaches 100% after 30 minutes. The survival rate for acute occlusion of the LAD can be increased by performing the occlusion distal to the main lateral branch at approximately two-thirds of the length of the artery. Ligation of the posterior vessels of the RCA creates a high incidence of heart block and other damage to the conduction system in contrast to ligation of the LAD. Partial occlusion of blood flow also increases the survival rate. Use of antiarrhythmics, such as bretylium, 5 mg/kg iv every 30 minutes as a slow injection, substantially decreases the risk of fatal arrhythmias. Pharmacologic agents and anesthetic recommendations are discussed in Chapter 2. Miniature swine appear to be more resistant to the development of arrhythmias than farm animals. Arrhythmias in farm animals may vary in incidence among herds, possibly because of heritable factors. Data are not available to support these observations.

The predominant surgical problem associated with instrumenting the coronary vessels is the development of vasoconstriction. The incidence of vasospasm can be decreased by careful surgical technique and the infusion of lidocaine iv following a bolus injection. Care should be taken to not damage the atria during manipulation of vessels such as the LCX (Rogers et al., 1988; Swindle et al., 1986).

Following manipulation of the coronary artery, the thoracotomy incision is closed in a routine manner. Animals should be monitored postoperatively with electrocardiograms, as well as the usual recommendations for cardiac surgery.

Vascular Aneurysms

Models of aortic aneurysm have been created in swine by making various-sized windows in the aorta and suturing in graft materials such as bovine pericardium. These can be variable in their effectiveness in producing aneurysmal sacs. A variety of aneurysms have been created using the neck vessels as a model of intracranial aneurysms. True aneurysms as they occur in humans have not been reported in swine (Chaloupka et al., 1994; Dawson et al., 1995; Guglielmi et al., 1991; Marinov et al., 1997; Massoud et al., 1994; Massoud et al., 1995; Turjman et al., 1994).

The work of Massoud et al. (1994, 1995) and Turjman et al. (1994) provides a detailed comparison of the various types of aneurysms (Fig. 9.18) and their surgical creation in porcine models and will be summarized here. Using a combination of procedures on unilateral external jugular veins, carotid arteries, and ascending cervical arteries, three types of bifurcation aneurysms, two types of terminal aneurysms, wide-necked aneurysms, and fusiform aneurysms were created. The surgical approach is the same as that described for access to the cervical vessels. Blood vessels were treated with heparinized saline to prevent coagulation and papaverine to prevent vasospasm.

Bifurcation Aneurysms

One type was created by harvesting a 5-cm segment of ascending cervical artery and a segment of the external jugular vein. One end of the external jugular vein was ligated to form a venous pouch. End-to-side anastomosis of the arterial graft was performed on a segment of the carotid artery. At the caudad anastomosis of the ascending cervical artery, the venous pouch was included in the anastomosis at the V-shaped notch created between the vessels. The cephalad portion of the arterial graft was looped around the venous pouch and anastomosed to the carotid artery. Blood flow to the carotid artery was restricted between the two arterial anastomoses with an incomplete ligature to increase blood flow through the bypass loop.

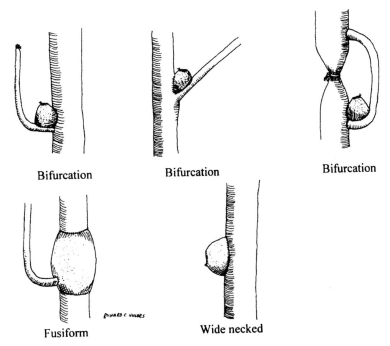

Bifurcation   Bifurcation   Bifurcation

Fusiform   Wide necked

FIGURE 9.18   Examples of surgically created bifurcation, fusiform, and wide-necked aneurysms.

A variation of the technique involved ligation of the ascending cervical artery at the caudal end and anastomosis as described above. This created a bifurcation aneurysm with flow continued in both the carotid and ascending cervical artery. A third type was created by suturing a venous pouch at the bifurcation of two cranial branches of the ascending cervical artery. This resulted in a smaller aneurysm in a smaller blood vessel.

Terminal Aneurysms

As above, a segment of the external jugular vein is isolated to be used as an aneurysmal sac. An additional 5-cm segment is isolated to be sewn to the carotid artery as a bypass loop. The venous pouch is sewn in the caudad notch of the bypass loop. When distended with blood, the aneurysm compresses the carotid artery, obviating the need for an incomplete ligature.

Another type is formed by the production of a carotid–bijugular fistula with an aneurysmal sac at the T junction. For this procedure, the external jugular vein is harvested for the aneurysm as before. The carotid artery on the same side has a 5-cm segment harvested, and two opposing elliptical arteriotomy sites are incised halfway along the segment. The carotid graft is sutured end-to-side to the carotid artery stump, and the aneurysmal pouch of the external jugular vein is sutured to the opposite arteriotomy. The ends of the carotid artery graft are then sutured end-to-side to the external jugular vein and the internal jugular vein. This will result in a rapid flow aneurysm with an arteriovenous fistula.

Fusiform Aneurysms

Fusiform aneurysms are produced by end-to-end anastomosis of the isolated external jugular vein segment to the carotid artery. A side branch may be added by anastomosing a segment of the anterior cervical artery in an end-to-side fashion with the external jugular vein segment on one end and ligating the other. The external jugular vein graft will dilate circumferentially and the side branch will fill with blood as well if it is added.

Wide-Necked Aneurysms

For this model, the external jugular vein segment is anastomosed end-to-side to the common carotid artery and the opposite end ligated. The model has had variations performed by suturing the venous pouch obliquely 45 degrees through the carotid artery to give a more acute angle and improve flow to prevent spontaneous thrombosis and minimize the Venturi effect (Dawson et al., 1995, Guglielmi et al., 1991).

Similar types of aneurysms can be produced in the aorta using bovine pericardium or venous grafts sutured over oval windows in the distal aorta (Fig. 9.19). All of the various aneurysms are prone to spontaneous thrombosis but may be used for acute and chronic evaluation of various endovascular devices to occlude them.

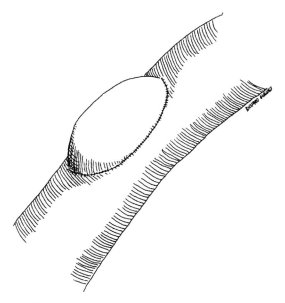

FIGURE 9.19   Aortic aneurysm.

Coarctation of the Aorta

Coarctation of the aorta may be created by surgically decreasing the size of the lumen of the aortic arch or descending aorta. Following a left thoracotomy in the fourth intercostal space, vascular clamps are applied to partially occlude the lumen proximally and distally to the ligamentum arteriosus. An elliptical excision of a portion of the aorta equal in length to one-half of the circumference of the aorta is performed. Continuous cardiovascular sutures are placed to close the edges of the ellipse (Fig. 9.20). After the clamps are removed, a defect that reduces the diameter of the aorta approximately 50% should be formed. Large-sized absorbable suture, such as 1 surgical gut or polydiaxonone ligatures, are placed around the narrowing of the wedge. The sutures are tied loosely, so that additional constriction of blood flow does not occur. The model may be used for angioplasty and/or stent placement (Lock et al., 1982; Morrow et al., 1994).

Cardiomyoplasty

Cardiomyoplasty procedures are utilized as interim cardiac assist procedures for heart failure. The procedure involves isolating and wrapping the latissimus dorsi muscle around the heart and stimulating it to contract like cardiac muscle (Fig. 9.21) (Borrego et al., 1996; Kratz et al., 1994).

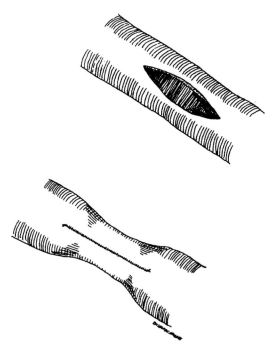

FIGURE 9.20   Coarctation of the aorta.

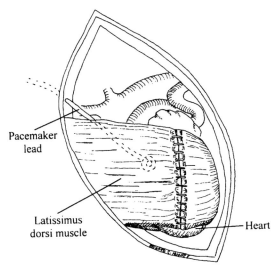

FIGURE 9.21   Cardiomyoplasty procedure.

In swine, the latissimus dorsi muscle is large and thick and receives its primary blood and nerve supply from the thoracodorsal artery and nerve that enter the muscle close to its insertion at the second rib. The origin of the muscle is broad and extends caudally to the last ribs. Because of the size of the muscle and the thoracic wall in swine, the procedure would be difficult to perform except in smaller animals. A long oblique incision over the fifth intercostal space is made and the skin is either undermined or an additional transverse incision is made to expose the origin of the muscle, which is transected. The muscle body is isolated to the area of insertion while preserving the neurovascular pedicle. After isolating the muscle, the fourth and/or fifth ribs are resected to allow space for the muscle to be inserted into the thoracic cavity. The pericardium is incised in such a manner as to allow the muscle to be wrapped around the heart. An epicardial sensor electrode is placed over the ventricle and muscular myostimulators are attached to the insertion of the muscle. The muscle is sutured with mattress sutures in such a way as to form a pocket around the ventricular region of the heart while preserving the blood and nerve supply to the muscle (Fig. 9.21).

Either prior to or after performing the procedure the skeletal muscle must be trained to develop a predominance of Type I muscle fibers, which are more resistant to fatigue. This is accomplished by resting the muscle for several weeks and then progressively stimulating it over several weeks to accomplish the task. Performing the procedure in a two-stage progression would involve isolating the muscle first and stimulating it prior to implanting it into the thorax.

This procedure impairs the mobility of swine and requires combination analgesic therapy with opioids and nonsteroidal antiinflammatory drugs to control the pain. The thoracic incision is closed in the usual manner.

Epicardial Pacemaker and Device Implantation

Epicardial pacemaker implantation may be performed to test pacemaker devices and leads (Brownlee et al., 1997; Gillette et al., 1991; Hughes and Bowman, 1986; Schumann et al., 1994; Smith et al., 1997; Tong et al., 1995) or used to create a model of dilated cardiomyopathy from rapid epicardial pacing (>180 beats per minute) (Hendrick et al., 1990; LeGrice et al., 1995; Spinale et al., 1990). The model of dilated cardiomyopathy results in congestive heart failure developing over several weeks and requires intensive postoperative care with diuretics for medical management. Endocardial pacemaker lead implantation and electrophysiology are discussed in Chapter 12. Other devices that may be required for implantation on the epicardium include sonomicrometry crystals for measurement of cardiac dimensions and flow transducers on the coronary arteries.

The surgical approach to the heart may either be through a left lateral thoracotomy in the fourth to fifth intercostal space or via a substernal or median sternotomy. The approach is dictated by the desired placement of the electrode or device. The left lateral thoracotomy allows access to the left coronary artery and its branches, as well as both the left and right ventricles. The median sternotomy allows access to different regions of the same structures and improved access to the epicardium. A substernal approach through the ventral midline of the abdomen and the ventral attachment of the diaphragm and pericardium allows access to the apex of the heart only. The relatively noninvasive substernal approach allows more rapid recovery without many of the complications associated with a thoracotomy.

Two basic types of pacemaker electrodes with some variations are used. They are generally either screw-in leads or sutured leads. The manufacturer's recommendations should be followed. Regardless of which lead is used, the coronary artery and its branches should be avoided during implantation. Because of the characteristics of the coronary circulation discussed above, damage of these vessels could result in an infarct. Pacemaker leads are implanted subcutaneously using the same principles of surgery that apply to chronic catheterization. In general, this means that the lead is tunneled through the subcutaneous tissue from the thorax to the subcutaneous site where the pulse generator is to be implanted. Pacemaker pockets can be made in the subcutaneous tissues of the side of the chest or preferably the neck or flank if the lead is long enough. The subcutaneous pockets need to be dissected carefully to avoid having seepage of blood from small vessels, which will consistently lead to hematomas and seromas. The subcutaneous pocket needs to be large enough so that the device to be implanted is easily placed and does not cause tension leading to necrosis and dehiscence. This is especially a problem on the chest wall. The implantation of pacemakers with endocardial pacemaker leads in the jugular furrow of the neck is discussed in Chapter 12. The skin incision should never be directly over or ventral to the implanted device. Implanted devices tend to gravitate ventrally in animals, and the incision is best made either cranial or caudal to the device to be implanted. The pacemaker pocket needs to be closed with subcutaneous and subcuticular sutures, ensuring that the dead space is closed adequately. Skin sutures are placed as required.

Implantation of sonomicrometry crystals and flow transducers follows the principles of surgery discussed above for ventriculotomy and coronary vessel procedures in myocardial infarction models.

Heart and Heart–Lung Transplantation

The pig has been utilized for all of the various forms of heart (Calne et al., 1976; Calne et al., 1978; Hall et al., 1986; Qayumi et al., 1991; Saito and Waters, 1994; Swindle et al., 1986; White and Lunney, 1979), heart–lung (Baumgartner et al., 1988; Harjula and Baldwin, 1987; Qayumi et al., 1990; Qayumi et al., 1993; Saito and Waters, 1994), and lung (see above) transplantation. However, swine are susceptible to apnea following total cardiopulmonary denervation and are usually reserved for acute and chronic heart and single-lung transplantation and for acute heart–double lung transplantation. The growth of the pig makes it useful for the growing heart model as described above (Brutel de la Riviere et al., 1983; Haworth and Hislop, 1981; Pae et al., 1981). A growing interest in the porcine model has developed because of the progress with xenotransplantation. It is likely that the pig will be the donor animal of choice for this procedure for multiple organs including the heart (Swindle, 1996).

The donor and recipient are operated on using a complete median sternotomy with a pericardial cradle for all of these procedures. Bretylium, 3-5 mg/kg, is useful as a preventative for cardiac arrhythmias in both the donor and the recipient (see Chapter 2).

Heart Transplant

Donor

The donor is prepared by dissection of the cranial and caudal vena cava. The pericardium between the aorta and pulmonary artery is dissected completely. The donor is heparinized (300 IU/kg), and cardiectomy is initiated. The cranial vena cava is ligated and divided caudal to the azygous vein. The caudal vena cava is ligated, and the aorta is cross clamped. The animal is exsanguinated, and the blood may be used for priming the bypass pump. Chilled cardioplegia solution (4°C) is infused into the aortic root, and the caudal vena cava is opened to allow drainage of the cardioplegia solution. The aorta and pulmonary arteries are transected distal to their first branches. The posterior wall of the left atrium is opened between the pulmonary veins and immersed in chilled preservation solution awaiting implantation.

Recipient

The recipient is prepared in a similar manner except the animal is placed on cardiopulmonary bypass. Venous bypass cannulae are passed through the right atrial appendage and snared in the cranial and caudal vena cavae. The arterial line is placed in the aorta or femoral artery. Bypass parameters may vary among experiments; however, cooling to 28°–30°C and flow rates of 50–80 ml/kg have been recommended.

The recipient cardiectomy is performed following cross clamping of the aorta with an incision that follows the atrioventricular groove. The incision should preserve the coronary sinus. The pulmonary artery and aorta are transected at the level of the commissures of the valves.

Implantation of the donor heart is performed with a series of continuous sutures with 5/0–6/0 nonabsorbable cardiovascular suture. The atria are anastomosed first. Descriptions of starting the anastomosis with either the left or right atrium have been published (Baumgartner et al., 1988; Saito and Waters, 1994). The heart must be rotated caudoventrally if the right atrium is anastomosed first, in order to accomplish anastomosis of the left atrium. The pulmonary artery and aorta are anastomosed next. Air is removed from the aorta prior to removing the cross clamp.

The cardiac rhythm is restored with internal defibrillation if it does not return spontaneously during rewarming and weaning from bypass. Isoproterenol infusion to effect is used postoperatively to provide a regular heart rate and blood pressure as the catecholamine-induced heart rate recovers. Protamine may be used judiciously at a slow infusion rate of 1 mg/100 U heparin if clotting is a problem. A double chest tube with a Y connection should be used postoperatively.

Heart–Lung Transplant

The donor and recipient are prepared in a similar manner as for heart transplantation, except that the trachea is divided cranial to the bifurcation and the recipient is left with the right atrium with a portion of the interatrial septum. The phrenic nerves are preserved on pedicles during the dissection. The pulmonary artery and veins remain intact with the transplantation block. With this technique, the anastomosis of the right atrium, trachea, and aorta are required for implantation into the recipient. The right lung is passed dorsally to the vena cava and phrenic nerve (Fig. 9.22). The donor vena cava is ligated.

Single-lung transplant (described above) provides an experimental model for evaluation of pulmonary transplant that is better than isolated double-lung transplant because of the physiologic problems associated with respirator apnea postoperatively in the pig. Consequently, double-lung transplant is not described.

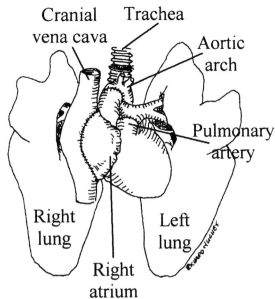

FIGURE 9.22   Heart-and-lung transplantation.

Miscellaneous Thoracic Procedures

Thoracic Duct Cannulation

Cannulation of the thoracic duct is performed to collect chyle for experimental studies (Fig. 9.23). The most frequent complication associated with collection of chyle is failure of the cannulation due to clotting shortly after the procedure. The reentry cannulation method described here may provide a longer collection period (Mendenhall et al., 1996).

The thoracic duct courses dorsal to the aorta and ventral to the hemiazygous vein from the base of the heart caudally to the cisterna-chyli, which it drains. The duct is dorsolateral to the aorta in the left side of the thorax until approximately the fifth rib, then it is more accessible from the right thorax. Cannulation is usually performed in the right seventh to eighth intercostal space. Variations in ductal anatomy may occur, such as branching ducts, which make the procedure more difficult.

Cannulation of the duct is performed in the same manner as cannulation of blood vessels described above. However, the duct is easily damaged and difficult to locate in fat animals and animals that have been fasted for a prolonged period of time. Feeding of liquids containing a high proportion of fatty substances prior to anesthesia may help to identify the duct.

The catheter needs to be small bore and composed of silicone or polyethyl-

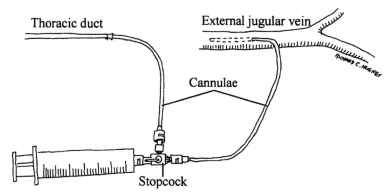

FIGURE 9.23   Cannulation of the thoracic duct with reentry into the external jugular vein.

ene. Coating with silicone or the use of heparin-impregnated catheters may be helpful to prevent catheter failure due to clotting. After cannulation, the catheter is passed through an intercostal space cranial to the cannulation site. It is tunneled subcutaneously in a cranial direction along the dorsum of the rib line. It is exteriorized several intercostal spaces cranial to the exit from the thorax. Chyle may be collected in this location, or the cannula can be placed into a reentry circuit to drain into the right external jugular vein. If it is drained back into the jugular vein, then a three-way valve is placed into the system at the exit site. The cannula is then passed subcutaneously to an incision into the right jugular furrow for cannulation into the jugular vein as described above for vascular cannulation. The incisions are closed in a routine manner. The cannula tract is kept open until collection of chyle is desired, and then the three-way valve is closed on the cranial side. Meticulous aseptic handling of the exteriorized catheter is indicated. In a closed system, the catheter should be heparinized if continuous flow into a collection site is not provided.

Postoperative care is routine.

Esophageal Surgery

Esophageal surgery is usually performed in the thorax or the neck. The techniques are described in this section, because, experimentally, it is likely that the thoracic approach will be the one most likely used.

The esophagus courses from the pharynx dorsal to the larynx. It begins to course to the left dorsolateral aspect of the trachea at approximately the fourth cervical vertebra. In the thorax, it passes dorsal to the tracheal bifurcation and to the right of the aortic arch. It enters the esophageal hiatus of the diaphragm and joins the stomach shortly after entering the abdominal cavity.

The esophagus can be surgically approached in the neck through a ventral midline incision with lateral retraction of the trachea. In the cranial thorax, it is best approached using a median sternotomy. It may also be approached using a lateral thoracotomy in the cranial thorax; however, access and dissection are more difficult. In the caudal abdomen, it is approached through either a right or left lateral thoracotomy from the fourth to the ninth intercostal spaces. The esophageal sphincter can be approached using a midline celiotomy incision with caudal retraction of the stomach and cranial retraction of the liver. At any location, care should be taken to avoid injury to the recurrent laryngeal nerves and vagal trunks, which are located in the proximity of the esophagus. Striated and smooth muscle are included in the tunica muscularis of swine.

The esophagus may be fistulated in the neck, have a pharyngostomy tube placed into the cervical region, have an esophagotomy or be anastomosed with or without a graft. The main problem associated with surgery of the esophagus is the retarded healing process because of the constant tension and peristalsis of the structure and the lack of a strong serosal layer to maintain sutures. The esophagus is usually closed in two layers. The inner layer is placed in the tunical mucosa and submucosa with continuous sutures using synthetic absorbable sutures. The outer muscular layers and adventitial layers are closed with simple interrupted or horizontal mattress sutures. For some chronic procedures, such as graft implantation, synthetic nonabsorbable sutures should be utilized. The surgical incisions are closed in the routine manner described for the region.

References

Bailie, M.B., S.K. Wixson, and M.S. Landi. 1986. Vascular access port implantation for serial blood sampling in conscious swine. Lab. Anim. Sci. 36(4): 431–433.

Baumgartner, W.A., R.J. Kirkman, L.R. Pennington, T.J. Pritchard, M.G. Sarr, and G.M. Williams. 1988. Organ transplantation. In Swindle, M.M., and Adams, R.J. (eds), Experimental Surgery and Physiology: Induced Animal Models of Human Disease. Baltimore: Williams and Wilkins, pp. 284–299.

Bloor, C.M., F.C. White, and R.J. Lammers. 1986. Cardiac ischemia and coronary blood flow in swine, In Stanton, H.C., and Mersmann, H.J. (eds), Swine in Cardiovascular Research, Vol. 2. Boca Raton: CRC Press, pp. 87–119.

Bloor, C.M., F.C. White, and D.M. Roth. 1992. The pig as a model of myocardial ischemia and gradual coronary occlusion. In Swindle, M.M. (ed), Swine as Models in Biomedical Research. Ames: Iowa State University Press, pp. 163–175.

Bobbie, D.L., and M.M. Swindle. 1986. Pulse monitoring, intramuscular, and intravascular injection sites in swine. In Tumbleson, M.E. (ed), Swine in Biomedical Research. New York: Plenum Press, pp. 273–277.

Borrego, J.M., A. Ordonez, A. Hernandez, and J. Perez. 1996. Neovascularization of the ischemic myocardium by cardiomyoplasty. In Tumbleson, M.E., and Schook, L.B. (eds), Advances in Swine in Biomedical Research, Vol. 2. New York: Plenum Press, pp. 653–661.

Brownlee, R.R., M.M. Swindle, R. Bertolet, and P. Neff. 1997. Toward optimizing a pre-shaped catheter and system parameters to achieve single lead DDD pacing. PACE 20(SPT1): 1354–1358.

Brutel de la Riviere, A., J.M. Quaegebeur, P.J. Hennis, G. Brutel de la Riviere, and G. Van Herpen. 1983. Growth of an aorta–coronary anastomosis. An experimental study in pigs. J Thorac. Cardiovasc. Surg. 86(3): 393–399.

Calne, R.Y., T.A. English, D.C. Dunn, P. McMaster, D.C. Wilkins, and B.M. Herbertson. 1976. Orthotopic heart transplantation in the pig. The pattern of rejection. Transplant. Proc. 8(1): 27–30.

Calne, R.Y., K. Rolles, D.J. White, D.P. Smith, and B.M. Herbetson. 1978. Prolonged survival of pig orthotopic heart grafts treated with cyclosporin A. Lancet 1(8075): 1183–1185.

Carew, T.E., R.P. Saik, K.H. Johansen, C.A. Dennis, and D. Steinberg. 1976. Low density and high density lipoprotein turnover following portocaval shunt in swine. J. Lipid Res. 17(5): 441–450.

Carroll, S.M., L.E. Nimmo, P.S. Knoepfler, F.C. White, and C.M. Bloor. 1995. Gene expression in a swine model of right ventricular hypertrophy. J. Mol. Cell. Cardiol. 27(7): 1427–1441.

Chaloupka, J.C., F. Vinuela, J. Robert, and J. Duckwiller. 1994. An in vivo arteriovenous malformation model in swine: Preliminary feasibility and natural history study. Am. J. Neuroradiol. 15(5): 945–950.

Corin, W.J., M.M. Swindle, J.F. Spann Jr., M. Frankis, W.W.R. Biederman, A. Smith, A. Taylor, and B.A. Carabello. 1988. The mechanism of decreased stroke volume in children and swine with ventricular septal defect and failure to thrive. J. Clin. Invest. 82(2): 544–551.

Dawson, R.C., A.F. Krisht, D.L. Barrow, G.J. Joseph, G.G. Shengelaia, and B. Bonner. 1995. Treatment of experimental aneurysms using collagen-coated microcoils. Neurosurgery 36(1): 133–140.

Dougherty, R.W. 1981. Experimental Surgery in Farm Animals. Ames: Iowa State University Press.

Drougas JG, S.E. Barnard, J.K. Wright, M. Sika, R.R Lopez, K.A. Stokes, P.E. Williams, and C.W. Pinson. 1996. A model for the extended studies of hepatic hemodynamics and metabolism in swine. Lab. Anim. Sci. 46(6): 648–655.

Dupont, J., W.V. Lumb, A.W. Nelson, J.P. Seegmiller, D. Hotchkiss, and H.P. Chase. 1985. Portocaval shunt as a treatment for hypercholesterolemia. Metabolic and morphological effects in a swine model. Atherosclerosis 58(1–3): 205–222.

Ehler, W.J., J.H. Cissik, V.C. Smith, and G.B. Hubbard. 1990. Evaluation of Gore-Tex graft material in the repair of right ventricular outflow tract defect. J. Invest. Surg. 3(2): 119–127.

Gadacz, T.R. 1988. Portal hypertension. In Swindle M.M., Adams, R.J. (eds), Experimental Surgery and Physiology: Induced Animal Models of Human Disease, Baltimore: Williams and Wilkins, pp. 250–253.

Gal, D., and J.M. Isner. 1992. Atherosclerotic Yucatan microswine as a model for novel cardiovascular interventions and imaging, In Swindle, M.M. (ed), Swine as Models in Biomedical Research. Ames: Iowa State University Press, pp. 118–140.

Gardner, T.J., and D.L. Johnson. 1988. Cardiovascular system. In Swindle, M.M., and Adams, R.J. (eds), Experimental Surgery and Physiology: Induced Animal Models of Human Disease. Baltimore: Williams and Wilkins, pp. 74–124.

Gaymes, C.H., M.M. Swindle, P.C. Gillette, M.E. Harold, and R.E Schumann. 1995. Percutaneous serial catheterization in swine: a practical approach. J. Invest. Surg. 8(2): 123–128.

Gillette, P.C., M.M. Swindle, R.P. Thompson, and C.L. Case. 1991. Transvenous cryoablation of the bundle of His. PACE 14(4) Pt1: 504–510.

Greenberg, S., C. McGowan, and T.M. Glenn. 1981. Pulmonary vascular smooth muscle function in porcine splanchnic arterial occlusion shock. Am. J. Physiol. 241(1): H33–34.

Guglielmi, G., F. Vinuela, J. Dion, and G. Duckwiler. 1991. Electrothrombosis of saccular aneurysms via endovascular approach. Part 2: Preliminary clinical experience. J. Neourosurg. 75(1): 8–14.

Hall, T.S., M. Borkon, W.A. Baumgartner, R. Scott Stuart, M.M. Swindle, E. Galloway, and B.A. Reitz. 1986. Use of Swine in heart transplantation research. In Tumbleson, M.E. (ed), Swine in Biomedical Research, Vol. 1. New York: Plenum Press, pp. 373–376.

Hand, M.S., R.W. Phillips, C.W. Miller, R.A. Mason, and W.V. Lumb. 1981. A method for quantitation of hepatic, pancreatic and intestinal function in conscious Yucatan miniature swine. Lab. Anim. Sci. 31(6): 728–731.

Harjula, A., and J.C. Baldwin. 1987. Lung transplantation in the pig with successful preservation using prostaglandin E-1. Appl. Cardiol. 2: 397.

Harvey, R.C., and E.F. Jones. 1982. A technique for bioinstrumentation of the thorax of miniature swine. Lab. Anim. Sci. 32(1): 94–96.

Haworth, S.G., and A.A. Hislop. 1981. Adaptation of the pulmonary circulation to extrauterine life in the pig and its relevance to the human infant. Cardiovasc. Res. 15(2): 108–119.

Hendrick, D.A., A.C. Smith, J.M. Kratz, F.A. Crawford, and F.G. Spinale. 1990. The pig as a model of tachycardia and dilated cardiomyopathy. Lab. Anim. Sci. 40(5): 495–501.

Horneffer, P.J., V.J. Gott, and T.J. Gardner. 1986. Swine as a cardiac surgical model. In Tumbleson, M.E. (ed), Swine in Biomedical Research, Vol. 1. New York: Plenum Press, pp. 321–326.

Hughes, H.C. 1986. Swine in cardiovascular research. Lab. Anim. Sci. 36(4): 348–350.

Hughes, H.C., and T.A. Bowman. 1986. Intracardiac electrophysiology of swine for design and testing of cardiac pacemakers. In Tumbleson, M.E. (ed), Swine in Biomedical Research, Vol. 1. New York: Plenum Press, pp. 327–331.

Jensen, D.M., G.A. Machicado, J.I. Tapia, G. Kauffman, P. Franco, and D. Beilin. 1983. A reproducible canine model of esophageal varices. Gastroenterology 84(3): 573–579.

Kahn, D., R. Hickman, H. Pienaar, and J. Terblanche. 1994. Liver transplantation in the pig. In Cramer, D.V., Podesta, L., and Makowka, L. (eds), Handbook of Animal Models in Transplantation Research. Boca Raton: CRC Press, pp. 75–86.

Kaplan, D.K., N. Atsumi, M.N. D'Ambra, and G.J. Vlahakes. 1995. Distal circulatory support for thoracic aortic operations—effects on intracranial pressure. Ann. Thorac. Surg. 59(2): 448–452.

Keech, G.B., M. Koide, B. Carabello, A.C. Smith, G. Defreyte, and M. Swindle. 1997. An adult canine model of progressive left ventricular pressure overload. J. Invest. Surg. 10(5): 295–304.

Kratz, J.M., W.S. Johnson, R. Mukherjee, J. Hu, F.A. Crawford, and F.G. Spinale. 1994. The relation between latissimus dorsi skeletal muscle structure and contractile function after cardiomyoplasty. J. Thorac. Cardiovasc. Surg. 107 (3): 868–878.

Lee, K.T. 1986. Swine as animal models in cardiovascular research. In Tumbleson, M.E. (ed), Swine in Biomedical Research, Vol. 3. New York: Plenum Press, pp. 1481–1496.

LeGrice, I.J., Y. Takayama, J.W. Holmes, and J.W. Covell. 1995. Impaired subendocardial function in tachycardia-induced cardiac failure. Am. J. Physiol. 268(5 Pt2): H1788–1794.

Litzke, L.F., and R. Berg. 1977. Quantitative-morphological studies of the heart of mini-lewe miniature swine. 2: Atrioventricular and semilunar valves. Arch. Exp.Veterin-armed 31(4): 547–556.

Lock, J.E., T. Niemi, B.A. Burke, S. Einzig, and W. Castaneda-Zuniga. 1982. Transcutaneous angioplasty of experimental aortic coarctation. Circulation 6(6): 1280–1286.

Marinov, G.R., Y. Marois, E. Paris, P. Roby, M. Formichi, Y. Douville, and R. Guidoin. 1997. Can the infusion of elastase in the abdominal aorta of the Yucatan miniature swine consistently produce experimental aneurysms? J. Invest. Surg. 10(2): 129–150.

Massoud, T.F., C. Ji, G. Guglielmi, F. Vinuela, and J. Robert. 1994. Experimental models of bifurcation and terminal aneurysms: Construction techniques in swine. Am. J. Neuroradiol. 15(5): 938–944.

Massoud, T.F., F. Turjman, C. Ji, F. Vinuela, G. Guglielmi, Y.P. Gobin, and G.R. Duckwiller. 1995. Endovascular treatment of fusiform aneurysms with stents and coils: Technical feasibility in a swine model. Am. J. Neuroradiol. 16(10): 1953–1963.

McKenzie, J.E. 1996. Swine as a model in cardiovascular research. In Tumbleson, M.E., and Schook, L.B. (eds), Advances in Swine in Biomedical Research, Vol. 1. New York: Plenum Press, pp. 7–18.

Mehran, R.J., M.A. Ricci, A.M. Graham, K. Carter, and J.F. Smyes. 1991. Porcine model for vascular graft studies. J. Invest. Surg. 4(1): 37–44.

Mendenhall, H.V., C. Horvath, M. Piechowiak, L. Johnson, and K. Bayer. 1996. An external thoracic duct venous shunt to allow for long-term collection of lymph and blood in the conscious pig. In Tumbleson, M.E., and Schook, L.E. (eds). Advances in Swine in Miomedical Research, Vol. 3. NY: Plenum Press, pp. 621–627.

Mitchell, S.E., J.H. Anderson, M.M. Swindle, J.D. Strandberg, and J. Kan. 1994. Atrial septostomy: Stationary angioplasty balloon technique. Experimental work and preliminary clinical applications. Pediatr. Cardiol. 15(1): 1–7.

Morrow, W.R., V.C. Smith, W.J. Ehler, A.F. Van Dellen, and C.E. Mullins. 1994. Balloon angioplasty with stent implantation in experimental coarctation of the aorta. Circulation 89(6): 2677–2683.

Murphy, J.G., R.S. Schwartz, W.D. Edwards, A.R. Camrud, R.E. Vliestra, and D.R. Holmes, Jr. 1992. Percutaneous polymeric stents in porcine coronary arteries: Initial experience with polyethylene terephthalate stents. Circulation 86(5): 1596–1604.

Nestruck, A.C., S. Lussier-Cacan, M. Bergseth, M. Bidallier, J. Davignon, and Y.L. Marcel. 1977. The effect of portocaval shunt on plasma lipids and lipoproteins in swine. Biochim. Biophys. Acta 488(1): 43–54.

Nicolau, D.P., Y.J. Feng, A.H.B. Wu, S.P. Bernstein, and C.H. Nightingale. 1996. Swine model of continuous arteriovenous hemofiltration. Lab. Anim. Sci. 46(3): 355–357.

Pae, W.E. Jr., J.L. Myers, J.A. Waldhausen, G.A. Prophet, and W.S. Pierce. 1981. Subclavian flap angioplasty. Experimental study in growing piglets. J. Thorac. Cardiovasc. Surg. 82(6): 922–927.

Purohit, D.M., M.M. Swindle, C.D. Smith, H.B. Othersen Jr., and J.M. Kazanovicz. 1993. Hanford miniature swine model for extracoporeal membrane oxygenation (ECMO). J. Invest. Surg. 6(6): 503–508.

Qayumi, A.K., W.R. Jamieson, D.M. Godin, S. Lam, K.M. Ko, E. Germann, and J. VandenBroek. 1990. Response to allopurinol pretreatment in a swine model of heart–lung transplantation. J. Invest. Surg. 3(4): 331–340.

Qayumi, A.K., W.R. Jamieson, L.J. Rosado, D.M. Lyster, M. Schulzer, B. McConville, K.D. Gillespie, and M.P. Hudson. 1991. Comparison of functional and metabolic assessments in preservation techniques for heart transplantation. J. Invest. Surg. 4(1): 93–102.

Qayumi, A.K., D.V. Godin, W.R. Jamieson, K.M. Ko, and A. Poostizadeh. 1993. Correlation of red cell antioxidant status and heart–lung function in swine pretreated with allopurinol (a model of heart–lung transplantation). Transplantation 56(1): 37–43.

Randsbaek, F., C.J. Riordan, J.H. Storey, W.D. Montgomery, W.P. Santamore, and E.H.

Austin III. 1996. Animal model of the univentricular heart and single ventricular physiology. J. Invest. Surg. 9(4): 375–384.

Ricci, M.A., R.J. Mehran, D. Petsikas, F. Mohamed, R. Guidoin, Y. Marois, N.V. Christou, A. Graham, and J.F. Symes. 1991a. Species differences in the infectability of vascular grafts. Invest. Surg. 4(1): 45–52.

Ricci, M.A., R. Mehran, N.V. Christou, F. Mohamed, A.M. Graham, and J.F. Smyes. 1991b. Species differences in the clearance of *Staphylococcus aureus* bacteremia. J. Invest. Surg. 4(1): 53–58.

Roberts, S.L., M. Gilbert, and J.H. Tinker. 1987. Isoflurane has a greater margin of safety than halothane in swine with and without major surgery or critical coronary stenosis. Anesth. Analg. 66(6): 485–491.

Rogers, G.P., D.M. Cromeens, S.T. Minor, and M.M. Swindle. 1988. Bretylium and diltiazem in porcine cardiac procedures, J. Invest. Surg. 1(4): 321–326.

Rysavy, J.A., G.E. Lund, J.E. Lock, J.L. Bass, S.S. Einzig, and K. Amplatz. 1986. A method for nonsurgical creation of patent ductus arteriosus and its applications in piglets. In Tumbleson, M.E. (ed), Swine in Biomedical Research, Vol. 1. New York: Plenum Press, pp. 351–361.

Saito, R., and P.F. Waters. 1994. Heart, lung, and heart-lung transplantation in the dog and the pig. In Cramer, D.V., Podesta, L.G., and Makowks, L. (eds), Handbook of Animal Models in Transplantation Research. Boca Raton, FL: CRC Press, pp. 161–172.

Schumann, R.E., M.M. Swindle, B.J. Knick, C.L. Case, and P.C. Gillette. 1994. High dose narcotic anesthesia using sufentanil in swine for cardiac catheterization and electrophysiologic studies. J. Invest. Surg. 7(3): 243–248.

Shimokawa S, H. Matsumoto, S. Ogata, T. Komokata, S. Nishida, T. Ushijima, H. Saigenji, Y. Moriyama, and A. Taira. 1996. A new experimental model for simultaneous evaluation of aortic and pulmonary allograft performance in a composite graft. J. Invest. Surg. 9(5): 487–493.

Smith, A.C., F.G. Spinale, B.A. Carabello, and M.M. Swindle. 1989. Technical aspects of cardiac catheterization of swine. J. Invest. Surg. 2(2): 187–194.

Smith, A.C., F.G. Spinale, and M.M. Swindle. 1990. Cardiac function and morphology of Hanford miniature swine and Yucatan miniature and micro swine. Lab. Anim. Sci. 40(1): 47–50.

Smith, A.C., L.J. Dungan, and M.M. Swindle. 1994. Induced heart defects; special considerations, pp. 76–130. NRC (National Research Council), Institute of Laboratory Animal Resources, Committee on Dogs. Dogs: Laboratory Animal Management. Washington, DC: National Academy Press.

Smith, A.C., B. Knick, M.M. Swindle, and P.C. Gillette. 1997. A technique for conducting non-invasive cardiac electrophysiology studies in swine. J. Invest. Surg. 10(1–2): 25–30.

Smith, A.C., C.H. Kline, R.P. Thompson, M.M. Swindle, and P.C. Gillette. In press. Pressure overload cardiac hypertrophy produced by pulmonary artery banding in Hanford miniature swine. J. Invest. Surg.

Sparrow, M.P. 1996. Bronchial function in the porcine lung—From the fetus to the adult. In Tumbleson, M.E., and Schook, L.B. (eds), Advances in Swine in Biomedical Research, Vol. 1. New York: Plenum Press, pp. 33–44.

Spinale, F.G., D.A. Hendrick, F.A. Crawford, A.C. Smith, Y. Hamada, and B.A. Carabello. 1990. Chronic supraventricular tachycardia causes ventricular dysfunction and subendocardial injury in swine. Am. J. Physiol. 259(1 Pt2) (Heart. Circ. Physiol. 28): H218–H229.

Stanton, H.C., and H.J. Mersmann (eds). 1986. Swine in Cardiovascular Research, Vols. 1–2. Boca Raton, FL: CRC Press.

Swindle, M.M. 1983. Basic Surgical Exercises Using Swine. Philadelphia: Praeger Press.

Swindle, M.M. 1986. Swine as models in thoracic surgery. In Powers, D.L. (ed.), Proceedings of the Second Annual Meeting of the Academy of Surgical Research. Clemson, SC: Clemson University Press, pp. 106–108.

Swindle, M.M. 1992. Swine as Models in Biomedical Research, Ames: Iowa State University Press.

Swindle, M.M. 1994. Anesthetic and perioperative techniques in swine: An update. Charles River Technical Bulletin 12(1): 1–4.

Swindle, M.M. 1996. Considerations of specific pathogen free (SPF) swine in xenotransplantation. J. Invest. Surg. 9(3): 267–271.

Swindle, M.M., and R.J. Adams. 1988. Experimental Surgery and Physiology: Induced Animal Models of Human Disease. Baltimore: Williams and Wilkins.

Swindle, M.M., and D.L. Bobbie. 1987. Comparative anatomy of the pig, Charles River Technical Bulletin 4(1): 1–4.

Swindle, M.M., P.J. Horneffer, T.J. Gardner, V.L. Gott, T.S. Hall, R.S. Stuart, W.A. Baumgartner, A.M. Borkon, E. Galloway, and B.A. Reitz. 1986. Anatomic and anesthetic considerations in experimental cardiopulmonary surgery in swine. Lab. Anim. Sci. 36(4): 357–361.

Swindle, M.M., A.C. Smith, and B.J.S. Hepburn. 1988. Swine as models in experimental surgery. J. Invest. Surg. 1(1): 65–79.

Swindle, M.M., D.B. Wiest, A.C. Smith, S.S. Garner, C.C. Case, R.P. Thompson, D.A. Fyfe, and P.C. Gillette. 1996. Fetal surgical protocols in Yucatan miniature swine. Lab. Anim. Sci. 46(1): 90–95.

Swindle, M.M., A.C. Smith, and J.A. Goodrich. 1998. Chronic cannulation and fistulation procedures in swine: A review and recommendations. J. Invest. Surg. 11(1): 7–20.

Tong, S.W., S. Ingenito, J.E. Anderson, N. Gootman, A.L. Sica, and P.M. Gootman. 1995. Development of a swine animal model for the study of sudden infant death syndrome. Lab. Anim. Sci. 45(4): 398–403.

Tong, S. S. Ingenito, I.D. Frasier, N. Gootman, and P.M. Gootman. 1996. Differential effects of left and right cariac sympathetic denervation on ventricular fibrillation threshold in developing swine. In Tumbleson, M.E., and Schook, L.B. (eds), Advances in Swine in Biomedical Research, Vol. 1. New York: Plenum Press, pp. 131–140.

Turjman, F., T.F. Massoud, C. Ji, G. Guglielmi, F. Vinuela, and J. Robert. 1994. Combined stent implantation and endosaccular coil placement for treatment of experimental wide-necked aneurysms: A feasibility study in swine. Am. J. Neuroradiol. 15(6): 1087–1090.

Verdouw, P.D., and J.M. Hartog. 1986. Provocation and suppression of ventricular arrhythmias in domestic swine. In Stanton, H.C., and Mersmann, H.J. (eds), Swine in Cardiovascular Research, Vol. 2. Boca Raton: CRC Press, pp. 121–156.

White, D., and J. Lunney. 1979. Transplantation in pigs. Transplant. Proc. 11(1): 1170–1173.

White, F.C., D.M. Roth, and C.M. Bloor. 1986. The pig as a model for myocardial ischemia and exercise. Lab. Anim. Sci. 36(4): 351–356.

White, C.J., S.R. Ramee, A.K. Banks, D. Wiktor, and H.L. Price. 1992. The Yucatan miniature swine: An atherogenic model to assess the early potency rates of an endovascular stent. In Swindle, M.M. (ed), Swine as Models in Biomedical Research. Ames: Iowa State University Press, pp. 156–162.

Wittnich, C., M.P. Belanger, B.S. Oh, and T.A. Salerno. 1991. Surgical model of volume overload-induced ventricular myocardial hypertrophy to study a clinical problem in humans. J. Invest. Surg. 4(3): 333–338.

10 HEAD AND NECK SURGERY, CENTRAL NERVOUS SYSTEM

General Principles

The use of swine in dental and neurological research has been relatively uncommon, probably due to the anatomy of the head, neck, and oral cavity (Figs. 10.1 and 10.2). Its use in oral and maxillofacial surgery has recently increased (Bermejo et al., 1993; Donovan et al., 1993; Drisco et al., 1996; North, 1988; Ouhayoun et al., 1992; Sims et al., 1997).

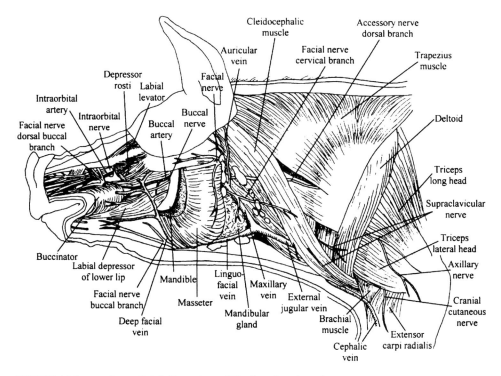

FIGURE 10.1   Superficial dissection of the head and neck.

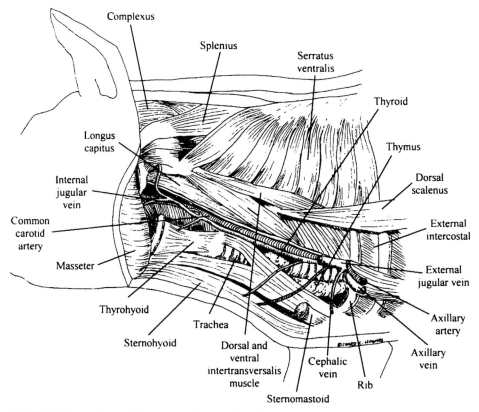

FIGURE 10.2   Deep dissection of the head and neck.

The dental formula for deciduous teeth in swine is 2(I 3/3, C 1/1, P 4/4) = 32. Permanent teeth have a dental formula of 2(I 3/3, C 1/1, P 4/4, M 3/3) = 44. Swine are born with the last incisors and canine teeth. The remainder of the incisors erupt between 2 weeks and 2 months of age. The premolars erupt between 4 days and 5 months. The molars are the first permanent teeth to erupt and appear between 4 months and 20 months of age. The incisors change between 8 and 20 months, the canines between 9 and 10 months, and the premolars between 12 and 15 months. The tooth eruption sequence of adult permanent teeth is $P_1/M_1/I_3/C/M_2/I_1/P_3/P_4/P_2/I_2/M_3.$ In the boar, the canine teeth become the tusks and require trimming two to four times a year in the adult. Growth of the tusks is delayed in females and castrated males. The newborn's canines are called "needle teeth" and are usually trimmed shortly after birth to prevent damage to the sow during nursing. The dental formulas are identical among farm and miniature breeds, and eruption dates are similar. A full set of permanent teeth is usually present around 18 months of age. The size of the teeth is similar to human, and the tooth eruption and exfoliation of the primary teeth can be followed in a normal time sequence (Hargreaves and Mitchell, 1969; Sisson and St. Clair, 1975a,b; Weaver et al., 1962).

There is a substantial difference in the conformation of the head and neck among different breeds. The snout of the Yucatan, Göttengen, Sinclair, and most other miniature pigs is considerably shorter than that of domestic farm breeds and the Hanford miniature pig. The heads of miniature breeds tend to be more rounded than that of the farm breeds and the Hanford, which has a head and snout shape similar to wild pigs. Selection of a breed for oral and maxillofacial surgery should include a consideration of the differences in head and neck conformation.

The bones of the cranium and the mandible are massive. The temporomandibular joint has been compared to other species and man in a detailed anatomic study (Bermejo et al., 1993). The authors concluded that the pig was an appropriate animal model to study temporomandibular joint abnormalities because it was most similar to humans. The pig has a reciprocally fitting meniscotemporal joint and a condylomeniscal joint of the condylar type. The size of the articular structures, the shape of the meniscus, and the omnivorous chewing characteristics of swine provided additional justification for the use of this model over that of rodents, rabbits, carnivores, and herbivores that were examined. Maxillofacial bone-healing studies have been performed in swine (North, 1988). Swine have also been found to have fluxes of autonomic tone in the nasal airway identical to humans (Campbell and Kern, 1981).

The salivary glands of the pig are the parotid, the mandibular, and the sublingual. The parotid gland enters the oral cavity opposite the upper fourth or fifth cheek tooth and may have accessory glands along the duct. The mandibular gland enters near the frenulum. The sublingual glands are located in bilateral chains and have multiple openings into the floor of the mouth. A series of minor buccal glands are located opposite the upper and lower cheek teeth. In the pig, the parotid gland is serous, the sublingual gland is mucoid, and the mandibular and buccal glands are mixed in secretions. Tonsils analogous to the palatine tonsils are embedded in the soft palate rather than in the lateral wall of the oropharynx as in other species. There is a pharyngeal diverticulum dorsal to the larynx in the caudal aspect of the nasopharynx; this structure may be damaged during the passing of gastric or endotracheal tubes. The thymus extends from the thorax to the level of the larynx in the pig. The thyroid gland has paired lobules that are fused on the ventral surface of the trachea near the thoracic inlet. The single pair of parathyroid glands are minute and are associated with the cranial end of the thymus (Sack, 1982; Schantz et al., 1996; Sisson and St. Clair, 1975a,b; Swindle and Bobbie, 1987).

The ophthalmic system of the pig has been previously reviewed and compared with other species of lab animals and the pertinent comparisons are summarized here (Adams, 1988). The pig has an open field of vision with a pupil and retina similar to man. The seven extraocular muscles are attached to the orbital wall in deep fossae. A nictitating membrane, Bowman's membrane and Descemet's membrane are present. A tapetum is absent. There may be either one or two puncta for lacrimal drainage. There is a deep gland of the third eyelid, Harder's gland. The ratio of body weight to eye weight is 2733:1.

A stereotaxic atlas of the pig brain (Fig. 10.3) has been published (Salinas-Zeballos et al., 1986). The atlas provides details for the anatomic placement of electrodes in the forebrain of neonatal swine 1–12 days old. A detailed description of the blood supply to the spinal cord and brain has also been published (Stodkilde-Jorgensen et al., 1986). The common carotid arteries leave the brachiocephalic trunk at the level of T1. The internal carotid artery provides most of the circulation to the brain. Vertebral arteries branch off the subclavian arteries at the level of C6–7 and supply the vertebrae, muscle, and spinal cord at each level. The cranial portion of the vertebral artery provides some blood supply to the medulla as well. In studies that interrupted the blood supply of the branches of the vertebral artery at C1–2, C4–5, and C7–T1, the latter produced the least hemodynamic and systemic changes. Venous plexi from the brain and plexus enter the internal jugular vein at the level of C1–2. The internal vertebral plexus enters the vertebral veins and drains into the azygous system at the level of C6. Venous drainage from the thoracic vertebrae enter the azygous veins cranial to the heart.

Principles of performing surgery on the head and neck of swine are the same as for other species. The principal problems involve the thickness of the cranium and the massive nature of the bones of the mandible and maxilla. Laryngeal and tracheal procedures are discussed in Chapter 9.

Dental Procedures/Tusk Trimming

The principles of performing oral and dental surgery are the same as for other species, except that exposure is limited for the premolars and molars because of the narrowness of the oral cavity opening. Retractors are necessary to keep

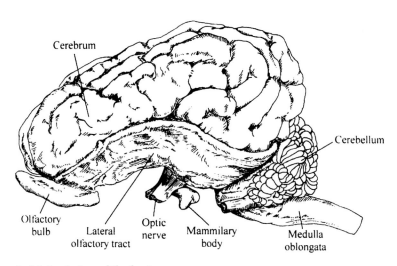

FIGURE 10.3   Left lateral view of the brain.

the mouth open for procedures on these teeth.

The tusks of the pig need to be trimmed periodically in adult animals, especially in boars, for personnel safety. In order to perform this procedure, pigs should have general anesthesia or chemical restraint. They may be trimmed in restraint slings with sedation. The roots of the canine teeth are deep and difficult to extract, consequently, the tusks are usually trimmed at the gum line using either Gigli wire or saws. In the adult male, this procedure needs to be performed every 3–6 months. Tusks are slower growing in castrated males and females and may not need to be trimmed. Veterinary advice should be sought to make this determination.

Dental extractions can be performed on the other teeth using standard methods of root elevation followed by extraction. Mucoperiosteal flaps may be reflected from the gingiva in the cranial aspects of the oral cavity using standard techniques of incision and retraction of the gingiva. Use of local anesthetics containing epinephrine as an adjunct to general anesthesia should aid hemostasis by the induction of local vasoconstriction. Oral incisions should be closed with absorbable sutures.

Maxillofacial/Craniotomy Procedures

Swine have been used as models for both soft tissue and bone healing, including studies of grafting and implantation of biomaterials (Bradley, 1982; Donovan et al., 1993; Kalkwarf et al., 1983; Ouhayoun et al., 1992; Robinson and Sarnat, 1955; Rosenquist and Rosenquist, 1982; Roth et al., 1984; Sims et al., 1997). Most of the studies have been performed on the mandible and temporomandibular joint. Surgical approaches will be described here.

The body of the mandible can be approached with the pig in dorsal recumbency. An incision made along the ventral aspect of the mandible will provide a relatively bloodless approach to the bone. Dorsal retraction of the skin and platysma muscle will expose the surface of the mandible. The facial vessels at the caudal end of the mandible should be avoided. The masseter muscle may be elevated with the periosteum to expose the lateral surface of the bone.

The temporomandibular joint may be approached using a lateral incision made dorsal to ventral from an area caudal to the ear and external auditory meatus to the ramus of the mandible following its caudal edge. This area may be readily palpated prior to making the incision. After incising the skin and platysma muscle, the dissection becomes difficult. Branches of the facial nerve, facial, temporal, and auricular arteries and veins should be retracted if possible. The parotid salivary gland should be retracted ventrally. The bodies of the parotidoauricularis muscle will have to be transected. The temporomandibular joint can then be accessed from a caudal direction under the zygomatic arch.

If greater exposure is required, the zygomatic arch will have to be transected, taking care not to damage the blood vessels underlying it.

The dorsolateral aspects of the skull can be approached using a midline incision with the pig in sternal recumbency. The nuchal crest of the pig is quite prominent and is the thickest part of the bone. The superficial muscles along the midline are incised and retracted with the skin. This is followed by incision and retraction of the periostum laterally from the midline. Using this approach the cranium, frontal sinus, parietal bone, and frontal bone may be approached.

The nasal bone, cranial aspects of the frontal sinus, and sinus cavity can be approached using a midline incision along the snout with the pig in sternal recumbency. The nasolabial muscles are incised with the skin and retracted subperiosteally and then retracted laterally. The nasal bone can be fractured along its suture lines for exposure of the nasal cavity.

These incisions may be closed routinely by repair of the bone with wires, screws, or dental acrylic if defects are created. The muscles, fascia, and skin are closed in a routine fashion.

Ocular Surgery

The eyes of the pig are deeply embedded in the sockets, especially in anesthetized animals, and exposure requires the use of ocular retractors. Swine have rarely been used in ophthalmic research despite some of their anatomic similarities to humans, but they have been used for corneal procedures (Adams, 1988). The surgical procedures and approaches are the same as for other species. Enucleation of the eye will be described in this section.

Allis tissue forceps are used to clamp the margins of the eyelids together. The eyelids are incised in a circumferential fashion beyond their margins, and blunt dissection is initiated at the edge of the orbicularis oculi and into the conjunctiva. After the conjunctiva is dissected to the attachments of the ocular muscles, they are transected. After transection of the muscles, the globe is bluntly dissected free of its attachments except for the ocular nerve, artery, and vein. The globe may be drained using needle aspiration at this point to increase exposure. Right-angle forceps are passed behind the globe, and those structures are clamped. The globe is excised on the proximal side of the forceps, and the vessels and nerve are ligated together followed by removal of the forceps. A biocompatible prosthesis may be inserted or the margins of the incision closed. Care should be taken prior to closure to ensure that all glandular structures have been excised and hemostasis is complete. The conjunctiva and skin are closed in a routine fashion.

Pharyngostomy Tubes

A pharyngostomy tube may be surgically implanted when there is a necessity to chronically administer food or medication without mastication. However, it is relatively easy to pass a stomach tube with a mouth gag while the pig is immobilized in a restraint sling. This method of nonsurgical intervention is recommended over the surgical procedure.

The pharynx and proximal esophagus is approached using a ventral midline incision over the larynx. Blunt dissection is continued through the midline and the esophagus is identified on the dorsum of the trachea by deviating laterally with the dissection when the sternohyoideus muscle is reached. After passing around the esophagus with elastic vessel loops, it is elevated, and a stab incision is made into the lumen. The proximal one-half to two-thirds of the muscle layers of the esophagus are striated muscle, which converts to smooth muscle in its distal length. A premeasured length of soft nasogastric tubing is passed into the stomach. The proper positioning can be determined when stomach gases are noted to be passing through the tube. The tubing is sutured in place with a purse-string suture. The tubing is tunneled subcutaneously to exit the skin behind the ear. A purse-string suture is placed in the exit site of the skin. The subcutaneous, muscle, and skin layers are closed routinely. The tubing may be taped to the ear for security.

Thyroidectomy

The approach to the thyroid gland (see Chapter 1, Fig. 1.25) is made with the pig in dorsal recumbency. A ventral midline incision is made cranial to the manubrium sterni in the last one-third to one-half of the neck (Swindle, 1983). The incision is continued between fascial planes of the sternohyoideus muscle until the thyroid is identified on the ventral surface of the trachea as a dark colored bilobular structure. The cranial and caudal thyroid artery and vein enter the gland from the dorsal surface and usually cannot be identified in advance. They are bisected and ligated during blunt dissection of the gland from the trachea. The fascial planes of the muscle, the subcutaneous tissues, and the skin are closed in a routine fashion.

Parathyroidectomy

The single pair of parathyroid glands (see Chapter 1, Fig. 1.25) (parathyroid gland III) are difficult to identify (Sack, 1982; Swindle and Bobbie, 1987). They are located on the cranioventral surface of the thymus gland caudolateral to the larynx. A line drawn between the angles of the mandible will provide the surgeon with an approximate location. Because the thymus changes in size with age the exact location of the dorsal end is variable. These grayish structures are minute (1–4 mm) but usually can be felt to be a definitive structure by rolling them between the thumb and forefinger.

They may either be approached using a ventral midline incision with lateral subcutaneous dissection or a ventral paramedian incision over the sternohyoideus and sternomastoideus muscles. Once the structures are identified, they are removed by blunt dissection. Histopathology is recommended to ensure that they have been removed. Alternatively, the dorsal pole of the thymus may be removed if the structures cannot be identified. Hemorrhage is minimal, and vessels usually do not require ligation. The muscle fascia, subcutaneous, and skin layers are closed routinely.

Hypophysectomy

The pituitary gland has been surgically removed in both fetal and adult animals (Drisko et al., 1996; Kraeling et al., 1986). The transsphenoidal and parapharyngeal approaches are difficult in swine because of the limitations in exposure through the open mouth and the extensive dissections involved from the ventral midline. The transfrontal, supraorbital approach has been used in the fetus and in gilts; however, the dissection in adult animals is much more difficult. The transorbital approach offers a minimally invasive technique in adult animals (Fig. 10.4).

The first step is to perform a right eye enucleation, including removal of the periosteum, as described above. A 5-mm burr hole is drilled caudodorsal and parallel to the optic canal. The site is located dorsomedial to the foramen or-

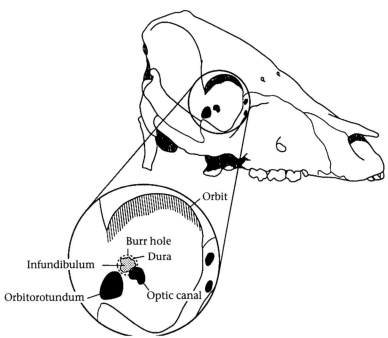

FIGURE 10.4   Hypophysectomy through the transorbital approach. *Reprinted with permission from Drisko et al., 1996. Transorbital approach to the porcine pituitary, J. Invest. Surg. 9(4): 305–311.*

bitorotundum. The drill is advanced carefully to the level of the dura overlying the juncture between the infundibulum and the infundibular stalk. Care should be taken to avoid the foramen orbitorotundum and the underlying internal carotid artery. If the hole requires enlargement, care should be taken to avoid damage to the underlying blood vessels and the optic chiasm. The dura is pulled away from the pituitary and a small hole is made with a dura twist hook. Use of suction and microdissection will allow the surgeon to visualize the pituitary. It can either be removed, transected, or cannulated at this point. When closing the incision, the burr hole is filled with bone wax to prevent leakage of cerebrospinal fluid. The socket can be filled with prosthetic material, such as dental acrylic, prior to closing the incision as described above for enucleation (Drisko et al., 1996).

The supraorbital frontal approach uses the surgical approach to the cranium described above. A section of the frontal and parietal bone is removed, and care must be taken to avoid damage to the frontal artery and vein. The exposure and craniotomy is performed to expose the left and one-half of the right cerebral hemispheres. The dura mater is incised taking care to avoid damaging the brain. A brain retractor is used to elevate the cerebral hemisphere and expose the region of the hypothalamus. The hypothalamus may be catheterized, transected, or removed as described above. The bone fragments are replaced, and the muscular, subcutaneous, and skin layers are closed in a routine manner. The authors recommended placement of a drain tube in the dorsum of the cranium for 48 hours postoperatively and 50 mg of cortisone pre- and postoperatively. Mineral mix was added to the ration of hypophysectomized gilts as a permanent dietary supplement (Kraeling et al., 1986).

Administration of 100 ml of 10% saline iv intraoperatively may help reduce brain size. Also, an increase in mortality was noted when nitrous oxide was used in the anesthetic protocol (Kraeling et al., 1986). Postoperatively, analgesics are required and the pig should be monitored closely to maintain homeostasis.

Spinal Cord Ischemia and Hemorrhage

Spinal cord ischemia can be a complication of aortic surgery (see Chapter 9) or vascular damage. Spinal cord damage usually becomes clinically relevant after 20 minutes of cross-clamp time in the suprarenal aorta but may be extended in the postrenal aorta. Thirty minutes of cross clamping of the thoracic aorta distal to the branching of the left subclavian aorta will consistently produce ischemic damage (Qayumi et al., 1997).

The model can be surgically produced by performing a left lateral thoracotomy (see Chapter 9) or a left flank celiotomy (see Chapters 4 and 7) to approach the aorta. The aorta may either be clamped with vascular clamps or encircled with an umbilical tape snare. Alternatively, selected dorsal branches of the aorta may be ligated. Experience from aortic anastomosis (see Chapter 9) demonstrates that this must be more than two continguent pairs of arteries.

Clamping of the prerenal aorta will produce hypertension that must be controlled with blood volume reduction or infusions of Na nitroprusside. Cross clamping of the aorta will also produce hypoperfusion of all of the distal organs with the potential of dysfunction. Animals may become paraplegic.

If this model is performed as a survival procedure, intensive care of the animal postoperatively is imperative. Housing the animal in deep wood-shaving bedding or on padding is necessary. Nutritional support may have to be administered.

Similar types of clinical syndromes occur with spinal cord hemorrhage (Ganz and Zwetnow, 1990) associated with decompression injury models at a simulated dive depth of 200 feet of seawater with decompression after 43 minutes at 60 feet of seawater per second (Broome et al., 1997; Dick et al., 1997). Approximately two-thirds of the swine will develop clinical neurologic syndromes related to petechia and ecchymoses in the spinal cord. Approximately 20% of the affected swine will die. Additional injuries due to dysbarism may occur and require treatment. This model avoids having to perform surgical procedures.

References

Adams, R.J. 1988. Opthalmic system. In Swindle, M.M., and Adams, R.J. (eds), Experimental Surgery and Physiology: Induced Animal Models of Human Disease. Baltimore: Williams and Wilkins, pp. 125–153.

Bermejo, A., O. Gonzalez, and J.M. Gonzalez. 1993. The pig as an animal model for experimentation on the temporomandibular articular complex. Oral Surg. Oral Med. Oral Pathol. 75(1): 18–23.

Bradley, P.F. 1982. A two-stage procedure for reimplantation of autogenous freeze-treated mandibular bone. J. Oral Maxillofac. Surg. 40(5): 278–284.

Broome, J.R., E.J. Dick, Jr., and A.J. Dutka. 1997. Neurological decompression illness in swine. Aviat. Space Environ. Med. 67: 207–213.

Campbell, W.M., and E.B. Kern. 1981. The nasal cycle in swine. Rhinology 19(3): 127–148.

Dick, E.J. Jr., J.R. Broome, and I.J. Hayward. 1997. Acute neurologic decompression illness in pigs: Lesions of the spinal cord and brain. Lab. Anim. Sci. 47(1): 50–56.

Donovan, M.G., N.C. Dickerson, J.W. Hellstein, and L.J. Hanson. 1993. Autologous calvarial and iliac onlay bone grafts in miniature swine. J. Oral Maxillofac. Surg. 51(8): 898–903.

Drisko, J.E., T.D. Faidley, D.F. Hora, Jr., G.W. Niebauer, W.P. Feeney, B.H. Friscino, and G.J. Hickey. 1996. Transorbital approach to the porcine pituitary. J. Invest. Surg. 9(4): 305–311.

Ganz, J.C., and N.N. Zwetnow. 1990. A quantitative study of some factors affecting the outcome of experimental epidural bleeding in swine. Acta Neurochir. (Wien) 102(3–4): 164–172.

Hargreaves, J.A., and B. Mitchell. 1969. Features of the dentition of the pig for experimental work. J. Dent. Res. 48 (21): 1103.

Kalkwarf, K.L., R.F. Krejci, A.R. Edison, and R.A. Reinhardt. 1983. Subjacent heat production during tissue excision with electrosurgery. J. Oral Maxillofac. Surg. 41(10): 653–657.

Kraeling, R.R., C.R. Barb, and G.B. Rampacek. 1986. Hypophysectomy and hypophysial stalk transection in the pig: Technique and application to studies of ovarian follicular development, In Tumbleson, M.E. (ed), Swine in Biomedical Research, Vol. 1. New York: Plenum Press, pp. 425–436.

North, A.F. 1988. Oral and maxillofacial surgery. In Swindle, M.M., and Adams, R.J. (eds), Experimental Surgery and Physiology: Induced Animal Models of Human Disease. Baltimore: Williams and Wilkins, pp. 173–203.

Ouhayoun J.P., A.H.M. Shabana, S. Issahakian, J.L. Patat, G. Guillemin, M.H. Sawaf, and N. Forest. 1992. Histological evaluation of natural coral skeleton as a grafting material in miniature swine mandible. J. Material Sci.: Material Med. 3(3): 222–228.

Qayumi A.K., M.T. Nanusz, D.M. Lyster, and K.D. Gillespie. 1997. Animal model for investigation of spinal cord injury caused by aortic cross-clamping. J. Invest. Surg. 10(1): 47–52.

Robinson, I.B., and B.G. Sarnat. 1955. Growth pattern of the pig mandible. Am. J. Anat. 96(41): 37–64.

Rosenquist, J.B., and K. Rosenquist. 1982. Effects of bone grafting on maxillary bone healing in the growing pig. J. Oral Maxillofac. Surg. 40(9): 566–569.

Roth, T.E. J.S. Goldberg, and R.G. Behrents. 1984. Synovial fluid pressure determinations in the temporomandibular joint. Oral Surg. Oral Med. Oral Pathol. 57(5): 583–588.

Sack, W.O. 1982. Essentials of Pig Anatomy and Harowitz/Kramer Atlas of Musculoskeletal Anatomy of the Pig. Ithaca, NY: Veterinary Textbooks.

Salinas-Zeballos, M.E., G.A. Zeballos, and P.M. Gootman. 1986. A stereotaxic atlas of the developing swine (Sus scrofa) forebrain. In Tumbleson, M.E. (ed), Swine in Biomedical Research, Vol. 2. New York: Plenum Press, pp. 887–906.

Schantz, L.D., K. Laber-Laird, S. Bingel, and M. Swindle. 1996. Pigs: Applied anatomy of the gastrointestinal tract. In Jensen, S.L., Gregersen, H., Moody, F., and Shokouh-Amiri, M.H. (eds), Essentials of Experimental Surgery: Gastroenterology. New York: Harwood Academic Publishers, pp. 2611–2619.

Sims, C.D., P.E.M. Butler, R. Casanova, M.A. Randolph, and M.J. Yaremchuk. 1997. Prolonged general anesthesia for experimental craniofacial surgery in fetal swine. J. Invest. Surg. 10(1–2): 53–57.

Sisson, S., and S.E. St. Clair. 1975a. Appendages. In Getty, R. (ed), Sisson and Grossman's The Anatomy of the Domestic Animals, 5th ed. Philadelphia: WB Saunders, pp. 1222–1230.

Sisson, S., and St. Clair, S.E. 1975b. Porcine digestive system. In Getty, R. (ed), The Anatomy of the Domestic Animals, 5th ed. Philadelphia: WB Saunders, pp. 1268–1282.

Stodkilde-Jorgensen, H., J. Frokiaer, H.J. Kirkeby, F. Madsen, and N. Boye. 1986. Preparation of a cerebral perfusion model in the pig: Anatomic considerations. In Tumbleson, M.E. (ed), Swine in Biomedical Research, Vol. 1. New York: Plenum Press, pp. 719–725.

Swindle, M.M. 1983. Basic Surgical Exercises Using Swine. Philadelphia: Prager Publishers.

Swindle, M.M., and D.L. Bobbie. 1987. Comparative anatomy of the pig. Charles River Technical Bulletin 4(1): 1–4.

Weaver, M.E., F.M. Sorenson, and E.B. Jump. 1962. The miniature pig as an experimental animal in dental research. Arch. Oral Biol. 7(1): 17–24.

11 MUSCULOSKELETAL SYSTEM/ORTHOPEDIC PROCEDURES

General Principles

The bones and musculature of the pig are massive, which is consistent with its use as a primary food source for humans. The cortex of the bones also tends to be thick compared to other animals, which serves to provide strength for supporting an animal that tends to have a heavy weight and a small stature. Diseases of the joints occur frequently, probably due to the rapid weight gain on an immature skeleton in young animals (Sack, 1982). Swine have seldom been used as models for musculoskeletal or orthopedic experiments because of the conformation of the muscles and skeletal axis. However, the proportion and distribution of muscles and bones that support and provide locomotion for the body are similar between farm and miniature pigs and they have been proposed as a model of growth of the system because of their rapid weight gain (Bobilya et al., 1991; Davies and Henning, 1986). They have also been used as models of bone healing and epiphyseal plate growth (Alitalo, 1979; Allan et al., 1990; Peltonen et al., 1984) and of congenital hip dislocation (Salter, 1968) and experimentally produced scoliosis (MacEwen, 1973). Recently there has been an increased interest in the model for the evaluation of grafting techniques (Donovan et al., 1993; Ouhayoun et al., 1992), bone implants (Buser et al., 1991), osteonecrosis (Swiontkowski et al., 1993), and osteoporosis (Boyce et al., 1995). The temporomandibular joint of swine has also been determined to be more similar to humans than many other species in a comparative macroscopic study (Bermejo et al., 1993).

Mammals have a predominance of Type II B muscle fibers

with a lesser extent of Type IIA and IIC fibers. Locomotion characteristics of swine, as well as most other quadrupeds, are also dissimilar from that of humans (Adams, 1988; MacEwen, 1973; Salter, 1968). An extensive dissection atlas of the musculoskeletal system of the domestic pig has been published (Sack, 1982).

There are differences in the closure of the epiphyses of the long bones among breeds of swine. The miniature pig breeds tend to have an earlier closure than domestic farm breeds, which typically have epiphyseal closure between 3 and 4 years of age (Sisson, 1975). Dates of epiphyseal closure for some of the breeds of miniature pigs are the following: Hanford, 2–4 years; Yucatan, 2–3 years; Yucatan micropig, 1.5–2 years.

Muscles may be transected, dissected between muscular fibers or preferably divided in the fascial plane between muscle bellies. The fascial sheath surrounding the muscle provides the predominant strength for holding sutures and must be included when suturing surgical incisions. Sutures may pass all the way through a muscle body and the sheath on both sides of the muscle or the muscular sheath can be sutured by itself (Swindle, 1983).

Amputation of a Digit

The principal digits of the pig are numbers III and IV. Vestigial digits, numbers II and V, form the dewclaws, which are positioned caudal to the principal digits. All terminate in hooves that may periodically have to be trimmed using hoof nippers on swine that are not housed on concrete floors or rough material that allows constant wear of the hoof. The dewclaws are non-weight bearing, and amputation of them does not result in any consequential debility to the pig. If the principal digits become injured or infected, they may require amputation. The pig will retain its locomotive ability as long as one of the pair is retained intact.

The digit is amputated in the joint between either the metacarpal bone and the proximal phalanx or between the proximal and middle phalanx depending upon the extent of the lesion. A horizontal incision is made across the dorsal aspect of the digit distal to the joint in which the amputation is to be performed. Two vertical incisions are made up the sides of the digit extending to the ventral surface of the joint in which the amputation is being performed. The dorsal flap is then bluntly dissected to the surface of the joint. The branches of the digital veins on the dorsal surface are ligated and the tendons severed at their insertions on the bones. A flap is then dissected on the palmar surface of the digit, and the vessels and tendons are similarly transected. The skin on the palmar surface is transected horizontally cranial to the joint. The joint is then disarticulated and amputated. The tendons and muscles are trimmed and tacked down across the ventral surface of the joint with stay sutures. The ventral aspect of the dorsal flap is sutured with simple interrupted sutures to the skin on the palmar surface of the joint. This will leave a skin flap that covers the joint from the dorsal to the palmar aspect of the joint.

The foot is bandaged leaving the intact digit uncovered. The animal should be housed in clean dry bedding and the bandage changed daily for the first few days following surgery.

Tendon and Ligament Repair

The major tendons that are substantial in size and accessible through superficial surgical dissection are the common calcaneus and the popliteus. The digital extensor and flexor tendons are also readily accessible on the distal portion of the metacarpal and metatarsal bones and on the cranial and palmar surfaces of the digits if small to midsized tendons are preferred. The patellar ligaments are the main superficial ligaments. These tendons and ligaments may be used in wound healing studies and may also require clinical repair due to trauma, especially of the digital extensor and flexor ligaments.

Methodology for suturing the ligaments is the same as for other species and has been described in the pig (Swindle, 1983). The common calcaneal tendon includes the tendons of the superficial flexor and the larger oval gastrocnemius tendon. It is approached with a caudal vertical incision along the distal end of the tibia ending at the tuber calcis. The popliteal tendon is approached using a similar incision along the caudal aspect of the humerus ending at the olecranon. The digital tendons can be palpated on the distal aspect of the legs and direct incisions made over them. The patellar ligaments can be approached using a vertical incision along the cranial aspect of the stifle joint, with the ventral patellar ligament being the most accessible.

After transecting the ligament or tendon, the edge is grasped with forceps and repaired using the Bunnell-Mayer technique (Fig. 11.1). Starting well back from the edge of the incised tendon, a transection suture is placed through the

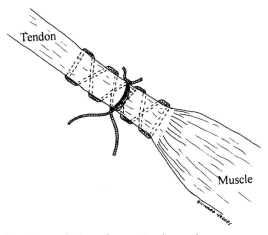

FIGURE 11.1   Suturing technique for repair of a tendon.

tendon from side-to-side using a double-armed suture with nonabsorbable material. The ends of the suture are left equidistant from the tendon. In an alternating pattern, the needles reenter the tendon at a 45-degree angle aimed distally. Sutures are continued distally in this crossing pattern until the outer edges of the severed tendon are exited. The same suture pattern is then placed in the distal end of the severed tendon. The ends of the sutures are tied along the lateral and medial edges of the tendon at the incised edge. The subcutaneous tissues and skin are closed in a routine fashion. Postoperatively, the limb may require immobilization in a plaster cast or require some other form of support for a short time.

Tail Amputation

Swine routinely traumatize the tails of less dominant animals when housed in groups. This may require corrective surgery. The tail is amputated between the bodies of the coccygeal vertebrae in the joint. It is best to amputate the entire length of the tail to prevent further trauma.

A V-shaped flap is made with the long ends of the flap on the dorsal and ventral aspects of the tail. The blood vessels along the ventral and lateral surfaces of the tail are identified and ligated. The tail is disarticulated in the joint, and the flap is sutured using a simple interrupted pattern.

Hernia Repair

Both umbilical and inguinal hernias occur spontaneously in swine. Inguinal hernias and retained testicles are more common on the left side (Bollwahn, 1992). Both conditions have a genetic predisposition.

For inguinal hernias, the pig is placed in dorsal recumbency. A skin incision is made directly over the inguinal canal, which can be readily palpated on a line drawn between the mid to cranial aspect of the cranial surface of the thigh and the midline. After the skin incision is made, the edges of the femoral ring are bluntly dissected away from the herniated tissues, which typically include omentum and fat without the intestines. The spermatic cord should not be damaged in this process. After the herniated tissue is free from attachments, it is bluntly replaced into the abdominal cavity. It may have to be held in place with a blunt instrument, or the pig's hindquarters directed upward, to move the herniated tissues and viscera away from the surgical site. The muscles surrounding the inguinal ring are sutured together with simple interrupted sutures using 2/0 or 3/0 nonabsorbable synthetic suture material. The inguinal canal should not be sutured tightly enough to constrict the blood flow to the blood vessels in the spermatic cord. The skin and subcutaneous tissues are closed in a routine manner.

An inguinal hernia may be created experimentally in small swine by making an incision over the inguinal ring and incising the muscles on the cranial edge of the ring. This relaxation of the ring should lead to herniation postsurgically and can be tested at the time of surgery by applying pressure to the abdomen to cause the viscera to herniate.

Umbilical hernias are usually closed around herniated omentum and fat and are rarely clinically relevant. The umbilical hernia may be closed after making a skin incision directly over the herniation and by either replacing or excising the eviscerated material. The umbilicus is closed with nonabsorbable sutures as described above.

Surgical Approaches to Bones and Joints

The surgical approaches (Figs. 11.2 and 11.3) to bones and joints of the pig can be determined by the surgeons using their knowledge of other species and by anatomic inspection and palpation of the animal prior to surgery. Surgical approaches to the major bones and joints that avoid major muscle dissection and vascular ligation are described here. Variations of these procedures may be dictated by the experimental protocol.

Foreleg

The shoulder joint is approached in the craniolateral aspect after flexion. The greater tubercle of the humerus is prominent and the caudal part is readily pal-

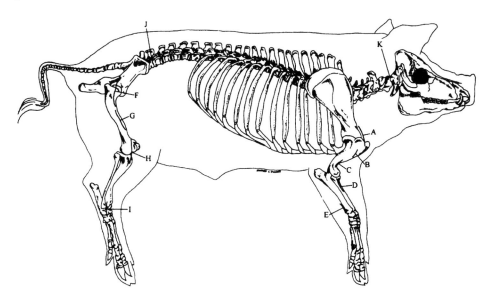

FIGURE 11.2   Surgical approaches to the bones and joints. *A*-Shoulder joint, *B*-Proximal humerus, *C*-Distal humerus, *D*-Proximal radius, *E*-Ulna, *F*-Hip joint, *G*-Femur, *H*-Stifle (knee) joint, *I*-Tarsocrural (hock) joint, *J*-Subarachnoid space injection site, *K*-Cisterna magna injection site.

pated. The incision is made between the cranial and caudal portions of the tubercle alongside the infraspinatus tendon. The infraspinatus tendon may have to be transected at its attachment in order to be retracted caudally. The infraspinatus nerve should be avoided.

The humerus is not readily approached surgically because of the massiveness of the musculature. Surgical approaches from the lateral aspect will probably involve transecting musculature. The proximal shaft can be approached between the brachiocephalic muscle and the distal portion of the deltoideus. The distal portion of the shaft can be approached between the brachiocephalic and biceps brachii muscles cranially and the lateral head of the triceps caudally. The radial nerve and deep branches of the brachial vessels should be avoided. The medial aspect is even more difficult to approach because of the close attachment of the leg to the trunk at that level. The distal shaft can be approached between the biceps brachii and the medial head of the triceps. The brachial artery and vein and the ulnar nerve should be avoided.

The elbow joint is approached from a medial aspect between the medial epicondyle of the humerus and the tuber olecrani of the ulna. The tensor fasciae antebrachii muscle will have to be partially transected and the medial head of

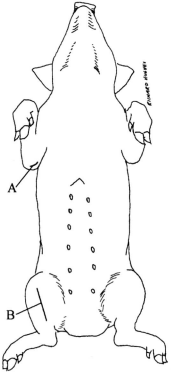

FIGURE 11.3   Surgical approaches to the bones and joints. *A*-Medial as part of elbow, *B*-Medial approach to tibia.

the triceps reflected. Laterally, the approach can be made by reflecting the lateral head of the triceps proximally and incising the anconeus muscle.

The radius can be approached from a lateral incision between the common digital extensor and the ulnaris lateralis. The distal shaft of the radius can be approached medially between the extensor carpi radialis and the pronater teres with caudal reflection of the digital flexors. The radial artery and vein and the median nerve should be avoided. The ulna is more accessible from the caudal aspect between the deep digital flexor and the ulnaris lateralis. The bones and joints of the distal limb can be readily palpated even in large swine and are easily approached from the cranial aspect.

Hindlimb

The approach to the femoral head and neck and acetabulum is difficult even in small pigs. The trochanter major can be palpated with difficulty below a line drawn from the tuber coxae and the tuber ischiadicum. A curved incision starting above this area and following the line of the femur is made to expose the juncture of the gluteus medius, the gluteus superficialis, and the tensor fasciae latae. Dissection through this juncture of fascia and tendinous attachments with retraction of the vastus lateralis and biceps femoris caudally will expose the greater trochanter and cranial aspect of the hip joint. Depending upon the experimental procedure, full exposure of the femoral head and neck and the joint will require cutting the tendinous attachments of these muscles and further deep dissection.

The femoral shaft can be exposed by an incision following the lateral aspect of the bone and dissecting between the fascia of the tensor fascia latae and the biceps femoris.

The stifle (knee) joint is approached from a craniolateral incision after flexion. The incision is made lateral to the patella and the patellar ligament through the infrapatellar fat pad. The tibia is subcutaneous on the medial aspect and can be surgically approached at any level with minimal difficulty. The medial saphenous artery, vein and nerve should be avoided.

The tarsocrural joint (hock) can be approached in either the lateral or medial aspect of the cranial border of the calcaneus. The malleolus of the fibula and the tuber olecrani can be palpated as landmarks and the incision line should be between them. On the lateral aspect, the saphenous vein should be avoided. On the medial aspect, the collateral ligaments and tendons are more prominent. The digits may be approached as described for the foreleg and the amputation described above.

Vertebral Column

The bones of the vertebral column of the pig are massive compared to many other species and the intervertebral spaces are relatively narrow. With the pig in sternal recumbency, the vertebra can be approached from a dorsal midline incision as in other species.

Injections into the subarachnoid space can be made between the last two lumbar vertebrae. The lateral wings of L5 are at the level of the tuber coxae. More cranial positions are difficult because of the conformation of the spinous processes of the vertebrae and the difficulty in flexing the vertebral column. The pig is positioned with the hindquarters hanging over the end of a table in order to flex the vertebrae. A spinal tap needle is slowly inserted until either cerebrospinal fluid drips from the needle or the position is confirmed radiographically (Boogerd and Peters, 1986; Punto, 1980). The cisterna magna can be accessed by flexing the pig's head off the table or over a sandbag. The space is narrow, and the needle should be directed cranioventrally until access is confirmed by dripping of cerebrospinal fluid.

A ventral midline approach can be made to the cervical and lumbar vertebrae. For the cervical vertebrae, the trachea and esophagus must be directed laterally and care taken not to damage the vagal sheath. The lumbar vertebrae can be approached from a ventral midline incision (Alitalo, 1979). The viscera must be retracted and packed off with laparotomy sponges within the abdomen. The aorta, vena cava, and branching vessels must be retracted laterally to expose the vertebrae underlying the ventral longitudinal ligament. Care should be taken to not damage the lymphatics in the region nor to ligate them if they are transected.

All of the musculoskeletal procedures should include the use of postoperative analgesics as part of the protocol. Use of phenylbutazone in combination with buprenorphine has been found to be superior to the use of either agent alone for procedures involving major muscular manipulations.

Bone Marrow Aspiration

Bone marrow aspiration to collect samples may be performed with standard bone marrow aspiration needles. The medial aspect of the proximal tibia approximately at the level of the tibial crest is a suitable site for obtaining bone marrow samples in all ages of swine (Figs. 11.3 and 11.4). Bone marrow may also be aspirated from the dorsal aspect of the tuber coxae (Fig. 11.5) and from the midsternum (Fig. 11.6). Sternal samples are best obtained from neonatal and juvenile animals. After aseptic preparation of the skin, the bone marrow aspiration needle with a stylet is inserted through the skin and muscle to the bone. It is then rotated back and forth while exerting forward pressure. A popping sensation will be felt when the needle penetrates the cortex. The stylet is removed, and the sample is collected with a syringe containing saline or preservative. The needle is removed when the sample is obtained. The same technique can be used to inject substances into the bone marrow. Bone marrow injections are absorbed in a similar manner to iv injections (Laber-Laird and Swindle, 1996).

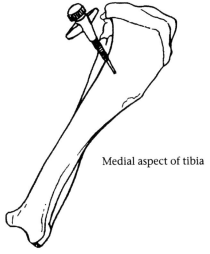

Medial aspect of tibia

FIGURE 11.4   Bone marrow aspiration site in medial aspect of tibia.

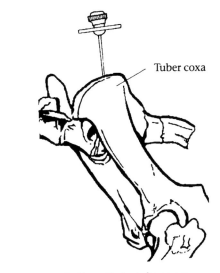

Tuber coxa

FIGURE 11.5   Bone marrow aspiration site in tuber coxa.

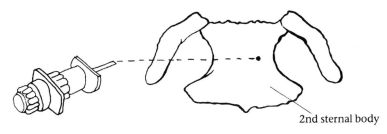

2nd sternal body

FIGURE 11.6   Bone marrow aspiration site in second sternal body.

References

Adams, R.J. 1988. Musculoskeletal system. In Swindle, M.M., and Adams, R.J. (eds), Experimental Surgery and Physiology: Induced Animal Models of Human Disease. Baltimore: Williams and Wilkins, pp. 10–41.

Alitalo, I. 1979. Ventral interbody implantation for fusion of the lumbar spine using polytetrafluoroethylene-carbonfiber and porous high density polyethylene: An experimental study in growing pigs. Acta Vet. Scand. 71(Suppl): 1–58.

Allan, D.G., G.G. Russell, M.J. Moreau, V.J. Raso, and D. Budney. 1990. Vertebral end plate failure in porcine and bovine models of spinal fracture instrumentation. J. Orthop. Res. 8(1): 154–156.

Bermejo, A., O. Gonzalez, and J.M. Gonzalez. 1993. The pig as an animal model for experimentation on the temporomandibular articular complex. Oral Surg. Oral Med. Oral Pathol. 75(1): 18–23.

Bobilya, D.J., M.G. Maurizi, T.L. Veum, and W.C. Allen. 1991. A bone biopsy procedure for neonatal pigs. Lab. Anim. 25(3): 222–225.

Bollwahn, W. 1992. Surgical procedures in boars and sows. In Leman, A.D., Straw, B.E., Mengeling, W.L., D'Allaire, S., and Taylor, D.J. (eds), Diseases of Swine, 7th ed. Ames: Iowa State University Press, pp. 782–793.

Boogerd, W., and A.C.B. Peters. 1986. A simple method for obtaining cerebrospinal fluid from a pig model of herpes encephalitis. Lab. Anim. Sci. 36(4): 386–388.

Boyce, R.W., D.C. Ebert, T.A. Youngs, C.L. Paddock, L. Mosekilde, M.L. Stevens, and H.J.G. Gundersen. 1995. Unbiased estimation of vertebral trabecular connectivity in calcium restricted ovariectomized minipigs. Bone 16(6): 637–642.

Buser, D., R.K. Schenk, S. Steinemann, J.P. Fiorellini, C.H. Fox, and H. Stich. 1991. Influence of surface characteristics on bone integration of titanium implants. A histomorphometric study in miniature pigs. J. Biomed. Mat. Res. 25(7): 889–902.

Davies, A.S., and M. Henning. 1986. Use of swine as a model of musculoskeletal growth in animals. In Tumbleson, M.E. (ed), Swine in Biomedical Research, Vol. 2. New York: Plenum Press, pp. 839–848.

Donovan, M.G., N.C. Dickerson, J.W. Hellstein, and L.J. Hanson. 1993. Autologous calvarial and iliac onlay bone grafts in miniature swine. J. Oral Maxillofac. Surg. 51(8): 898–903.

Laber-Laird, K.E., and M.M. Swindle. 1996. Techniques for serial bone marrow aspirations in growing Yucatan minipigs. Contemp. Top. Lab. Anim. Sci. 35(4): 73.

MacEwen, G.D. 1973. Experimental scoliosis. Clin. Orthop. 93: 69–74.

Ouhayoun J.P., A.H.M. Shabana, S. Issahakian, J.L. Patat, G. Guillemin, M.H. Sawaf, and N. Forest. 1992. Histological evaluation of natural coral skeleton as a grafting material in miniature swine mandible. J. Mat. Sci.: Mat. Med. 3(3):222–228.

Peltonen, J., I. Alitalo, E. Karaharju, H. Helio. 1984. Distraction of the growth plate. Experiments in pigs and sheep. Acta Orthop. Scand. 55(3): 359–362.

Punto, L. 1980. Lumbar leptomenigeal and radicular reactions after the subarachnial injection of water-soluble contrast media, meglumine iocarmate and metrizamide: An experimental study in the pig. Acta Vet. Scand. 73(Suppl): 1–52.

Sack, W.O. 1982. Essentials of Pig Anatomy and Harowitz/Kramer Atlas of Musculoskeletal Anatomy of the Pig. Ithaca, NY: Veterinary Textbooks.

Salter, R.B. 1968. Etiology, pathogenesis and possible prevention of congenital dislocation of the hip. Can. Med. Assoc. J. 98(20): 933–945.

Sisson, S. 1975. Appendages. In Getty R. (ed), Sisson and Grossman's The Anatomy of the Domestic Animals, 5th ed. Philadelphia: WB Saunders, pp. 1222–1230.

Swindle, M.M. 1983. Basic Surgical Exercises Using Swine. New York: Praeger Publishers.

Swiontkowski, M.F., S. Tepic, B.A. Rahn, J. Cordey, and S.M. Perren. 1993. The effect of fracture on femoral head blood flow. Osteonecrosis and revascularization studied in miniature swine. Acta Orthop. Scand. 64(2): 196–202.

12 CARDIOVASCULAR CATHETERIZATION LABORATORY PROCEDURES

Introduction

Swine have been used extensively in procedures involving the use of cardiovascular catheterization laboratories, fluoroscopic imaging, and interventional radiology techniques (Gaymes et al., 1995; Smith et al., 1989; Swindle et al., 1992; Swindle et al., 1994). The anatomy and surgical procedures involving the cardiovascular system have been discussed in Chapter 9. The relationship of the vessels entering and exiting the heart is illustrated here (Fig. 12.1). Recommended anesthetics for cardiovascular protocols and methods of prevention of cardiac arrhythmias are discussed in Chapter 2. The purpose of this chapter is to provide practical guidance to the use of swine in catheterization and fluoroscopy laboratories.

Peripheral Vascular Access for Cardiovascular Catheters

Access to the femoral and neck vessels (see Chapter 9, Figs. 9.10–9.12) via surgical cutdown procedures has been discussed in detail in Chapter 9. The technique of catheterization of these vessels using percutaneous techniques (Seldinger technique) (Fig. 12.2) for cardiovascular research has been published (Gaymes et al., 1995; Smith et al., 1989). Advantages of percutaneous techniques include minimal damage to the catheterized vessels, a shorter healing time than surgical procedures, and an increased likelihood that serial catheterizations can be performed in the same animal. The technique of

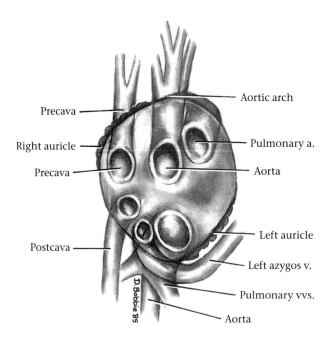

FIGURE 12.1   Relationship of the blood vessels entering and exiting the heart cap.
Reprinted with permission from Swindle et al., 1986, Anatomic and anesthetic considerations in experimental cardiopulmonary surgery in swine, Lab. Anim. Sci. 36(4): 357–361.

locating and accessing blood vessels for percutaneous catheterization is discussed here.

The femoral vessels are located with the pig in dorsal recumbency and the legs restrained caudolaterally. If the legs are stretched too tightly, it will be more difficult to determine the location of the vessels than if the hip joint remains slightly flexed. The medial saphenous artery may be routinely palpated as it crosses the medial aspect of the stifle (knee) joint. The arterial pulse may be palpated until it enters the deep muscles of the leg to join the femoral artery between the cranial sartorius and caudal gracilis muscles in the femoral canal (see Chapter 9, Fig. 9.12). The femoral canal is palpated and the vessels are located lateral to the edge of the sartorius muscle. The femoral pulse is difficult to palpate, even in smaller animals, and the anatomic guide to location is usually more reliable.

A saline filled 19-gauge 1.5-inch percutaneous needle is inserted through the caudal edge of the sartorius muscle approximately one-third to one-half the distance from the entrance of the median saphenous artery into the femoral canal and the hip joint. The needle should enter the skin at a 45-degree angle in a craniolateral direction. The needle is advanced slowly until blood appears in the needle or the passage through the vessel is felt by a pop-

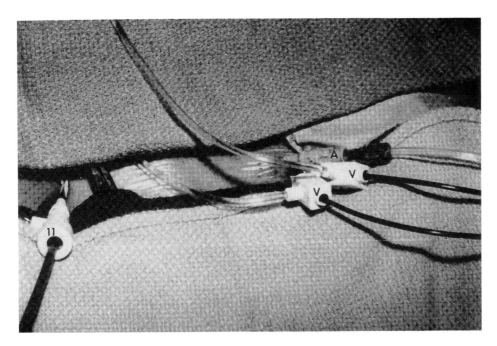

FIGURE 12.2   Percutaneous catheterization of the femoral vessels. 11—long sheath in
right femoral vein, *A*—Percutaneous dilator in left femoral artery, *V*—
Percutaneous sheaths in left femoral vein. *Reprinted with permission from
Gaymes et al., 1995, Percutaneous serial catheterization in swine: A practical
approach, J. Invest. Surg. 28(2): 123–128.*

ping sensation. The tip of the needle is manipulated until a free flow of blood
is obtained. Venous and arterial blood may be distinguished by pressure and
color. The vein is usually encountered first, is caudal, and slightly overlaps the
artery. The nerve is cranial to the artery. If the vessel cannot be catheterized
percutaneously after three tries with the needle, a surgical cutdown should be
performed because of the high probability of vasospasm.

When the vessel is accessed as indicated by bleeding, a 0.021 guidewire is inserted into the needle with the soft tip first. It is advanced cranially to the site
of interest using fluoroscopy for guidance. A skin nick is made at the site of
needle entry, and the needle is removed, leaving the wire in place. A dilator inside a 5- to 7-French (Fr) sheath with a side arm is passed over the guidewire. It
is advanced into the vessel using a gentle back-and-forth rotational movement. The dilator and sheath should be wet and filled with saline prior to their
introduction. After full advancement and demonstration of blood reflux, the
dilator and guidewire are removed, and the sheath is flushed with heparinized
saline. Two sheaths may be placed in the same vessel by passing a second
guidewire into the first sheath, removing the sheath, and passing two smaller
dilators and sheaths over the individual wires. It is also possible to catheterize
both the artery and vein on the same side. The medial saphenous artery, but

not the vein, can be catheterized with a smaller needle and guidewire and can accommodate up to a 5-Fr catheter in 25- to 30-kg swine. It is possible to insert a small guidewire and cannulate the central cardiovascular system from this vessel. However, digital pressure will have to be applied at the juncture of the saphenous artery and the femoral artery to facilitate passage of the angle of the juncture between the vessels by directing the tip of the catheter more deeply.

It is possible to pass up to 11 French sheaths in 15-kg swine. However, use of the smallest possible size is advisable, because larger catheters are more likely to cause permanent damage to the vessels. Five to 9-French sheaths suffice for most procedures. When the sheath and catheters are removed, digital pressure should be applied for approximately 5 minutes to prevent the formation of a hematoma. If the animal has been systemically heparinized, the activated clotting time (ACT) should be allowed to return to baseline before removal of the sheath. The skin can usually be repaired with a single suture.

The external jugular vein, internal jugular vein, and carotid artery can be catheterized using a similar technique (see Chapter 1, Fig. 1.12). Larger sheath sizes can be used, especially in the external jugular vein. The pig is placed in dorsal recumbency and the forelegs are restrained caudally. The anatomic locations for percutaneous needle insertion can be identified. A triangle is identified with the cranial surface of the first rib as the base and the apex forming in the jugular furrow. At the middle of this triangle along the lateral aspect of the jugular furrow, the needle is inserted through the juncture of the sternohyoideus and sternomastoideus muscles. This location is approximately one-quarter of the distance between the manubrium sterni and the ramus of the mandible. The carotid arterial pulse and/or the wings of the cervical vertebrae can usually be palpated, even in large swine, along the lateral aspect of the trachea. The internal jugular vein, carotid artery, and vagus nerve are located in a sheath on the floor of the cervical vertebrae. Depending upon whether the catheterization direction is cranial or caudal, the needle is still inserted at an angle in the appropriate direction.

Other vessels, such as the auricular and cranial abdominal vessels, can be cannulated to gain access into the central circulation in large swine, depending upon the indications for catheterization. These techniques, as well as the chronic catheterization techniques previously described, can be modified for any size pig.

Hemodynamics

Hemodynamic measurements may be taken using the cardiovascular catheterization techniques described above, using fluoroscopic guidance to see the catheter placement and by noting the morphology of the pressure waves (Fig. 12.3). Standard-sized catheters used for measurements in humans, such as Swan-Ganz catheters, in the 5- to 7-Fr range of sizes, work for most laboratory swine. The length of the catheter to be used should be determined in advance. As a general rule, pediatric lengths work best in swine. Echocardiography can also be used as a noninvasive technique for obtaining some measurements. Chronic cardiovascular catheterization, as described in Chapter 9, may be performed if it is desirable to take hemodynamic measurements without sedation. Peripheral cuff measurements from the tail or the medial saphenous artery can also be used for limited measurements of systemic pressure. Physiologic and monitoring equipment used for other species is appropriate for swine.

Pulse oximetry is a useful technique for monitoring swine for oxygenation. Human finger cuffs may be used on the dewclaws, tail, ear, or tongue. If the soft tissues are chosen, the cuff will periodically have to be repositioned because of vascular compression. Arterial blood gases may be measured using the same techniques that are applicable to humans and other species.

Hemodynamic values are affected by age, weight, breed, measurement technique, body temperature, ventilation, anesthetic administration, and pathologic conditions. Consequently, comparison to normal values in the literature

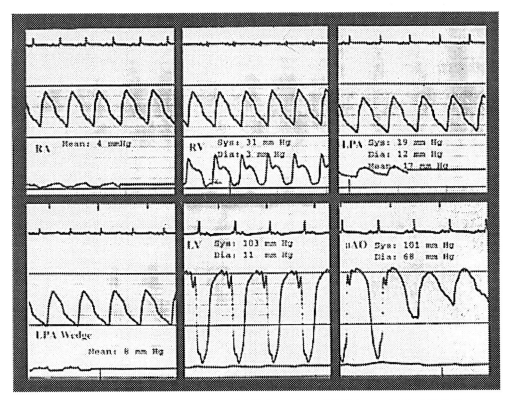

FIGURE 12.3   Pressure wave recording. *RA*-Right atrium, *RV*-Right ventricle, *LPA*-Left pulmonary artery, *LPA wedge*-Left pulmonary artery wedge, *LV*-Left ventricle, *AO*-Aorta.

should be made with caution. In cases of measurements taken under anesthesia, it is not always possible to reproduce the exact anesthetic level from the description in the literature. If possible, each animal should be used as its own control and experimental measurements compared to the baseline. As a general rule, sexually mature miniature swine have hemodynamics that closely resemble those of adult humans.

The animals should be matched for age, body weight (BW), and breed, if possible. Hemodynamic values should be indexed to body surface area (BSA). Formulas are based upon dissection and measurement of the skin of farm pigs. One formula, BSA = 0.097 × body weight in $kg^{0.633}$ (Brody and Kibler, 1944), should be used with caution because the conformation of farm pigs has changed substantially since the time of that publication. The formulas were recalculated more recently to reflect those differences. Kelley et al. (1973) provided two formulas: BSA (cm^2) = 734 $(BW_{kg})^{0.656}$ and BSA (cm^2) = 3996 + 110(BW_{kg}). The first is a geometric formula and correlates better with other formulas than the second linear formula. Wachtel et al. (1972) used a different formula to calculate BSA in miniature swine, which were determined to be different from farm pigs. That formula is: BSA (m^2) = 0.121 $BW_{kg}^{0.575}$.

Another formula was determined for BSA in neonatal swine less than 2 kg (DeRoth and Bisaillon, 1979). That formula is: BSA(cm^2) = 337.2 + 0.553 BW(g). The formulas that are most applicable to current research are probably the Kelley formula: BSA(cm^2) = 734 $BW_{kg}^{0.656}$ or BSA(m^2) = 0.0734 BW$_{kg}$ for farm pigs and the Wachtel formula BSA(m^2) = 0.121 $BW_{kg}^{0.575}$ for miniature breeds. The neonatal formula may be useful for some studies.

All anesthetic protocols have some effects on hemodynamics; however, they can be minimized as discussed in Chapter 2. A complete review of the effects of hemorrhagic shock on the hemodynamics of domestic farm swine as well as hemodynamic methods has been published (Hannon, 1992; McKirnan et al., 1986). In addition the effects of age on hemodynamics in domestic farm swine under pentobarbital anesthesia has been published (Buckley et al., 1979) and comparison to different breeds of swine, dogs, and humans (Benharkate et al., 1993; McKenzie, 1996; Vogl et al., 1997). In general, blood pressure increases and heart rate decreases with age. Some examples of hemodynamic values and cardiac sizes from the literature are listed in Tables 12.1-12.4.

Comparisons were made among 4-month-old Hanford miniature swine, Yucatan miniature swine, and Yucatan microswine under a surgical plane of isoflurane anesthesia (Smith et al., 1990). Table 12.1 compares hemodynamic values and Table 12.2 compares cardiac morphometrics from this study.

Table 12.3 contains measurements that were made in 20- to 22-week-old Yucatan micropigs under isoflurane anesthesia (Corin et al., 1988).

Table 12.4 contains measurements that were made in domestic farm swine, 10–15 kg, without anesthesia. They previously had chronic atrial lines implanted (Smith et al., 1989).

Table 12.1.   Hemodynamic parameters for three groups of miniature swine

	Hanford	Minipig	Micropig
Heart rate (bpm)	105 ± 7	112 ± 3	106 ± 5
Left ventricle			
Systolic pressure (mmHg)	116 ± 4[b,c]	58 ± 2	59 ± 3
Diastolic pressure (mmHg)	4 ± 1	3 ± 1	6 ± 2
Right ventricle			
Peak pressure (mmHg)	30 ± 1[b]	24 ± 2	27 ± 2
Diastolic pressure (mmHg)	4 ± 1[b]	2 ± 1	5 ± 1[a]
Mean arterial pressure (mmHg)	89[b,c]	48 ± 3	53 ± 2
Mean pulmonary artery pressure (mmHg)	19 ± 1[b]	15 ± 1[a]	20 ± 2
Right atrial pressure (mmHg)	9 ± 1[b,c]	3 ± 1[a]	6 ± 1
Pulmonary capillary wedge pressure (mmHg)	12 ± 1	12 ± 2	11 ± 1

NOTE: All values are reported as mean ± standard error of the mean.
[a] Significant ($p < 0.05$) difference between minipig versus micropig.
[b] Significant ($p < 0.05$) difference between minipig versus Hanford.
[c] Significant ($p < 0.05$) difference between micropig versus Hanford.
SOURCE: Reprinted with permission from Smith et al., 1994, Cardiac function and morphology of Hanford miniature and Yucatan miniature and micro swine, Lab. Anim. Sci. 40(1): 47–50.

Table 12.2.   Cardiac morphometrics for three groups of miniature swine

	Hanford	Minipig	Micropig
Heart weights (g)			
Total	117 ± 4[b,c]	61 ± 2	53 ± 2
Right ventricular (RV) free wall	23 ± 1[b,c]	13 ± 1	11 ± 1
Left ventricular (RV) free wall	39 ± 1[b,c]	23 ± 1	19 ± 1[a]
Wall thickness (cm)			
Right ventricular	4.1 ± 0.1	4.4 ± 0.2	4.5 ± 0.2
Left ventricular	10.4 ± 0.3	11.2 ± 0.3	10.2 ± 0.3
Heart weight/body weight	4.6 ± 0.1[b,c]	5.7 ± 0.1	5.5 ± 0.1
LV weight/body weight	1.5 ± 0.1[b,c]	2.2 ± 0.1	2.0 ± 0.1
RV weight/body weight	0.9 ± 0.1[b,c]	1.2 ± 0.1	1.2 ± 0.1

NOTE: All values are reported as mean ± standard error of the mean.
[a] Significant ($p < 0.05$) difference between minipig versus micropig.
[b] Significant ($p < 0.05$) difference between minipig versus Hanford.
[c] Significant ($p < 0.05$) difference between micropig versus Hanford.
SOURCE: Reprinted with permission from Smith et al. 1994, Cardiac function and morphology of Hanford miniature and Yucatan miniature and micro swine, Lab. Anim. Sci. 40(1): 47–50.

Table 12.3.   Yucatan swine data

QP/QS	Controls (mean ± SEM)
Age (weeks)	21 ± 1
Wt (kg)	21 ± 2
HR (beats per minute)	116 ± 13
LVMI (g/kg)	2.4 ± 0.4
EDVI (ml/kg)	1.9 ± 0.5
ESVI (ml/kg)	0.8 ± 0.3
EF (%)	0.58 ± 0.08
IP (mmHg)	81 ± 8
PAP (mmHg)	21 ± 10
PCW (mmHg)	4 ± 4
V_2 (ml/m/kg)	2.6 ± 0.3
FSVI (ml/kg)	1.1 ± 0.26
CI (liters/min/kg)	0.12 ± 0.03
SVRI (dyn $\cdot$ s/cm$^5 \cdot$ kg)	152 ± 71
PVRI (dyn $\cdot$ s/cm$^5 \cdot$ kg)	37 ± 17
EDS (dyn/cm^2)	9 ± 5
ESS (dyn/cm^2)	111 ± 28
Emax	2.2 ± 0.7
Emax$_c$	84 ± 27
V_{cf50} (circ/sec)	1.04 ± 0.14
V_{cf100} (circ/sec)	0.68 ± 0.14

NOTE: QP/QS, ratio of pulmonary to systemic blood flow; Wt, body weight; HR, heart rate; LVMI, left-ventricular muscle mass index; EDVI, end-diastolic volume index; ESVI, end-systolic volume index; EF, ejection fraction; IP, incisural pressure; PAP, mean pulmonary artery pressure; PCW, pulmonary capillary wedge pressure; V_2, oxygen consumption; FSVI, forward stroke volume index; CI, systemic cardiac index; SVRI, systemic vascular resistance index; PVRI, pulmonary vascular resistance index; EDS, end-diastolic stress; ESS, end-systolic stress; Emax, maximum systolic elastance; Emax$_c$, Emax corrected for end-diastolic volume; V_{cf50}, V_{cf100}, mean velocity of circumferential fiber shortening at a common end-systolic stress of 50 and 100 kdyn/cm^2.

SOURCE: Reprinted with permission from Corin et al. 1988, Mechanisms of decreased forward stroke volume in children and swine with ventricular septal defect and failure to thrive, J. Clin. Invest. 82: 544–551.

Table 12.4.   Weekly catheterization results of chronic atrial line implantation: control of animals[a]

	Week 1
Left Ventricle	
Ejection fraction (%)	59 ± 1
End-diastolic volume (cc)	54 ± 4
Peak systolic pressure (mmHg)	104 ± 4
End-diastolic pressure (mmHg)	2 ± 1
Right Ventricle	
Ejection fraction (%)	53 ± 3
End-diastolic (cc)	56 ± 4
Peak systolic pressure (mmHg)	24 ± 1
End-diastolic pressure (mmHg)	2 ± 1

[a]Data presented as means ± standard error of the means. There was no significant difference in weekly values ($p < 0.75$, $n = 4$).

SOURCE: Reprinted with permission from Smith et al. 1989, Technical aspects of cardiac catheterization of swine. J. Invest. Surg. 2(2): 187–194.

Angioplasty Balloon Techniques/Intravascular Device Implantations/Atherosclerosis

Swine have been used for testing angioplasty balloon techniques, implantation of intravascular devices, and interventional radiology procedures (Gal and Isner, 1992; Grifka et al., 1993; Lock et al., 1982; Lock et al., 1985; Lund et al., 1984; Mitchell et al., 1994; Morrow et al., 1994; Murphy et al., 1992; Randsbaek et al., 1996; Rashkind et al., 1987; Rogers et al., 1988; Swindle et al., 1992; White et al., 1992). The techniques of using these devices involve the procedures described above for vascular access and the procedures for surgical approaches to peripheral vessels and cannulations described in Chapter 9. Models of aneurysm for endovascular device closure are also discussed in the same chapter. The anatomic depictions of the vessels in the angiography section of this chapter and the magnetic resonance imaging images in Chapter 14 may be of use in designing protocols and approaches for these procedures. Sizes of the heart and blood vessels may be estimated from these images. The manufacturer's directions for use of these devices should be followed.

Angioplasty balloon techniques (Fig. 12.4) have been utilized to reopen intracardiac and intravascular shunts in neonates, to provide models of shunt patency for device closure, to produce left-to-right shunts for volume overload cardiac hypertrophy, and to study the effects of angioplasty on stenosed valvular structures and atherosclerotic lesions (Lock et al., 1985; Lund et al., 1984; Mitchell et al., 1994; Rashkind et al., 1987; Smith et al., 1997). Transient decreases in systemic blood pressure will probably be noted with the inflation of angioplasty balloons. The angioplasty balloon should be filled with contrast material to observe inflation better and to observe for leaks. Catheters filled with air may cause air embolism if the balloon ruptures.

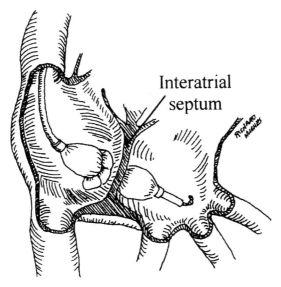

FIGURE 12.4   Method of using angioplasty balloon catheter inflation to create a shunt.

Atrial septostomy has been performed in 18- to 27-kg domestic swine to produce a patent foramen ovale. A transseptal catheter was advanced from the femoral vein to cross the closed fossa ovalis. After exchanging the catheter with an angioplasty balloon catheter, the balloon was inflated three times with 3–4 atmospheres of pressure for 10–15 seconds. No reclosures of the septum were noted with balloon sizes greater than 12 mm during long-term studies. Histologically, the septums healed with collagenous scar tissue and reendothelization (Mitchell et al., 1994).

Five-kilogram domestic swine were used to create a model of patent ductus arteriosus (PDA). A 0.035-inch guidewire was passed distal to the aortic arch from the right femoral artery. A 5-French curved catheter was advanced over the guidewire, and the guidewire was advanced across the PDA into the right ventricle. The catheter was exchanged for a 6-mm diameter angioplasty balloon. The balloon was inflated to 8–10 atmospheres of pressure for 2–5 minutes. No reclosures of the PDA were noted in long-term studies (Lund et al., 1984). This method offers an alternative to keeping the PDA open with multiple injections and long-term infusions of prostaglandins (Starling et al., 1978).

Models of atherosclerosis (Fig. 12.5) can be produced by inflation of angioplasty balloons in the artery and denudation of the endothelium by pulling back on the inflated balloon in swine fed an atherogenic diet (Attie et al., 1992; Gal and Isner, 1992; Lee et al., 1986; Rogers et al., 1988; White et al., 1992). The denudation procedure should be repeated two to three times. Fogarty embolectomy catheters (5–6 Fr) may be used for this technique after being inflated to 6–8 atmospheres of pressure. Other angioplasty catheters can also be used. Animals must be fed an atherogenic diet of 0.5%–4.0% cholesterol. The cholesterol is added as a supplement in lard, or atherogenic food oils and fats are mixed in standard diets. Alternatively, diets may be commercially prepared by food manufacturers. No universal standard for the amount of cholesterol to be included in the diet has been developed, but it is likely that 2% cholesterol is adequate for most studies. The diet should be fed to the animals starting 2 weeks prior to the procedure. The diet has to be continued for up to 12 weeks following the procedure to have radiographically visible occlusal lesions. Swine fed atherogenic diets alone may not develop significant atherogenic lesions within a year. The arteries most utilized in these techniques are the coronaries and the iliacs. The iliacs are approached from catheters introduced into the carotid artery and the coronaries from the femoral artery. Anesthetic and ancillary drug administration for coronary artery catheterization is discussed in Chapter 2.

Gal and Isner (1992) concluded that the Yucatan micropig may be a more favorable model for the development of these lesions than other miniature swine and domestic swine after comparing their results with the literature. The model can then be tested for balloon angioplasty of the occlusal lesions, atherectomy techniques, stent implantation, and local and systemic drug therapies.

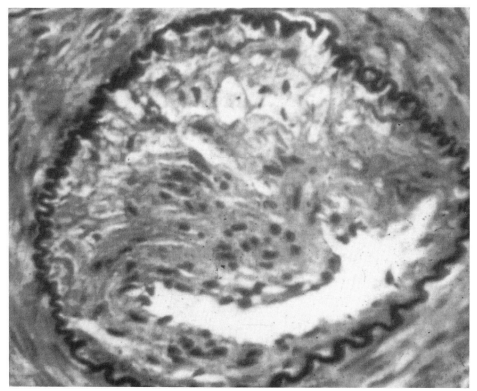

FIGURE 12.5   Coronary arterial atherosclerotic plaque. (Hematoxylin and Eosin stain, ×100)

Yucatan microswine, weighing 14–33 kg, had the following diameter measurements in vivo: iliac arteries, 5 mm; femoral arteries, 3.5 mm; popliteal arteries, 2.0 mm (Gal and Isner, 1992).

Yucatan miniature swine, weighing 10–20 kg, had the following measurements in vivo: coronary arteries, 2.0–3.5 mm; iliac artery, 2.5–4.0 mm (White et al., 1992).

Hanford miniature swine, weighing 15 kg, had coronary artery diameters of 2.0–2.5 mm (Rogers et al., 1988).

Necropsy measurements of the diameters of various arteries and veins were collected by the author. In vivo, it can be expected that these vessel sizes can be expanded. The measurements recorded were the following.

Yucatan micropig (29 kg): Aortic arch—1.2 cm, Abdominal aorta—6 mm, External iliac artery—2 mm, Internal iliac artery—1 mm, Portal vein—1.0 cm, Postcava—2 cm

Yucatan miniature pig (109 kg): Aortic arch—1.1 cm, Abdominal aorta—6 mm, External iliac artery—4 mm, Internal iliac artery—3 mm, Renal artery—2 mm

Hanford miniature pig (43.6 kg): Aortic arch—1.3 cm, Abdominal aorta—4 mm, External iliac artery—3 mm, Internal iliac artery—2 mm, Postcava, 4 mm

Landrace domestic pig (70 kg): Aortic arch—1. 2 cm, Abdominal aorta—5 mm, External iliac artery—4 mm, Internal iliac artery—3 mm, Renal artery—2 mm, Carotid artery—3.5 mm, Coronary artery—3.0 mm

Expandable stents can be placed in atherogenic and normal arteries to provide patency and for local drug delivery. The technique involves placing an expandable stent over an inflatable balloon and then inflating the balloon after the stent is in the proper location. The balloon is then deflated and the catheter removed. Stents are most commonly employed to study percutaneous transluminal coronary angioplasty (PCTA) but have also been used for other vascular models such as surgically produced coarctation of the aorta or iliac artery stenosis (Gal and Isner, 1992; Grifka et al., 1993; Lock et al., 1982; Morrow et al., 1994; Murphy et al., 1992; White et al., 1992).

A model of restenosis of the coronary artery following balloon angioplasty or stent implantation has been developed in swine (Murphy et al., 1992; Willette et al., 1996). The model may be produced by either overinflation with a balloon angioplasty catheter of 25%–75% (20 seconds, 10 atmospheres of pressure) repeated three times. Neointimal formation occurs in approximately 50% of the miniature or domestic swine subjected to this procedure. The implantation of various stents reliably produces 100% neointimal formation. The stent needs to be oversized (> 30%) in the coronary artery (Willette et al., 1996). The restenosis following the procedure may be noted in as short as 2 weeks but consistently occurs in 4–6 weeks with some stents.

In one of the investigations, it was noted that pigs developed postinfarction ventricular aneurysm similar to the clinical syndrome in humans. The infarctions and aneurysms occurred in all animals that developed occlusion following implantation of the stent. This model provides distinct advantages to surgical implantation of graft material into windows created in the ventricular wall. It can be performed without a thoracotomy and provides a more similar pathogenesis to the human situation (Murphy et al., 1992).

Postoperative and/or intraoperative antithrombotic therapy may be necessary in the models of stent implantation and is discussed in Chapter 2.

Electrophysiology

Swine have been used as models for study of cardiac electrophysiology and cardiac arrhythmias (Gillette et al., 1991; Hughes, 1986; Schumann et al., 1993; Schumann et al., 1994; Smith et al., 1997; Verdouw and Hartog, 1986).

The anatomy of the conduction system of the porcine heart has been compared to other species, including humans (Bharati et al., 1991; Truex and

Smythe, 1965). The principal difference between the porcine conduction system and that of humans is the presence of large numbers of adrenergic and cholinergic nerve fibers in the AV node and bundle branches. Nerve cells are lacking in the fibers. The Purkinje fibers are large, well differentiated, and easily identifiable in the endocardium (Fig. 12.6). Humans have some nerve fibers, no ganglia, and smaller Purkinje fibers. Swine may have more of a neuromyogenic rather than predominantly a myogenic component to the conduction system because of these differences.

The sinus rhythm rate and conduction system velocity rates vary depending upon the age and weight of the pig; in smaller pigs, they are more rapid. In general, heart rates are more rapid than for humans of equivalent maturity. Heart conduction system rates are also affected by the anesthetic protocol. Long QT segments, with the T wave sometimes becoming superimposed with the following p wave, may be observed in deep surgical anesthesia. Ketamine-midazolam or sufentanil infusions (see Chapter 2) may be used to shorten the QT interval if required (Schumann et al., 1993; Schumann et al., 1994). Swine have been demonstrated to have similar enough conduction system parameters

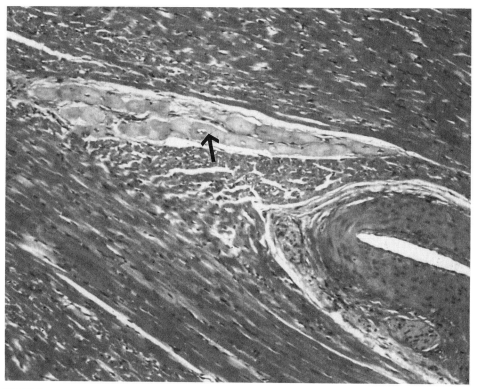

FIGURE 12.6   Histology of the heart demonstrating large Purkinje cells (*arrow*). (×100, Hematoxylin and Eosin Stain)

(Fig. 12.7) to be used for pacemaker testing (Brownlee et al., 1997; Hughes, 1986; Smith et al., 1997) and for study of ventricular arrhythmias (Verdouw and Hartog, 1986). Arrhythmias following myocardial infarction are discussed in Chapters 2 and 9. The electrophysiologic (EP) testing techniques of Gillette and Garson (1981) and Gillette and Griffin (1986) have been modified for use in swine (Smith et al., 1997). Noninvasive programmable stimulation (NIPS) that performs EP using a telemetry system has also been successfully used in Hanford miniature swine (Smith et al., 1997).

Examples of intracardiac electrophysiologic parameters in anesthetized domestic swine used for pacemaker testing are listed in Table 12.5 and 12.6.

The NIPS program is summarized below:

1. Verify programming parameters of the pacemaker. Surface electrocardiogram should be recorded simultaneously.
2. Retrieve diagnostic data collected by the NIPS.
3. Intracardiac electrogram is checked for proper lead placement.
4. The stimulation threshold is determined for atrial and ventricular leads by pacing at 50 msec shorter than the shortest sinus rhythm cycle.
5. AAI and VVI modes are used to perform pacing stimulation protocols for the atrium and ventricle separately.
6. Pacing procedures:
    (a) 8 beats of burst pacing (300 msec) and determination of the rate at which 2:1 block occurs (decrease cycle by 10 msec each time).
    (b) Deliver a single premature beat into the paced chamber (SPRA/V). Start at 400 msec for 8 beats and deliver a premature beat at 380 msec. Decrease the interval of premature beat delivery by 20 msec until 300 msec. The interval at which the premature beat was introduced is decreased by 10 msec until capture discontinues. The shortest interval without capture of either chamber is the atrial or ventricular effective refractory period (AERP or VERP).
    (c) Deliver two premature beats into the paced chamber (DPPRA/V) after 8 beats of 400 msec. The two premature beats are introduced at a cycle length 50 msec greater than AERP or VERP. The introduction of each premature beat is decreased by 10-msec intervals until it no longer captured. The protocol is concluded when AERP or VERP is reached.
7. Reprogram the pacemaker to DDD mode for previous pacing parameters.

Table 12.7 contains values recorded from this technique in Hanford miniature swine (Smith et al., 1997).

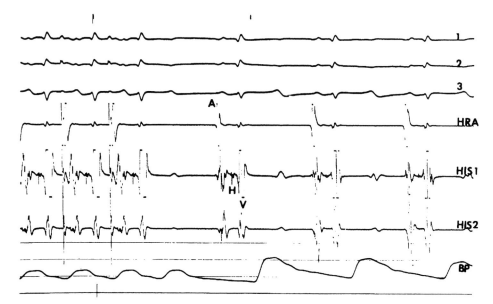

FIGURE 12.7   Surface and intracardiac electrocardial recordings. *1, 2, 3*-Surface leads, *HRA*-High right atrium, *HIS 1* and *HIS 2*-distal and proximal bundle of His catheter recordings, *BP*-Blood pressure, *A*-Atrium, *H*-Bundle of His spike, *V*-Ventricle. *Reprinted with permission from Gaymes et al., 1995, Percutaneous serial catheterization in swine: A practical approach, J. Invest. Surg. 8(2): 123–128.*

Table 12.5.   Threshold voltage (volts) requirements: domestic swine 25–30 kg

Electrode location	Mean pulse duration (msec)	Pig (range)
SA node	1.0	0.36–0.58
	0.5	0.58–0.96
Atrial appendage	1.0	0.26–0.60
	0.5	0.27–1.21
Right ventricle	1.0	0.15–0.35
	0.5	0.23–0.51
Left ventricle	1.0	0.17–0.43
	0.5	0.31–0.69

SOURCE: Reprinted with permission from Hughes, 1986, Swine in cardiovascular research, Lab. Anim. Sci. 36(4): 348–350.

Table 12.6.   Threshold current (mA) requirements: domestic swine 25–30 kg

Electrode location	Mean pulse duration (msec)	Pig (range)
SA node	1.0	0.81–1.25
	0.5	1.54–2.70
Atrial appendage	1.0	0.37–1.55
	0.5	0.47–2.87
Right ventricle	1.0	0.24–0.74
	0.5	0.43–1.21
Left ventricle	1.0	0.38–0.80
	0.5	0.72–1.44

SOURCE: Reprinted with permission from Hughes, 1986, Swine in cardiovascular research, Lab. Anim. Sci. 36(4): 348–350.

Table 12.7. Noninvasive programmable stimulation values for Hanford miniature swine

	VTHRESH	VBURST	VERP	DPPRV S2	S3	ATHRESH	ABURST	AVNERP	AERP	DPPRA S2	S3
Mean	0.07	220.98	228.51	226.45	163.01	0.25	233.55	249.88	210.25	221.15	166.73
Standard deviation	0.07	29.01	20.54	19.54	27.22	0.20	35.09	27.91	30.51	34.53	33.77
Range, minimum	0.03	140.00	180.00	170.00	110.00	0.03	160.00	210.00	150.00	140.00	100.00
Range, maximum	0.45	290.00	320.00	330.00	260.00	1.00	370.00	340.00	320.00	310.00	270.00

Refer to the description of electrophysiologic testing in text for explanation of pacing protocols.

NOTE: VTHRESH, ventricular threshold; VBURST, ventricular burst pacing; VERP, ventricular effective refractory period; DPPRV, double premature beats into paced right ventricle; S2, first premature beat; S3, second premature beat; ATHRESH, atrial threshold; ABURST, atrial burst pacing; AVNERP, AV node effective refractory period; AERP, atrial effective refractory period; DPPRA, double premature beats into paced right atrium.

SOURCE: Reprinted with permission from Smith et al., 1997, A technique for conducting noninvasive cardiac electrophysiology studies in swine, J. Invest. Surg. 10(1–2): 25–30.

Pacemaker Implantation/Endocardial Pacemaker Leads

The technique for epicardial pacemaker implantation is described in Chapter 9. In this section the implantation of endocardial pacemaker leads and the implantation of the pulse generator in the neck is described.

Hanford miniature swine weighing more than 45 kg have similar intracardiac measurements to the human heart and single pass 11- to 13-cm pacemaker leads designed for adult humans can be inserted for testing (Figs. 12.8 and 12.9) (Brownlee et al., 1997). Smaller swine of the same breed have been used for pacemaker implantation after conduction system ablation (Gillette et al., 1991; Smith et al., 1997). Both single pass leads and separate atrial and ventricular leads have been used for dual chamber pacing. The angle of entry into the heart is different in swine, as it is in other quadrupedal animals, and adjustments in the technique of passing a lead into the heart using fluoroscopic guidance must be made.

A left external jugular cutdown surgery is performed as described in Chapter 9. The pacemaker generator will be implanted in the pocket formed by this surgery (Figs. 12.10 and 12.11); consequently, dorsal dissection between the muscle planes along the path of the external jugular vein to accommodate the device will be required. Elastic vessel loops are applied to the external jugular vein and a venotomy is made with iris scissors. The pacemaker leads are passed into the heart through the venotomy. The ventricular lead is implanted first if two leads are required. Either screw-in or tined lead tips will work in the ventricle; however, screw-in leads work best in the atrium.

When the ventricular lead tip is observed at the tricuspid valve the insertion wire is retracted 1–5 cm so that the tip of the lead is floppy and can be manipulated through the valve. The internal guidewire can be slightly curved along the distal end to facilitate the manipulation. Depending upon the location of the lead tip either a counterclockwise or a clockwise twist is performed on the lead while inserting it through the valve. The tendency of the lead will be to pass into the post cava, and multiple insertion attempts to correct the angle usually have to be made. Once the lead tip is in the ventricle, the tip will pass into the pulmonary outflow tract if it is passed between tendinous chordae. The goal of the insertion is to implant it into the apex. This can be accomplished by inserting the internal guidewire fully into the pacemaker lead after it has been passed into the ventricle.

For single pass leads after the ventricular tip is secured, the electrodes are placed close to the entrance of the precava into the atrium. For atrial screw-in leads the implantation site should be the high right atrium. Care must be taken when inserting this lead to avoid overmanipulation that will dislodge the ventricular lead. The internal guidewire is retracted slightly to place the lead in the proper location using a counterclockwise twist. The tip is then screwed into the atrial wall.

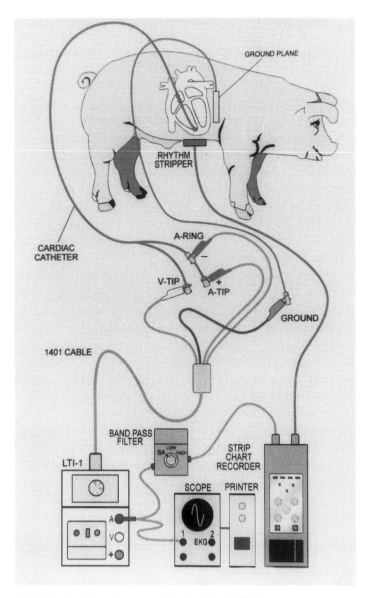

FIGURE 12.8   Atrial lead testing. *Courtesy of Cardiac Control Systems.*

After the electrode tips are implanted, they are tested to ensure that appropriate impedance and threshold values are obtained. The manufacturers instructions for the electrodes should be followed and similar electrophysiology values to humans can be expected with implantation of these devices in swine (Brownlee et al., 1997; Hughes, 1986; Smith et al., 1997). The phrenic nerve runs along the course of the pre- and postcava, and diaphragmatic stimulation may occur with improper positioning of the lead electrodes or too high a threshold value. The pacemaker leads are secured in place with nonabsorbable

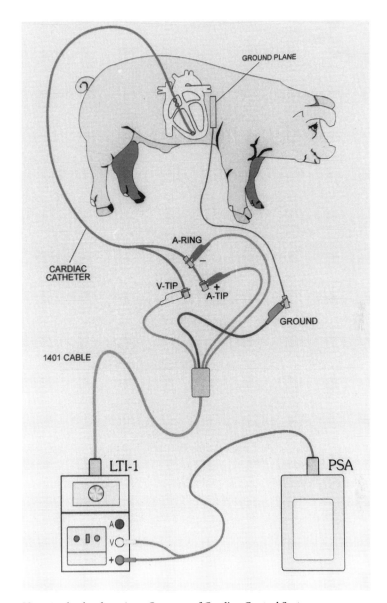

FIGURE 12.9   Ventricular lead testing. *Courtesy of Cardiac Control Systems.*

suture ligatures around the proximal and distal venotomy sites and around the suture sleeves on the leads. The pacemaker generator is attached, and excess lead material is coiled around the device. The device is implanted into the pocket, and its placement is checked to ensure that it is not stimulating the skeletal muscle in the region. The pocket is enclosed by suturing the muscles over the pacemaker generator. The closure between the sternohyoideus and the sternomastoideus muscles should completely cover the device. Leaving dead space in the pocket will lead to seroma formation. The fascial layers are

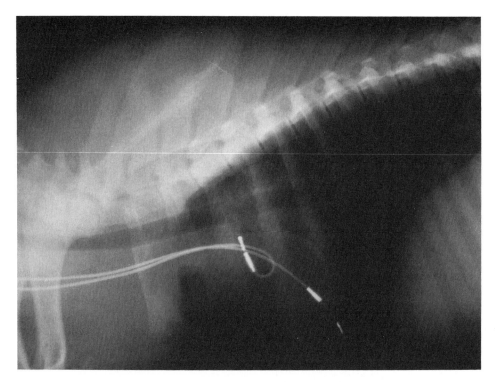

FIGURE 12.10   Lateral radiograph of placement of atrial and ventricular leads. The pacemaker generator has been implanted in the neck.

closed using synthetic absorbable sutures, and a subcuticular suture pattern is used to close the skin.

Pacemaker wand telemetry systems should be able to communicate with the device through the skin and muscle if it is held next to the skin. Some manipulation of the wand may be necessary to achieve the desired communication. The wand should be checked in its ability to communicate with the pacemaker generator prior to closing the muscle layers.

Conduction System Ablation

Conduction system ablation is used to study electrophysiology of the heart, techniques for ablation of aberrant conduction system pathways and the function of cardiac pacemakers. Heart block and regional ablation of the conduction system of the heart has been produced in animals by traumatic damage to the area of interest using surgical techniques. These have included cutting, thermal damage, tight sutures, and injection of formalin into the SA node, AV node, bundle of His, and bundle branches. Some of these techniques involve the use of a right atriotomy, and most have a high failure rate (Gardner and Johnson, 1988). Transvenous ablation of the conduction system has been developed using catheter delivery of cryothermia (Fig. 12.12), radiofrequency, di-

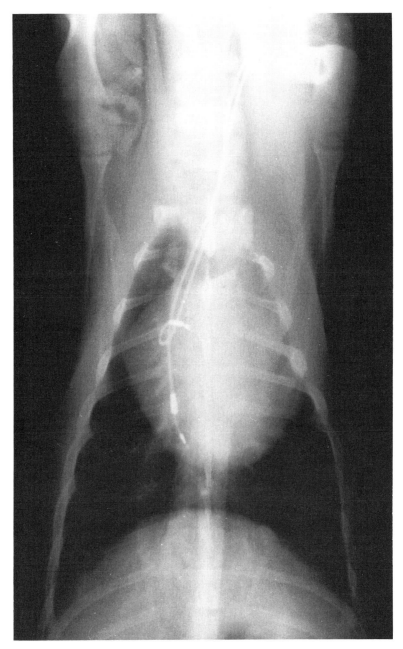

FIGURE 12.11   Ventrodorsal radiograph of placement of atrial and ventricular leads.

rect current and laser trauma to the conduction system. These methods have been utilized in swine (Fujino et al., 1991; Fujino et al., 1993; Gillette et al., 1991; Smith et al., 1997).

The technique of transvenous ablation involves the positioning of intracardiac tripolar electrode catheters into the heart to record electrical signals of the

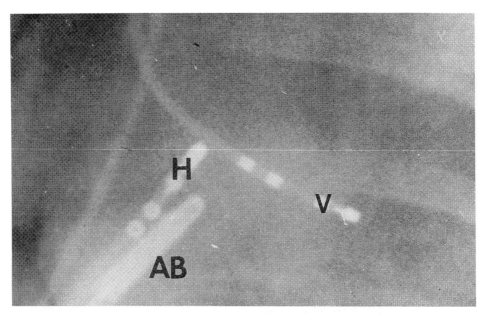

FIGURE 12.12   Cryoablation catheter at the bundle of His (*AB*). The other catheters are electrodes for recording the intracardiac electrogram (*H* and *V*).

heart. The area of interest is positioned between two of the electrodes. An ablation catheter is guided fluoroscopically until the tip of the catheter can be seen at the area of interest, and the energy to ablate the conduction system is delivered using the applicable generator. Recordings of the electrical signals of the heart will indicate when a lesion has been delivered. When producing heart block, it is necessary to provide ventricular pacing. Currently, the two most common types of energy-delivery systems in use are radiofrequency and cryothermia. The catheters are usually introduced into the heart from the femoral vessels, as described above.

The catheter size, amount of energy delivered, length of delivery of energy, and necessity to repeat the procedure varies depending upon the type of ablation selected and the design characteristics of the catheter and equipment. From our experience, the following examples are given for cryoablation and radiofrequency ablation in 14- to 22-kg Hanford pigs. Cryoablation of the bundle of His: 11-Fr catheter, –60°C, 180 seconds, three freeze-and-thaw cycles. Radiofrequency ablation of the bundle of His: 5-Fr catheter, 50-watt energy output, 70°–90°C, 30 seconds, repeated once.

Angiography

Angiography may be performed in swine in a similar fashion to other species. The angiographic images included in this section are provided to give anatomic guidance of structures of major importance in research in swine (Figs. 12.13–12.27). They were taken in 16-kg Yorkshire swine with iodine contrast solution (iohexol 350 mg/ml). An 8-Fr 110-cm Cordis catheter (inside dimension, 1.2 mm) with side holes was used. A Cordis automated injector was set at a volume of 14 ml, a delay of 0.15 sec, a pressure of 490 psi, and a rate of 14 ml/sec. The coronary arteriograms were taken using 7-Fr Judkins left and right coronary artery catheters with the same contrast material in a 43-kg Hanford pig. Instead of an automated injector, 10 ml of contrast solution was injected manually during cinefluorography. The size marker in the films is an 18-ga 1.5-inch hypodermic needle.

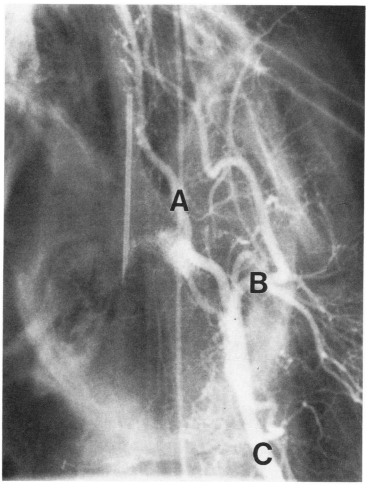

FIGURE 12.13   Ventrodorsal view of a cerebral angiogram with the catheter placed in the carotid artery. *A*-Rostral cerebral artery, *B*-External carotid artery and branches, *C*-Internal carotid artery.

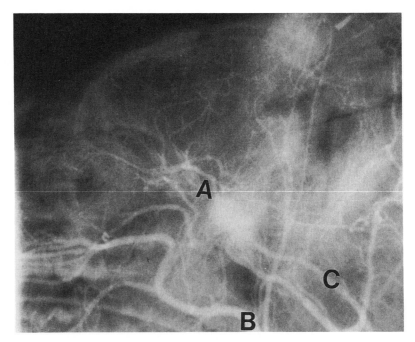

FIGURE 12.14   Lateral view of a cerebral angiogram with the catheter placed in the carotid artery. *A*-Rostral cerebral artery, *B*-Facial artery, *C*-Internal carotid artery.

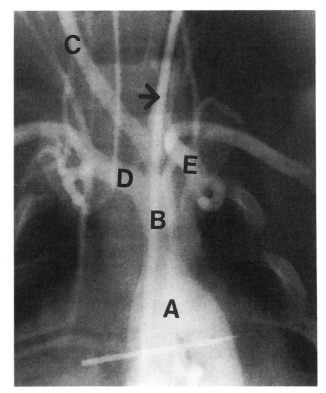

FIGURE 12.15   Ventrodorsal view of the arteries of the cranial thorax and neck with the catheter (*arrow*) placed at the aortic root. *A*-Aorta, *B*-Brachiocephalic trunk, *C*-Right carotid artery, *D*-Right subclavian artery, *E*-Left subclavian artery.

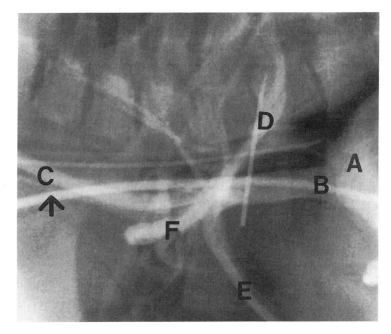

FIGURE 12.16   Lateral view of the arteries of the cranial thorax and neck with the
catheter (*arrow*) placed at the aortic root from the left carotid artery.
A-Aorta, *B*-Brachiocephalic trunk, *C*-Right carotid artery, *D*-Costo-
cervical trunk, *E*-Internal thoracic artery, *F*-Left subclavian artery.

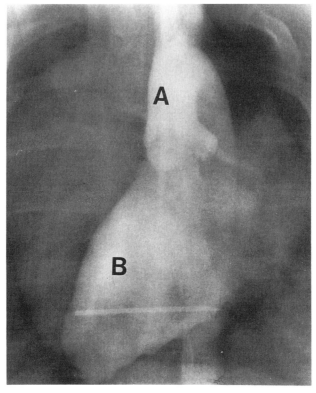

FIGURE 12.17   Ventrodorsal view of the left ventricular chamber. *A*-Aorta, *B*-Left
ventricle.

250

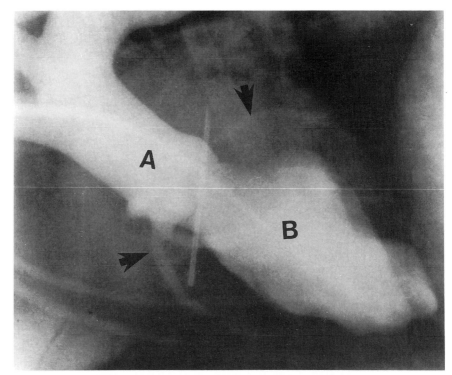

FIGURE 12.18   Lateral view of the left ventricular chamber. The coronary arteries are apparent (*arrows*). *A*-Aorta, *B*-Left ventricle.

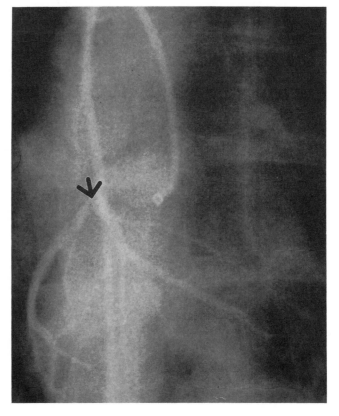

FIGURE 12.19   Left coronary (*arrow*) arteriogram, ventrodorsal view.

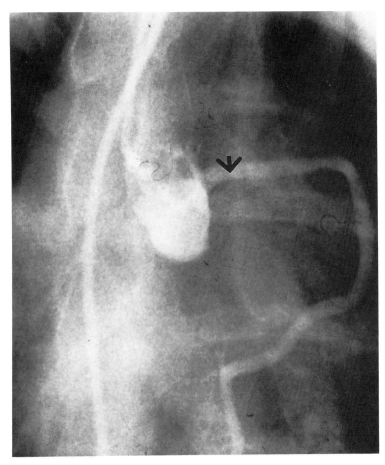

FIGURE 12.20   Right coronary (*arrow*) arteriogram, ventrodorsal view.

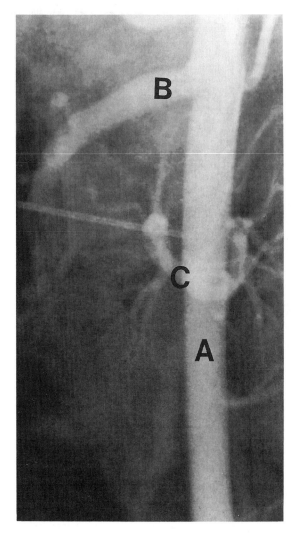

FIGURE 12.21   Ventrodorsal view of the root of the coeliac and cranial mesenteric arteries. *A*-Aorta, *B*-Celiac artery, *C*-Cranial mesenteric artery.

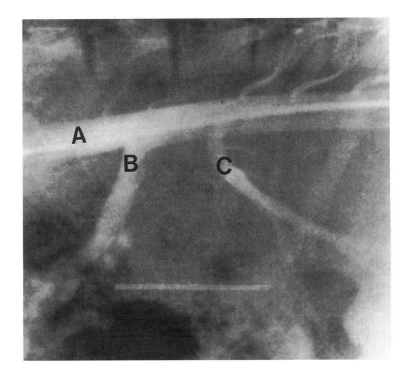

FIGURE 12.22   Lateral view of the root of the coeliac and cranial mesenteric arteries.
A-Aorta, *B*-Celiac artery, *C*-Cranial mesenteric artery.

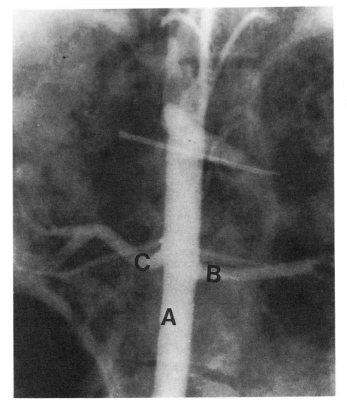

FIGURE 12.23   Ventrodorsal view of the renal arteries. *A*-Aorta, *B*-Right renal artery,
C-Left renal artery.

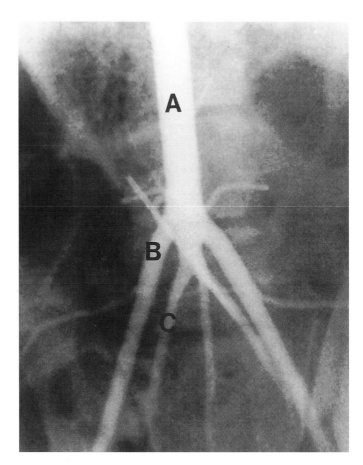

FIGURE 12.24   Ventrodorsal view of the iliac arteries. *A*-Aorta, *B*-External iliac artery, *C*-Internal iliac artery.

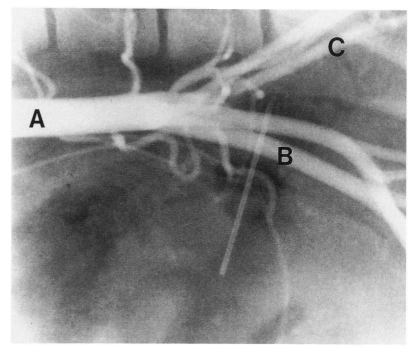

FIGURE 12.25   Lateral view of the iliac arteries. *A*-Aorta, *B*-External iliac artery, *C*-Internal iliac artery.

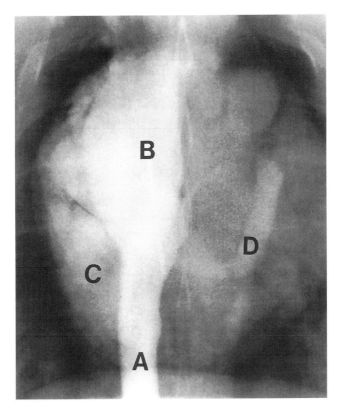

FIGURE 12.26   Ventrodorsal view of the right side of the heart. *A*-Caudal vena cava, *B*-Right atrium, *C*-Right ventricle, *D*-Reflux of contrast into the coronary sinus and left azygous (hemiazygous) vein.

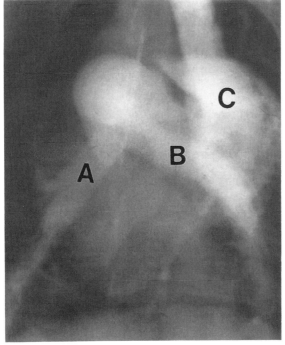

FIGURE 12.27   Ventrodorsal view of the pulmonary veins. *A*-Right pulmonary artery, *B*-Left pulmonary artery, *C*-Left atrium.

Echocardiography

Echocardiography can be challenging in swine because of the narrow intercostal spaces and wide ribs. Standard equipment used in humans can be utilized for porcine studies. Echocardiographic images of domestic, miniature, and fetal swine have been published. The figures in this chapter (Figs. 12.28–12.35) are examples of images of the heart in an 8-month-old female Hanford miniature pig weighing 36.5 kg.

M mode echocardiograph

Dimensions (cms)
controls

RVEDD: 0.9   (0.9-1.3)

LVEDD: 3.1   (1.9-2.6)

%FS: 0.29 (0.32-0.40)

IVS: 0.4   (0.3-0.5)

LVPW: 0.3   (0.3-0.5)

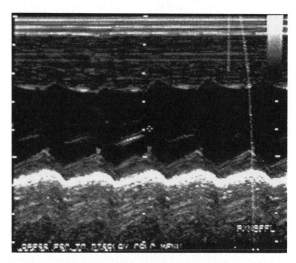

FIGURE 12.28   M mode echocardiogram. *RVEDD*-Right ventricular end diastolic dimension, *LVEDD*-Left ventricular end diastolic dimension, *%FS*-Fractional shortening, *IVS*-Interventricular septum, *LVPW*-Left ventricular posterior wall.

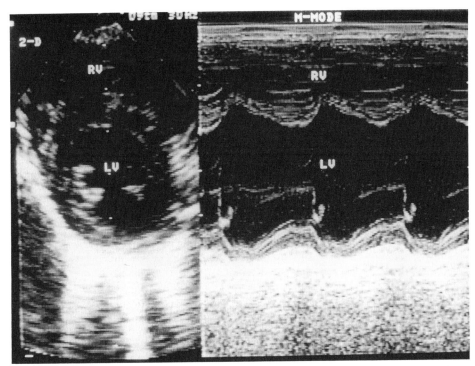

FIGURE 12.29   2D Directed M mode echocardiogram short axis view, *LV*-Left ventricle, *RV*-Right ventricle.

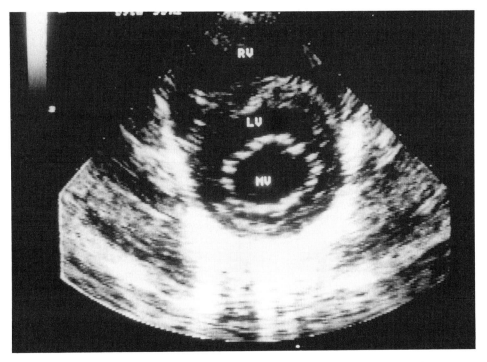

FIGURE 12.30   2D Short axis view echocardiogram, *RV*-Right ventricle, *LV*-Left ventricle, *MV*-Mitral valve.

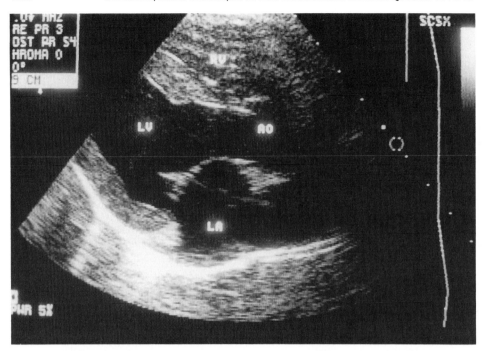

FIGURE 12.31   2D Long axis view (parasternal) echocardiogram, *LV*-Left ventricle, *AO*-Aorta, *LA*-Left atrium.

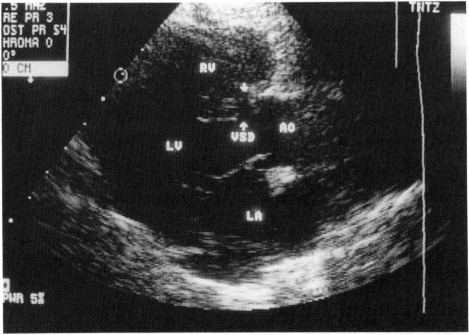

FIGURE 12.32   2D Long axis view echocardiogram of a pig with a ventricular septal defect (*VSD*), *RV*-Right ventricle, *LV*-Left ventricle, *AO*-Aorta, *LA*-Left atrium.

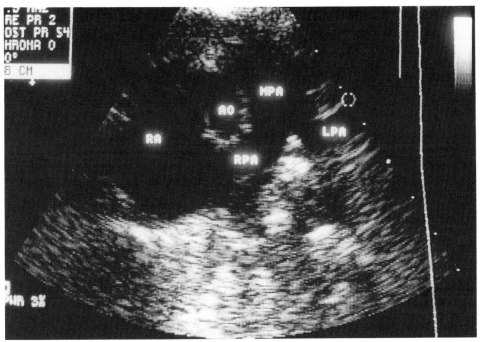

FIGURE 12.33   2D Short axis view (great vessels). *AO*-Aorta, *MPA*-Main pulmonary
                  artery, *LPA*-Left pulmonary artery, *RPA*-Right pulmonary artery,
                  RA-Right atrium.

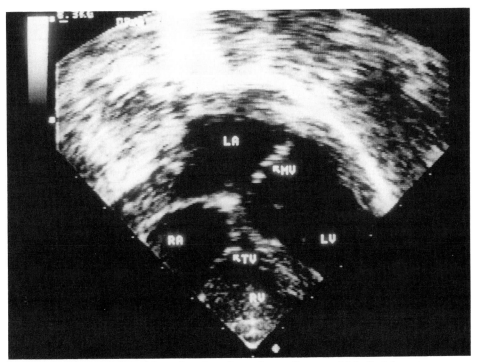

FIGURE 12.34   2D Apical four chamber view echocardiogram. *LA*-Left atrium,
                  MV-Mitral valve, *RA*-Right atrium, *LV*-Left ventricle, *RV*-Right ventricle,
                  TV-Tricuspid valve.

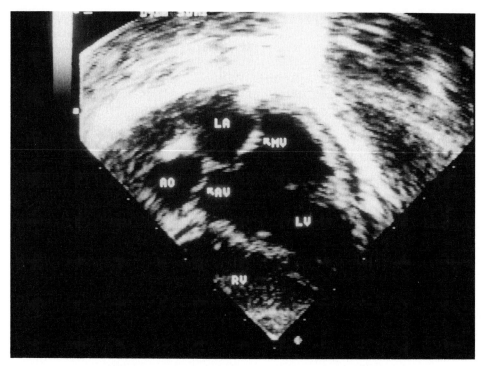

FIGURE 12.35   2D Apical four chamber long axis view. *LA*-Left atrium, *AO*-Aorta, *MV*-Mitral valve, *AV*-Aortic valve, *LV*-Left ventricle, *RV*-Right ventricle. *2D echos courtesy of Pediatric Cardiology, MUSC.*

References

Attie, A.D., R.J. Aiello, and W.J. Checovich. 1992. The spontaneously hypercholesterolemic pig as an animal model of human hypercholesterolemia. In Swindle, M.M. (ed), Swine as Models in Biomedical Research, Ames: Iowa State University Press, pp. 141–155.

Benharkate, M., V. Zanini, R. Blanc, O. Boucheix, F. Coyez, J.P. Genevois, and M. Pairet. 1993. Hemodynamic parameters of anesthetized pigs: A comparative study of farm piglets and Gottingen and Yucatan miniature swine. Lab. Anim. Sci. 43(1): 68–72.

Bharati, S., M. Levine, K. Shoei, S. Huang, B. Handler, G.V.S. Parr, R. Bauernfeind, and M. Lev. 1991. The conduction system of the swine heart. Chest 100(1): 207–212.

Brody, S., and H.H. Kibler. 1944. Table for measuring the body surface area of swine. Missouri University Agricultural Experimental Station Research Bulletin 380.

Brownlee, R.R., M.M. Swindle, R. Bertolet, and P. Neff. 1997. Toward optimizing a preshaped catheter and system parameters to achieve single lead DDD pacing. PACE 20(5, Pt 1): 1354–1358.

Buckley, N.M., P.M. Gootman, P. Brazeau, B.P. Matanic, I.D. Frasier, and E.L. Gentles. 1979. Cardiovascular function in anesthetized miniature swine. Lab. Anim. Sci. 29(2): 200–208.

Corin, W.J., M.M. Swindle, J.F. Spann, Jr., M. Frankis, W.W.R. Biederman, A. Smith, A. Taylor, and B.A. Carabello. 1988. The mechanism of decreased stroke volume in children and swine with ventricular septal defect and failure to thrive. J. Clin. Invest. 82(2): 544–551.

DeRoth, L.A., and A. Bisaillon. 1979. Determination of body surface area in neonatal swine. Lab. Anim. Sci. 29(2): 249–250.

Fujino, H., R.P. Thompson, P.G. Germroth, M.M. Swindle, C.L. Case, and P.C. Gillette. 1991. Histological comparison of cryothermia and radiofrequency catheter ablation in swine. Circulation 84(4)II: 514.

Fujino, H., R.P. Thompson, P.G. Germroth, M.E. Harold, M.M. Swindle, and P.C. Gillette. 1993. Histological study of chronic catheter cryoablation of atrioventricular conduction in swine. Am. Heart J. 125(6): 1632–1637.

Gal, D., and J.M. Isner. 1992. Atherosclerotic Yucatan microswine as a model for novel cardiovascular interventions and imaging. In Swindle, M.M. (ed), Swine as Models in Biomedical Research. Ames: Iowa State University Press, pp. 118–140.

Gardner, T.J., and D.L. Johnson. 1988. Cardiovascular system. In Swindle, M.M., and Adams, R.J. (eds), Experimental Surgery and Physiology: Induced Animal Models of Human Disease. Baltimore: Williams and Wilkins, pp. 74–124.

Gaymes, C.H., M.M. Swindle, P.C. Gillette, M.E. Harold, and R.E Schumann. 1995. Percutaneous serial catheterization in swine: a practical approach. J. Invest. Surg. 8(2): 123–128.

Gillette, P.C., and A. Garson, Jr. (eds). 1981. Pediatric Cardiac Dysrhythmias. New York: Grune and Stratton.

Gillette, P.C., and J.C. Griffin (eds). 1986. Practical Cardiac Pacing. Baltimore: Williams and Wilkins.

Gillette, P.C., M.M. Swindle, R.P. Thompson, and C.L. Case. 1991. Transvenous cryoablation of the bundle of His. PACE 14(4 Pt1): 504–510.

Grifka, R.G., G.W. Vick III, M.P. O'Laughlin, T.J. Myers, W.R. Morrow, M.R. Nihill, D.L. Kearney, and C.E. Mullins. 1993. Balloon-expandable intravascular stents: Aortic implantation and later furthur dilation in growing mini-pigs. Am. Heart J. 126(4): 979–984.

Hannon, J.P. 1992. Hemorrhage and hemorrhagic shock in swine. A review. In Swindle, M.M. (ed), Swine as Models in Biomedical Research. Ames: Iowa State University Press, pp. 197–245.

Hughes, H.C. 1986. Swine in cardiovascular research. Lab. Anim. Sci. 36(4): 348–350.

Kelley, K.W., S.E. Curtis, G.T. Marzan, H.M. Karara, and C.R. Anderson. 1973. Body surface area of female swine. J. Anim. Sci. 36(5): 927–930.

Lee, K.T., D.N. Kim, and W.A. Thomas. 1986. Atherosclerosis in swine. In Stanton, H.C., and Mersmann, H.J. (ed), Swine in Cardiovascular Research, Vol. 1. Boca Raton, FL: CRC Press, pp. 33–48.

Lock, J.E., T. Niemi, B.A. Burke, S. Einzig, and W. Castaneda-Zuniga. 1982. Transcutaneous angioplasty of experimental aortic coarctation. Circulation 6(6): 1280–1286.

Lock, J.E., J.L. Bass, G. Lund, J.A. Rysavy, and R.V. Lucas, Jr. 1985. Transcatheter closure of patent ductus arteriosus in piglets. Am. J. Cardiol. 55(6): 826–829.

Lund, G., J. Rysavy, A. Cragg, E. Salomonowitz, Z. Vlodaver, W.C. Zuniga, and K. Amplatz. 1984. Long-term patency of the ductus arteriosus after balloon dilatation: An experimental study. Circulation 69(4): 772–775.

McKenzie, J.E. 1996. Swine as a model in cardiovascular research. In Tumbleson, M.E., and Schook, L.B. (eds), Advances in Swine in Biomedical Research, Vol. 1. New York: Plenum Press, pp. 7–18.

McKirnan, M.D., F.C. White, B.D. Guth, and C.M. Bloor. 1986. Exercise and hemodynamic studies in swine. In Stanton HC, and Mersmann, H.J. (ed), Swine in Cardiovascular Research, Vol. 2. Boca Raton: FL: CRC Press, pp. 105–120.

Mitchell, S.E., J.H. Anderson, M.M. Swindle, J.D. Strandberg, and J. Kan. 1994. Atrial septostomy: Stationary angioplasty balloon technique. Experimental work and preliminary clinical applications. Pediatr. Cardiol. 15(1): 1–7.

Morrow, W.R., V.C. Smith, W.J. Ehler, A.F. Van Dellen, and C.E. Mullins. 1994. Balloon angioplasty with stent implantation in experimental coarctation of the aorta. Circulation 89(6): 2677–2683.

Murphy, J.G., R.S. Schwartz, W.D. Edwards, A.R. Camrud, R.E. Vliestra, and D.R. Holmes, Jr. 1992. Percutaneous polymeric stents in porcine coronary arteries: Initial experience with polyethylene terephthalate stents. Circulation 86(5): 1596–1604.

Randsbaek, F., C.J. Riordan, J.H. Storey, W.D. Montgomery, W.P. Santamore, and E.H. Austin III. 1996. Animal model of the univentricular heart and single ventricular physiology. J. Invest. Surg. 9(4): 375–384.

Rashkind, W.J., C.E. Mullins, W.E. Hellenbrand, and M.A. Tait. 1987. Nonsurgical closure of patent ductus arteriosus: Clinical application of the Rashkind PDA occluder system. Circulation 75(3): 583–592.

Rogers, G.P., D.M. Cromeens, S.T. Minor, and M.M. Swindle. 1988. Bretylium and diltiazem in porcine cardiac procedures, J. Invest. Surg. 1(4): 321–326.

Schumann, R.E., M. Harold, P.C. Gillette, M.M. Swindle, and C.H. Gaymes. 1993. Prophylactic treatment of swine with bretylium for experimental cardiac catheterization. Lab. Anim. Sci. 43(3): 244–246.

Schumann, R.E., M.M. Swindle, B.J. Knick, C.L. Case, and P.C. Gillette. 1994. High dose narcotic anesthesia using sufentanil in swine for cardiac catheterization and electrophysiologic studies. J. Invest. Surg. 7(3): 243–248.

Smith, A.C., F.G. Spinale, B.A. Carabello, and M.M. Swindle. 1989. Technical aspects of cardiac catheterization of swine. J. Invest. Surg. 2(2): 187–194.

Smith, A.C., F.G. Spinale, and M.M. Swindle. 1990. Cardiac function and morphology of Hanford miniature swine and Yucatan miniature and micro swine. Lab. Anim. Sci. 40(1): 47–50.

Smith, A.C., J.L. Zellner, F.G. Spinale, and M.M. Swindle. 1991. Sedative and cardiovascular effects of midazolam in swine. Lab. Anim. Sci. 41(2): 157–161.

Smith, A.C., B. Knick, M.M. Swindle, and P.C. Gillette. 1997. A technique for conducting non-invasive cardiac electrophysiology studies in swine, J. Invest. Surg. 10(1–2): 25–30.

Starling, M.B., J.M. Neutze, R.L. Elliott, I.M. Taylor, and R.B. Elliott. 1978. The effects of some methyl prostaglandin derivatives on the ductus arteriosus of swine in vivo. Prostaglandins Med. 1(4): 267–281.

Swindle, M.M., R.P. Thompson, B.A. Carabello, A.C. Smith, C. Green, and P.C. Gillette. 1992. Congenital cardiovascular disease. In Swindle, M.M. (ed), Swine as Models in Biomedical Research. Ames: Iowa State University Press, pp. 176–184.

Swindle, M.M., A.C. Smith, K. Laber-Laird, and L. Dungan. 1994. Swine in biomedical research: Management and models. ILAR News 36(1): 1–5.

Truex, R.C., and M.Q. Smythe. 1965. Comparative morphology of the cardiac conduction tissue in animals. Ann. NY Acad. Sci. 127: 19–23.

Verdouw, P.D., and J.M. Hartog. 1986. Provocation and suppression of ventricular arrhythmias in domestic swine. In Stanton, H.C., Mersmann, H.J. (eds), Swine in Cardiovascular Research, Vol. 2. Boca Raton: CRC Press, pp. 121–156.

Vogl, H.W., A.E. Colletti, and E.J. Zambraski. 1997. Nitric oxide inhibition causes an exaggerated pressor response in Yucatan miniature swine. Lab. Anim. Sci. 47(2)161–166.

Wachtel, T.L., G.R. McCahan, Jr., W.I. Watson, and M. Gorman. 1972. Determining the surface areas of miniature swine and domestic swine by geometric design. A comparative study. USAARL Report 73-5, Fort Rucker, AL.

White, C.J., S.R. Ramee, A.K. Banks, D. Wiktor, and H.L. Price. 1992. The Yucatan miniature swine: An atherogenic model to assess the early potency rates of an endovascular stent. In Swindle, M.M. (ed), Swine as Models in Biomedical Research, Ames: Iowa State University Press, pp. 156–162.

Willette, R.N., H. Zhang, C. Louden, and R.K. Jackson. 1996. Comparing porcine models of restenosis. In Tumbleson, M.E., and Schook, L.B. (eds), Advances in Swine in Biomedical Research, Vol. 2. New York: Plenum Press, pp. 595–606.

13 ENDOSCOPIC/ LAPAROSCOPIC SURGERY

M. M. Swindle, R. H. Hawes, and W. Knapple

Introduction

Minimally invasive surgery (Fig. 13.1), especially celioscopic and thoracoscopic techniques, is capable of replacing many of the open operations described in this textbook. Although the field has only recently been developed, these techniques have replaced many open surgical procedures in humans, because they offer the advantages of decreased morbidity, shortened recovery, and an improved cosmetic effect. However, performing these procedures requires the learning of a new set of skills beyond those of open surgery. New techniques and instruments develop so rapidly that their use in experimental and clinical settings out paces their documentation in the literature. Porcine models have been important in both the development of these techniques and in the training of surgeons (Bailey et al., 1991; Freeman, 1994; Kopchok et al., 1993; Lyons and Sosa, 1992; Soper and Hunter, 1992).

Endoscopic techniques have advanced beyond diagnosis into treatment and implantation of devices. These therapeutic techniques also require advanced skills beyond those of diagnostic endoscopy. Here again, the porcine model has been and will be important in both teaching and development of new techniques (Freys et al., 1995; Ma and Fang, 1994; Noar, 1995; Pasricha et al., 1995; Rey and Romanczyk, 1995).

It is beyond the scope of this chapter to describe every technique that can be performed either endoscopically or laparoscopically. Rather, this text will discuss the general principles of performing these techniques, because development of new

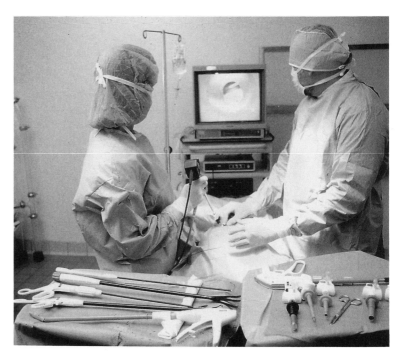

FIGURE 13.1   Operating room for laparoscopic surgery technique.

techniques and instruments is frequently the purpose of the research protocol.

Methodologies of prepping and anesthetizing the animals for these proce-dures, as well as the anatomy, are discussed in the various system chapters and in Chapter 2. However, some of the intraoperative and preoperative proce-dures, such as the fasting techniques, are essential for these procedures and are repeated within some of the sections in this chapter.

Endoscopic/Bronchoscopic Surgery

Endoscopic procedures refer to the nonsurgical examination and therapeutic interventions in hollow and viscus organs using catheters with visualization capabilities. Technological advances in these procedures make the use of ani-mal models essential in both the training and development of new techniques. Training protocols should include inanimate models, computer simulations, and/or necropsy specimens as part of the program prior to performing the techniques in live animals. Porcine models in the 20–34 kg weight range are ac-ceptable as models for most of the endoscopic instruments in clinical practice (Freys et al., 1995; Ma and Fang, 1994; Noar, 1995; Pasricha et al., 1995; Rey and Romanczyk, 1995).

The porcine model has both advantages and disadvantages as a model for these techniques (Figs. 13.2–13.6). The porcine stomach is in a tighter J-shaped curve than the human stomach, and a muscular outpouching, the torus pyloricus, is located adjacent to the pylorus (Freys et al., 1995; Rey and Romanczyk, 1995). The biliary papilla is located 1–2 cm distal to the pylorus and is separate from the pancreatic ductal papilla. The orifice of the pancreatic duct is located 7–12 cm distal to the biliary papilla and is extremely difficult to distinguish from inside the duodenum, although it is readily located surgically. Function of the sphincter of Oddi and the pressures within the biliary system (see Chapter 5) are similar to that of humans (Noar, 1995; Pasricha et al., 1995). The pig is reported to have differences in the amplitude of phasic contractions with significantly lower values than humans (Noar, 1995). The functions of the pancreas and pancreatic duct (see Chapter 6) are similar to humans, even though the gross anatomy is different (Mullen et al., 1992; Pasricha et al., 1995; Stump et al., 1988). The spiral colon and lack of a true sigmoid flexure also provide differences in anatomy from the human (see Chapter 4).

Endoscopic retrograde cholangiopancreatography (ERCP) is a technique (Figs. 13.7 and 13.8) for which the pig may have particular usage, even with the differences in anatomy noted above (Gholson et al., 1990; Noar, 1995). The pig is the primary model for biliary sphincterotomy and biliary stenting. Nonhuman primates and cats have a common opening for the biliary and pancreatic duct, however, cats are too small for most equipment and appropriately sized primates, such as the baboon (Siegel and Korsten, 1989), are expensive and difficult to obtain. The dog also has problems with availability, and size of the

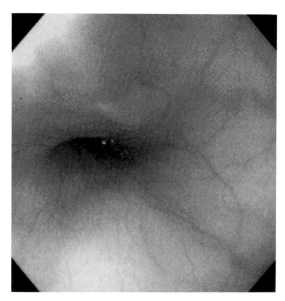

FIGURE 13.2   Endoscopic view of the esophagus.

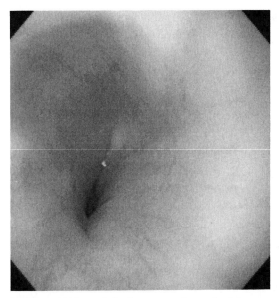

FIGURE 13.3   Endoscopic view of the lower esophageal sphincter.

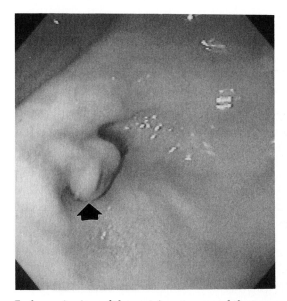

FIGURE 13.4   Endoscopic view of the gastric antrum and the torus pyloricus (*arrow*).

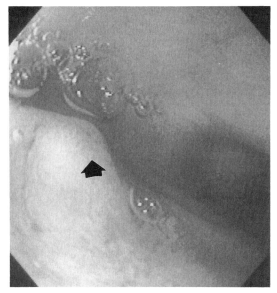

FIGURE 13.5   Endoscopic view of the biliary papilla (*arrow*).

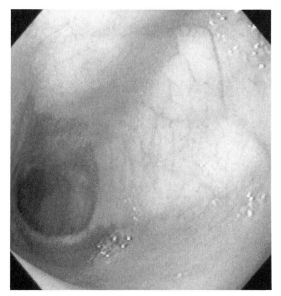

FIGURE 13.6   Endoscopic view of the duodenum.

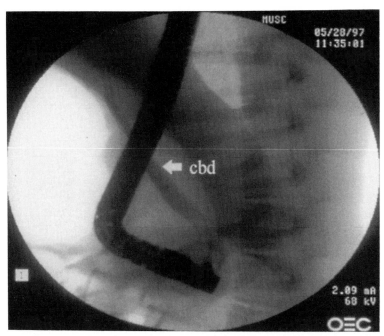

FIGURE 13.7   Retrograde cholangiogram of the common bile duct (*cbd*).

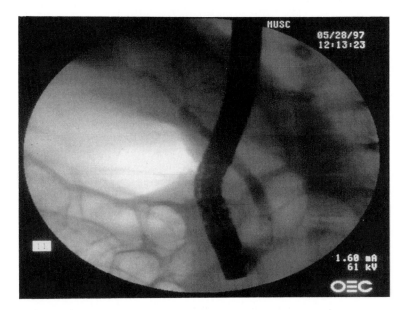

FIGURE 13.8   Retrograde cholangiogram of the common bile duct with retrograde flow
into the hepatic biliary system.

structures can vary substantially among animals of the same weight because of breed differences. However, the dog has been uniquely useful in some procedures, such as the development of a model of esophageal varices (Jensen et al., 1983).

Implantation of gallstones has been performed in swine to make a more realistic model (Griffith et al., 1989). Endoscopic procedures have been modified for mandibular angle surgery (Ma and Fang, 1994) and for retroperitoneal adrenalectomy (Brunt et al., 1993).

The basic technique of gastrointestinal endoscopy involves careful passage of the lubricated endoscopic device into the area of interest using air insufflation anterior to the passage of the tube to accommodate the device without trauma to the animal.

Animals should be fully anesthetized and intubated (see Chapter 2). Fasting instructions and methods of bowel evacuation for gastrointestinal procedures are discussed in Chapter 4. Fasting for 48 hours in a cage without contact bedding is essential for these procedures. It is not desirable to eliminate water unless it is of importance to a particular gastric procedure. Electrolyte/glucose and/or protein supplements as described in Chapter 4 may be given as liquid diets during the 48-hour fast without producing significant residue. This also provides the animals with a form of nutrition that will prevent them from being compromised physiologically for these procedures.

Care should be taken to avoid passing the device into the pharyngeal diverticulum when entering the esophagus. The minimal amount of insufflation that is necessary for observation and passage of the device should be used. Glucagon is administered iv intraoperatively to prevent peristalsis. It is administered in 0.25- to 0.5-mg dosages by slow injection as required. It is essential to use a veterinary mouth gag to prevent the sharp teeth from damaging the tip of the endoscopes.

It is also essential in endoscopic procedures to avoid overinsufflation (> 8 mmHg) of the gut lumen. This can produce a vagal response resulting in cardiac arrest. Insufflation should be performed slowly and judiciously as required for observation rather than continually administering air.

When the endoscope enters the stomach, the pylorus is located close to the entrance of the esophagus after manipulating through the J-shaped stomach (Figs. 13.3–13.5). The torus pyloricus is a landmark for the biliary orifice and pylorus. The pylorus is entered in the usual fashion. The bile duct orifice can usually be located readily 1–2 cm distal to the torus pyloricus. Observation of bile at the papilla is common. It is entered with a counterclockwise rotation. The pancreatic orifice is indistinct but can be located in most animals with experience (Noar, 1995; Pasricha et al., 1995). The small intestine may be observed using the same methodologies as for other species. Air or saline tonometry can be used to estimate gastrointestinal mucosal carbon dioxide tension in swine (Salzman et al., 1994).

Entering the animal rectally for colonoscopy requires the same caution as for oral entry to avoid rupture of the colon. The colon may be observed in the same manner as for other species, with the exception of the spiral colon, which is located in the left upper quadrant of the abdomen (see Chapter 6).

Laryngoscopy and bronchoscopy can also be performed in swine. The anatomy is discussed in Chapter 9. Two precautions are necessary when using this technology. The epiglottis and larynx are very prone to spasm and edematous swelling with manipulation. The lateral ventricles of the larynx are also easily ruptured resulting in subcutaneous emphysema. The larynx should always be sprayed with topical anesthetics, and appropriate-sized devices should be used to prevent trauma. Swine are also very susceptible to vagal stimulation and bradycardia with manipulation of the airway. Animals should always be atropinized during the entire procedure (see Chapter 2). Isoproterenol is useful to prevent bronchospasm.

Laparoscopic/Celioscopic/Thoracoscopic Surgery

The minimally invasive surgical techniques that are rapidly developing will replace many of the open surgical techniques now in clinical practice. The porcine model has proved to be invaluable in both training and development. The basic techniques involve insufflating a body cavity with CO_2, placing trocars, and using camera guidance to perform surgical techniques with specialized instruments through the trocars. Specialized suturing and instrument-handling techniques, different from those of open surgery, are required.

When using swine for training, nonsurvival techniques are preferred, because they allow the surgeon the chance to perform multiple procedures and do not require close attention to aseptic techniques. Some laboratories have used survival surgery for training and returned the animals to the food chain. In this case, an approved program of postoperative care and careful attention to drug withdrawal times must be maintained and documented to avoid violations of federal law as administered by the United States Department of Agriculture (USDA). It is also highly recommended that training programs be conducted only in facilities with an approved USDA registration as a research institution. The liability of conducting training sessions outside of registered research facilities is not worth the risk of either potential violations of Federal law or problems with public relations. New regulations being written by the USDA to include farm animals will probably make this precaution a necessity. Training courses should include the use of inanimate models and/or computer simulations prior to performing the techniques on live animals. Most procedures and instruments can be utilized in swine weighing 25–35 kg. Reviews of recommendations for training of surgeons have been published (Bailey et al., 1991; Freeman, 1994; Kopchok et al., 1993; Lyons and Sosa, 1992; Soper and Hunter, 1992).

Swine are usually positioned in dorsal recumbency for these procedures, but the positioning may have to be varied for retroperitoneal and thoracic procedures. The positioning of the trocars and the insufflation needle depends upon the procedure being performed. Standard positions are described here as an example (Fig. 13.9). A Veress needle is positioned at the umbilicus and the abdomen is inflated to 12–14 mmHg with CO_2. As a minimum, a trocar is required for insertion of a camera, usually near the umbilicus, so that the procedure can be viewed on a TV screen and a second trocar is required to insert and manipulate the surgical instruments. As many as four secondary trocars for instrumentation may be required, depending upon the procedure and types of instruments. Instrumentation trocars are positioned so that the area of surgical interest can be seen and manipulated with the least interference with surrounding structures.

Insufflation of the abdomen and thorax causes hemodynamic changes, and

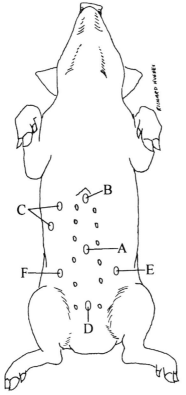

FIGURE 13.9   Examples of laparoscopic surgical trocar sites. *A*-Site for placement of Veress needle and camera trocar, *B*-Large trocar site for upper abdominal procedures, *C*-Site for small trocars in paramedian and lateral positions for upper abdominal procedures, *D*-Large trocar site for lower abdominal procedures, *E,F*-Sites for small trocars for caudal abdominal procedures.

monitoring the intraabdominal pressure is essential. Creating a pneumoperi-toneum with CO_2 increases the arterial pCO_2 and reduces the pH. It has been demonstrated that using helium as the gas eliminates this respiratory acidosis (Leighton et al., 1993). Both the reverse Trendelenburg position and the in-crease in intraabdominal pressure caused by insufflation reduce the venous blood flow from the lower limbs, which could predispose to venous thrombo-sis and pulmonary embolism (Jorgensen et al., 1994). The effects of insuffla-tion during thoracoscopy are even more dramatic. Significant decreases in car-diac index, mean arterial pressure, stroke volume, and left ventricular stroke work index were noted with pressures greater than 5 mmHg. In the same study, central venous pressure increased (Jones et al., 1993). In pigs, 25–35 kg, rou-tinely used for these procedures, the mediastinum is thin and easily ruptured, and precautions should be taken both with the use of insufflation and the placement of chest tubes (see Chapter 9). The diaphragmatic communication between the peritoneal and pleural cavities in young swine is easily ruptured, and gas in either cavity is likely to penetrate the other cavity if the pressure is high enough (Freeman, 1994; Swindle et al., 1988).

At the end of the procedure, the cavity is examined for hemostasis and proper tissue apposition. Following desufflation, the peritoneum, muscle, and skin layers penetrated by the trocars are closed with sutures or staples.

Freeman (1994) has written a succinct synopsis of the most common tech-niques used for training in swine, and that publication, in conjunction with the technical descriptions provided by others, will be used as examples of the types of technical variations that are used in performing various laparoscopic surgical techniques.

Cholecystectomy

Two 5-mm and one 10- or 12-mm trocars are inserted into the cranial ab-domen. The gallbladder (Fig. 13.10) is bluntly dissected to the cystic duct and ligated. The gallbladder is removed through the large trocar and may be emp-tied with suction prior to removal (Pasricha et al., 1995; Rodriguez et al., 1993; Soper et al., 1991; Soper et al., 1993). The open technique is described in Chap-ter 5.

Small Intestinal Anastomosis

Four 10- or 12-mm trocars are inserted in the paramedian position over the area of interest. The standard techniques of identification of a segment, isola-tion, and anastomosis are described in Chapter 4 and are performed with la-paroscopic instruments, sutures, and staples. The anastomosis must be checked for patency, and the mesenteric defect closed with this technique as well. The excised segment is removed through one of the trocars after closure.

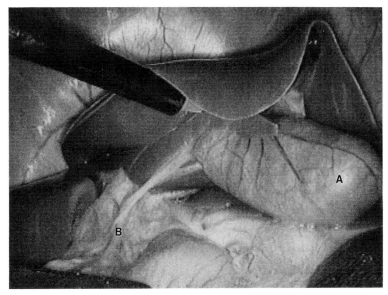

FIGURE 13.10   Laparoscopic views. *A*-Gallbladder, *B*-Common bile duct.

Laparoscopic techniques have been demonstrated to be as effective as open techniques when wound healing and complications were compared (Fleshman et al., 1993; Noel et al., 1994; Olson et al., 1995; Pietrafitta et al., 1992; Soper et al., 1993).

Colonic Anastomosis

As for small intestinal anastomosis, four secondary 10- or 12-mm trocars are positioned in the paramedian position; however, they are in the caudal abdomen. A staple anastomosis is performed after mobilization of the segment to be excised. Both intracorporeal and extracorporeal techniques have been utilized. For the extracorporeal technique, the proximal segment is externalized through the right lower quadrant. The circular stapler may be placed through the anus if the anastomotic site is distal. Colonic anastomosis using these techniques has been demonstrated to be as effective as the open techniques described in Chapter 4 (Fleshman et al., 1993; Noel et al., 1994; Olson et al., 1995; Pietrafitta et al., 1992; Soper et al., 1993).

Vagotomy and Hiatal Procedures

Four 5-mm or 10- or 12-mm trocars are used in the cranial abdomen. The vagus nerve can be identified along the margin of the esophagus, or selective vagotomy procedures at the level of the stomach can be performed (Fig. 13.11). Hiatal hernias can be created and repaired as well as the performance of fundo-

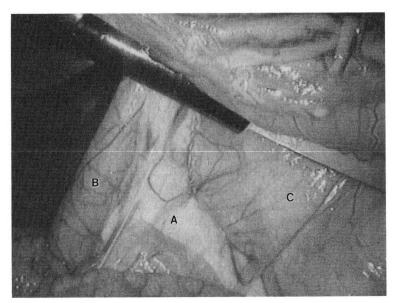

FIGURE 13.11   Laparoscopic views. *A*-Pancreas, *B*-Duodenum, *C*-Stomach.

plications. Procedures in this region require atropinization of the animal to prevent vagal, induced bradycardia. Pneumothorax is also a potentially fatal complication associated with the dissection and must be monitored by the anesthetist and relieved with chest tubes, if necessary (Freeman, 1994; Josephs et al., 1992).

Nephrectomy

Either a paramedian or a retroperitoneal approach may be made to the kidney with three 10- or 12-mm trocars (Fig. 13.12). After dissection and ligation of the blood vessels, the kidney may be removed with a larger trocar or a specimen retrieval bag after morcellation (Chiu et al., 1992; Kerbl et al., 1993). The open techniques are described in Chapter 7.

Inguinal Herniorrhaphy

Spontaneous inguinal hernias of swine or dissected inguinal rings (Fig. 13.13) of male swine may be used as models. Two secondary 10- or 12-mm trocars are introduced in the caudal abdomen. For this procedure the edges of the peritoneum around the inguinal ring are dissected free from the inguinal ring and a prosthetic mesh is inserted and stapled in place. The insufflation pressure is reduced to facilitate proper alignment of the tissues prior to placing the last staples and closure of the peritoneum (Layman et al., 1993). The inguinal ring may also be repaired using a preperitoneal approach. From the midline, the

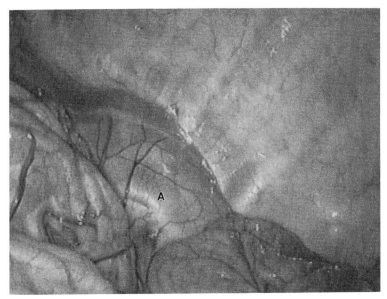

FIGURE 13.12   Laparoscopic view. *A*-Right kidney.

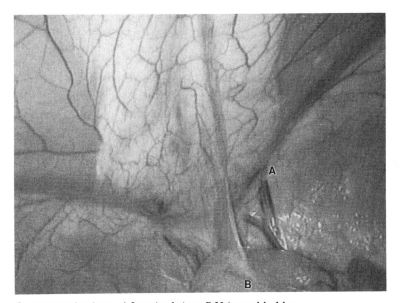

FIGURE 13.13   Laparoscopic views. *A*-Inguinal ring, *B*-Urinary bladder.

trocars are inserted without penetration of the peritoneum. After insufflation, the operating trocars are inserted lateral to the midline below the umbilicus and cranial to the pubis (Freeman, 1994). Inguinal hernias are discussed in Chapter 11.

Appendectomy

The pig does not have an appendix, however, one can be created as an acute model for training purposes from a loop of small intestine or uterine horn. For this procedure, two 10- or 12-mm trocars are introduced on either side of the midline. A loop of the structure has its blood supply ligated, and pretied loop ligatures are placed at the base of the loop (Freeman, 1994).

Splenectomy

The spleen may be removed after placing four secondary 10- or 12-mm trocars in the cranial abdomen. The vascular supply is ligated or stapled and the organ reduced in size with a morcellation device prior to removal. The spleen can be removed through a 33-mm trocar site (Freeman, 1994). Splenectomy is discussed in Chapter 4.

Adrenalectomy

With the pig in ventral recumbency, a unilateral adrenalectomy may be performed in the retroperitoneal space. Trocars are placed in the flank without penetrating the peritoneum, and the retroperitoneal space is insufflated. After ligation of the blood vessels and removal of the structure through 10- or 12-mm trocars, the retroperitoneal space is desufflated and closed in a routine fashion. Care should be taken to avoid penetration of the diaphragm from this position with a trocar (Brunt et al., 1993). Adrenalectomy is discussed in Chapter 7.

Urinary Bladder Procedures

Urinary procedures are discussed in Chapter 7. Laparoscopic urinary incontinence procedures have been described (Ou et al., 1993; Vancaillie, 1993). Two or three 10- or 12-mm trocars are placed in the right and left caudal quadrants of the abdomen. After tissue dissection to expose the urethra, a mesh or sutures are placed in the perivaginal tissue and anchored to Cooper's ligament.

Reproductive Procedures

The uterus of the pig is bicornuate with a small body (see Chapter 8). The anatomy of the structure is dissimilar to human anatomy, and the goat is the preferred model for uterine body procedures and hysterectomy (Freeman, 1994). However, the porcine model may be used for ovarian and Fallopian tube procedures, such as ovariectomy and tubal ligation.

Thoracoscopy

Because of the precautions described above and in Chapter 9, the procedure should not be performed with insufflation of the thoracic cavity. Rather, single lung ventilation can be performed after unilateral intubation of the right main stem bronchus. Auscultation can be used to confirm the correct placement of the tube. Pneumothorax on the left side will be produced when the trocars are inserted and the lung collapses. Depending upon the procedure that is performed, the trocars can be inserted into the appropriate intercostal spaces with the pig in dorsal, ventral, or lateral recumbency (Freeman, 1994).

Laparoscopic Ultrasonography

A semiflexible ultrasound transducer introduced through a laparoscopic port has been utilized to visualize abdominal structures. The transducer uses both gray-scale and color Doppler techniques to observe normal structures, to aid dissection and also to diagnose abnormalities, such as gallstones. In this study, a 9.6-mm diameter catheter with a 5.0–7.5 mHz transducer was found to be applicable in both miniature swine and humans (Liu et al., 1995).

If the surgeries are performed as survival procedures, appropriate postoperative care must be administered, including the use of postoperative analgesics. Discomfort may be associated secondary to the introduction of CO_2 into the peritoneal cavity. Animals should also be monitored for respiratory acidosis and the potential of a tension pneumothorax.

References

Bailey, R.W., A.L. Imbembo, and K.A. Zucker. 1991. Establishment of a laparoscopic cholecystectomy training program. Am. Surg. 57(4): 231–236.

Brunt, L.M., E.P. Molmenti, K. Kerbl, N.J. Soper, A.M. Stone, and R.V. Clayman. 1993. Retroperitoneal endoscopic adrenalectomy: An experimental study. Surg. Laparoscop. Endoscop. 3(4): 300–306.

Chiu, A.W., M.T. Chen, W.J. Huang, S.T. Young, C. Cheng, S.W. Huang, C.L. Chu, and L.S. Chang. 1992. Laparoscopic nephrectomy in a porcine model. Eur. Urol. 22(3): 250–254.

Fleshman, J.W., L.M. Brunt, R.D. Fry, E.H. Birnbaum, C.L. Simmang, A. Mazor, N. Soper, L. Freeman, and I.J. Kodner. 1993. Laparoscopic anterior resection of the rectum using a triple stapled intracorporeal anastomosis in the pig. Surg. Laparoscop. Endoscop. 3(2): 119–126.

Freeman, L.J. 1994. Laparoscopic surgery courses, In Smith, A.C., and Swindle, M.M. (eds), Research Animal Anesthesia, Analgesia and Surgery. Greenbelt, MD: Scientists Center for Animal Welfare, pp. 15–24.

Freys, S.M., J. Heimbucher, and K.H. Fuchs. 1995. Teaching upper gastrointestinal endoscopy: The pig stomach. Endoscopy 27(1): 73–76.

Gholson, C.F., J.M. Provenza, R.C. Silver, and B. Bacon. 1990. Endoscopic retrograde cholangiography in the swine: A new model for endoscopic training and hepatobiliary research. Gastrointest. Endoscop. 36(6): 600–603.

Griffith, S.L., B.T. Burney, F.J. Fry, and T.D. Franklin, Jr. 1989. A large animal model (swine) to study the diagnosis and treatment of cholelithiasis. Invest. Radiol. 24(2): 110–114.

Jensen, D.M., G.A. Machicado, J.I. Tapia, G. Kauffman, P. Franco, and D. Beilin. 1983. A reproducible canine model of esophageal varices. Gastroenterology 84(3): 573–579.

Jones, D.R., G.M. Graeber, G.G. Tanguilig, G. Hobbs, and G.F. Murray. 1993. Effects of insufflation on hemodynamics during thoracoscopy. Ann. Thorac. Surg. 55(6): 1379–1382.

Jorgensen, J.O., R.B. Gillies, N.J. Lalak, and D.R. Hunt. 1994. Lower limb venous hemodynamics during laparoscopy: An animal study. Surg. Laparosc. Endoscop. 4(1): 32–35.

Josephs, L.G., J.H. Arnold, and J.L. Sawyers. 1992. Laparoscopic highly selective vagotomy. J. Laparoendoscopic Surg. 2(3): 151–153.

Kerbl, K., R.S. Figneshau, R.V. Clayman, P.S. Chadhoke, L.R. Kavoussi, D.M. Albala, and A.M. Stone. 1993. Retroperitoneal laparoscopic nephrectomy: Laboratory and clinical experience. J. Endourol. 7(1): 23–26.

Kopchok, G.E., D.M. Cavaye, S.R. Klein, M.P. Mueller, J.L. Lee, and R.A. White. 1993. Endoscopic surgery training: Application of an in vitro trainer and in vivo swine model J. Invest. Surg. 6(4): 329–337.

Layman, T.S., R.P. Burns, K.E. Chandler, W.L. Russell, and R.G. Cook. 1993. Laparoscopic inguinal herniorrhaphy in a swine model. Am. Surg. 59(1): 13–19.

Leighton, T.A., S.Y. Liu, and F.S. Bongard. 1993. Comparative cardiopulmonary effects of carbon dioxide versus helium pneumoperitoneum. Surgery 113(5): 527–531.

Liu, J.B., R.I. Feld, B.B. Goldberg, D.J. Barbot, L.N. Nazarian, D.A. Merton, N.M. Rawool, F.E. Rosato, C.A. Winkel, and D.R. Gillum. 1995. Laparoscopic gray-scale and color Doppler US: Preliminary animal and clinical studies. Radiology 194(3): 851–857.

Lyons, J.M., and R.E. Sosa. 1992. Laparoscopy: New applications of an established technique. Urol. Nurs. 12(1): 2–8.

Ma, S., and R.H. Fang. 1994. Endoscopic mandibular angle surgery—A swine model. Ann. Plastic Surg. 33(5): 473–475.

Mullen, Y., Y. Taura, M. Nagsta, K. Miyazawa, and E. Stein. 1992. Swine as a model for pancreatic beta-cell transplantation. In Swindle, M.M. (ed), Swine as Models in Biomedical Research. Ames: Iowa State University Press, pp. 16–34.

Noar, M.D. 1995. An established porcine model for animate training in diagnostic and therapeutic ERCP. Endoscopy 27(1): 77–80.

Noel, P., H. Fagot, J.M. Fabre, C. Mann, F. Quenet, F. Guillon, H. Baumel, and J. Domergue. 1994. Resection anastomosis of the small intestine by celioscopy in swine. Comparative experimental study between manual and mechanical anastomosis. Ann. Chir. 48(10): 921–929.

Olson, K.H., E.G. Balcos, M.C. Lowe, and M.P. Bubrick. 1995. A comparative study of open, laparoscopic intracorporeal and laparoscopic assisted low anterior resection and anastomosis in pigs. Am. Surg. 61(3): 197–201.

Ou, C.S., J. Presthus, and E. Beadle. 1993. Laparoscopic bladder neck suspension using hernia mesh and surgical staples. J. Laparoendosc. Surg. 3(6): 563–566.

Pasricha, P.J., T.G. Tietjen, and A.N. Kalloo. 1995. Biliary manometry in swine: A unique endoscopic model for teaching and research. Endoscopy 27(1): 70–72.

Pietrafitta, J.J., L.S. Schultz, J.N. Graber, and D.F. Hickok. 1992. An experimental technique of laparoscopic bowel resection and anastomosis. Surg. Laparosc. Endosc. 2(3): 205–211.

Rey, J.F., and T. Romanczyk. 1995. The development of experimental models in the teaching of endoscopy: An overview. Endoscopy 27(1): 101–105.

Rodriguez, J., K. Kensing, C. Cardenas, and P. Stoltenberg. 1993. Laparoscopy-guided subhepatic cholecystostomy: A feasibility study in swine. Gastrointest. Endosc. 39(2): 176–178.

Salzman, A.L., K.E. Strong, H.L. Wang, P.S. Wollert, T.J. Vandermeer, and M.P. Fink. 1994. Intraluminal balloonless air tonometry—A new method for determination of gastrointestinal mucosal carbon dioxide tension. Crit. Care Med. 22(1): 126–134.

Siegel, J.H., and M.A. Korsten. 1989. ERCP in a nonhuman primate. Gastrointest. Endosc. 35(6): 557–559.

Soper, N.J., and J.G. Hunter. 1992. Suturing and knot tying in laparoscopy. Surg. Clin. North Am. 72(5): 1139–1152.

Soper, N.J., J.A. Barteau, R.V. Clayman, and M.J. Becich. 1991. Safety and efficacy of laparoscopic cholecystectomy using monopolar electrocautery in the porcine model. Surg. Laparosc. Endosc. 1(1): 17–22.

Soper, N.J., L.M. Brunt, J. Fleshman, Jr., D.L. Dunnegan, and R.V. Clayman. 1993. Laparoscopic small bowel resection and anastomosis. Surg. Laparosc. Endosc. 3(1): 6–12.

Stump, K.C., M.M. Swindle, C.D. Saudek, and J.D. Strandberg. 1988. Pancreatectomized swine as a model of diabetes mellitus. Lab. Anim. Sci. 38 (4): 439–443.

Swindle, M.M., A.C. Smith, and B.J.S. Hepburn. 1988. Swine as models in experimental surgery. J. Invest. Surg. 1(1): 65–79.

Vancaillie, T.G. 1993. Laparoscopic bladder neck suspension. In Winfield, H.N. (ed), Atlas of the Urologic Clinics of North America—Urologic Laparoscopic Surgery. Philadelphia: WB Saunders, pp. 73–86.

14 CONSIDERATIONS IN XENOGRAFIC AND TRANSGENIC TECHNOLOGIES

Introduction

Xenotransplantation procedures involving both whole organs and tissues will probably be developed to a level of clinical relevance within the next decade. Transgenic technologies will continue to be involved in the development of organs that would be resistant to the host rejection phenomena. Most likely, a combined strategy of transgenic manipulation and improvement in immunosuppressive agents will be required to achieve success. Xenografic tissue implants, such as islet cells for diabetic patients, are likely to be developed prior to whole-organ transplantation of such organs as the heart, liver, and kidneys. Swine are generally considered to be the most probable species to be utilized in clinical xenografic procedures. Primates are likely to be utilized only during initial experimental procedures because of supply, public health, and ethical considerations.

The technical aspects of the surgery involved in the xenotransplant procedures are the same as those described previously in the various system chapters in this textbook. Other considerations include ethical aspects, public health considerations, husbandry practices, and pre- and postsurgical monitoring procedures for both donors and recipients. Swine to nonhuman primate transplantations, especially baboons, are the most likely experimental procedures to be utilized during development of these procedures. For artificial organs and tissue or cellular implantations of porcine origin, other species, such as the dog, may be used during some aspects of development if the xenografic devices provide a barrier to immunologic insult from the recipient.

The Institute of Medicine and the Food and Drug Administration held public hearings in 1995 and 1998 to discuss the various aspects of xenotransplantation and to develop draft guidelines (Institute of Medicine, 1996; Public Health Service, 1996), which are currently being revised, for the procedures. The emphasis of these proceedings is related to the public health considerations.

Ethical Considerations

Millions of swine per year are consumed as food by the human population, and they are not an endangered species. These two considerations combined with the physiologic, immunologic, and zoonotic disease considerations make swine the predominant choice as a donor animal for xenografic procedures. More of the general population would have an ethical concern with the use of primates. The entire captive population of some species of primates, such as baboons, could be consumed by the clinical requests within a few years. The ethical considerations of xenografic transplant have been reviewed (Institute of Medicine, 1996; Prentice et al., 1994).

The shortage of human donors of whole organs has not kept up with the demand, and patients routinely die while on waiting lists for organ transplants. This problem could be greatly alleviated, if not eliminated, by a significant increase in the number of humans willing to donate organs. This solution has obvious advantages over the development of xenografic organ donations; however, it is unlikely to be successful because of the reluctance of surviving family members to donate organs. However, campaigns to increase the number of organ donors should be conducted to decrease the need for xenografts.

Tissue transplants have an additional consideration. They are being developed for diseases, such as diabetes, because of the potential improvement in therapy that could be derived from not having to control the disease with insulin injections. The potential for curative therapy with these xenografic therapies is a significant consideration in their development.

The risk/benefit ratio of these therapies must include a consideration of the potential for transmission of zoonotic diseases, which is minimal with swine compared to species such as nonhuman primates.

With all of these considerations, it is probable that the majority of the human population will accept the necessity of using swine as xenografic donors with minimal moral and ethical reservations.

Immunologic and Physiologic Considerations

The immunologic and physiologic considerations associated with xenografic transplantation have been summarized in the Institute of Medicine study

(1996) and in the scientific literature (Binns and Pabst, 1996; Cramer and Makowka, 1994; Kaufmann et al., 1995; Lin and Platt, 1996; Matthews and Beran, 1996; Pursel et al., 1996; Smith and Beattie, 1996). The outline in the Institute of Medicine study is followed in this section.

Phylogenetically distant species experience hyperacute rejection phenomena when donor endothelium is attacked by circulating antibodies. These xenoreactive antibodies attach to the endothelium of the discordant organ, and the complement system is activated. Within a few hours, the vascularized graft develops edema and hemorrhage followed by clotting, which decreases the blood supply to the transplanted organ. Techniques that reduce circulating antibodies, such as plasmapheresis or immunoabsorption, prolong the period of time that is required for the hyperacute rejection to occur.

Acute vascular rejection is a delayed response occurring days to weeks following the transplant. This delayed reaction is likely to be a sequela of hyperacute rejection caused by genetic up-regulation of different genes in the endothelium of the graft. T-cell immune responses related to the major histocompatibility complex (MHC), as occurring in allografts, are likely to be the next phase of rejection to be overcome. These complex reactions may be successfully overcome with immunosuppressive drugs.

Chronic rejection occurs months to years following the transplant procedure and is the result of combined humeral and cellular responses. This phenomenon occurs in allografts, but no xenografic procedure has been successful for a long-enough period of time to determine whether or not it will occur with xenografts.

Cellular grafts can be protected from the chronic rejection phenomenon by protection against circulating antibodies using encapsulation or protective filtration of the cells. Whole-organ transplantation offers more formidable obstacles. Research approaches to prevention of the various types of rejection include pharmaceutical development of immunosuppressive agents, modification of the source tissue, modification of the host immune system, and encapsulation/protection methodologies for the donor tissue or organ.

Donor modification includes transgenic modification, gene knockout, blocking of complementary fragments of ribonucleic acid (antisense RNA), and antibody masking. All of these technologies are being evolved to block the immune response of the host. Transgenic modification is currently the most advanced of the methods (Pinkert, 1994).

The host response may be modified by bone-marrow chimerism or microchimerism phenomena discovered in long-term transplant recipients and caused by gradual lymphocytic release from transplanted tissue. Bone-marrow chimerism has not been tried between swine and humans. It would involve ablation of the host bone marrow and replacement with bone marrow from the donor animal. The procedure was unsuccessful in a single trial with baboon-to-human chimerism. This is the procedure that stimulated the Institute of Medicine study (1996).

Semipermeable barriers for encapsulation of tissues and cells are currently feasible but are unlikely to be developed for whole-organ transplantation without new technology.

Regulatory Guidelines

The Public Health Service (PHS) *Guideline on Infectious Disease Issues in Xenotransplantation* (PHS, 1996) outlines regulatory considerations in a draft form for xenotransplantation of cells, tissues, and organs. This document is currently being revised following meetings in 1998. A draft guideline was also published by the World Health Organization (WHO, 1996), and it has recently been revised into two documents (WHO, 1998a,b).

The PHS Guideline deals mainly with potential public health issues. The guideline provides recommendations for protocol approval, animal sources, clinical issues, and the need for a national registry and archive.

The protocol issues include the composition of the xenotransplant team, the site, the protocol review, health surveillance plans, and the need for informed consent. The transplant team should include an infectious disease physician with knowledge of zoonoses, a veterinarian with expertise in zoonotic disease and animal husbandry, a transplant immunologist, a hospital epidemiologist or infection control specialist, and the director of the clinical microbiology laboratory at the transplantation site, in addition to the transplant surgical team. The transplantation site has to be accredited and associated with the Organ Procurement and Transplantation Network. The protocol has to be reviewed by the institutions Animal Care and Use Committee, the Biosafety Committee, and the Institutional Review Board for Human Research. All of these committees must have expertise in zoonotic diseases and disease control. In addition, these protocols may be subject to regulation by the Food and Drug Administration. The protocol must include a plan for screening of the animal, organ, and the source herd. It also must include provisions for written informed consent and education of the recipient.

The major portion of the document related to regulation of animal sources of xenotransplant materials. Animals have to be bred and reared in captivity, herds have to be closed and serologically screened, and tissues and organs from slaughterhouses cannot be used. Biomedical research animal facilities should be accredited by the Association for the Assessment and Accreditation of Laboratory Animal Care (AAALAC) International to ensure compliance with all federal guidelines. The facility has to maintain and follow detailed standard operating facilities for quarantine and disease surveillance. Standard laboratory animal procedures for sanitation of facilities need to be followed, and the feed source and quality should be controlled to prevent the use of rendered products. Preclinical screening of the herd for potential zoonoses is required. Herd health maintenance programs include both prevention and treatment of potential zoonotic problems. The use of sentinel animals is suggested for monitoring serology, microbiology, and necropsy studies. Individual animals to be used as donors must also be screened. Biopsies of the actual xenograft are recommended.

The clinical issues deal with the safety of the recipient and the medical personnel and require lifetime monitoring and archiving. It also requires educating the recipient about informing close contacts. The archived information must be made available to a national archiving registry.

The World Health Organization (1996, 1998a,b) prepared similar draft documents. However, they recommend the use of gnotobiotic animals that have been Cesarian derived and maintained in barrier facilities. Recognizing the impracticality of this source of animals, they provide for the use of animals from a similar health and husbandry situation as that described in the PHS document. They provide a criteria list for developing an exclusion list of infectious agents for xenografic organ donation. Their criteria for the clinical arena is similar to the PHS document, however, it is not in as much detail.

These guidelines are so intense as to preclude the conduction of xenotransplants in other than major medical centers with accredited laboratory animal programs. Very few commercial producers of swine could provide the required husbandry without substantial modification of their facilities and programs.

Public Health Considerations

Pig-to-human xenotransplantation carries little risk compared to other species, such as primates. A proposed set of practical considerations on herd maintenance and surveillance has been published (Swindle, 1996) and revised recently (Swindle, in press). Viruses with the highest potential for zoonotic infection in immunocompromised recipients or damage to tissue and cellular xenotransplants include swine influenza, human influenza, encephalomyocarditis virus, porcine rotavirus, porcine reovirus, parainfluenza virus, porcine adenovirus, porcine circovirus, porcine pneumovirus, hepatitis E, pseudorabies, and porcine retrovirus. The incidence of occurrence and potential of pathogenicity vary widely among these infectious agents. The primary agents of concern are the influenza viruses.

Bacterial pathogens and commensals that are of concern include those of the following genera: *Salmonella, Pasteurella, Brucella, Erysipelothrix, Streptococcus, Campylobacter, Staphylococcus, Coxiella, Leptospira,* and *Mycobacterium.* The pathogenicity of these organisms varies widely depending upon the species and serotype.

Parasitic organisms should also be considered in the screening. *Balantidium coli* is the primary protozoal organism of concern. Nematodes can generally be controlled by anthelmintics; however, some, such as *Ascaris suum,* can also be associated with visceral larval migrans and damage of donor organs such as the liver.

The potential list of pathogens is much longer and includes organisms such as dermatomycoses, and immunocompromised patients may experience infection from organisms not previously associated with zoonotic disease. Summaries of the infectious risks associated with xenotransplantation have been published (Cooper et al., 1991; Kalter and Heberling, 1994; Michaels and Simmons, 1994; Ye et al., 1994). Specific pathogen-free (SPF) swine, as discussed in Chapter 1, could be used as a starter herd source for animals; however, they would not be considered to be of a pathogen-free status necessary for xenotransplantation by current guidelines. There is a suggestion that a term such as "xenografic-defined flora animals" should be used rather than SPF to differentiate these two standards (Swindle, 1996).

Management and Husbandry Strategies

Management and husbandry strategies are discussed in the PHS guidelines (1996) and by Swindle (1996; in press). AAALAC-accredited biomedical research facilities with Class II biosafety facilities are more likely to be capable of handling the quarantine and disease-control standards required for xenotransplantation. The standard operating procedures for husbandry and the construction of the facilities should be adequate to meet these guidelines in such accredited research facilities. Their standards could be used as a guideline for the development of xenografic transplant facilities for housing donor herds of animals.

The use of a sentinel animal system of monitoring herds, similar to those used in rodent facilities for biomedical research, should be instituted. The use of multiple rooms with an all-in/all-out management system for batch procurement of tissues and organs is probably the most practical method to ensure compliance.

Other Considerations

Besides the immunologic and zoonotic problems to be overcome through research and management techniques, there are other issues to be considered. Swine may have congenital defects or genetic diseases, such as malignant hyperthermia. There are also nonflexible regulations related to the shipment of swine and porcine tissues between states and countries that are in effect for agricultural and economic control purposes. Swine used for xenografts will also have to either receive an exception to these regulations or be in compliance depending upon the destination locale (Swindle, 1996).

It is likely that guidelines will continue to be revised as additional scientific meetings and public forums are held on the subject. The NY Academy of Sciences recently held such a meeting in March 1998 and has plans to publish the proceedings in the *Annals of the NY Academy of Sciences*.

References

Binns, R.M., and R. Pabst. 1996. The functional structure of the pig's immune system, resting and activated. In Tumbleson, M.E., and Schook, L.B. (eds), Advances in Swine in Biomedical Research, Vol. 1. New York: Plenum Press, pp. 253–266.

Cooper D..K.C., Y. Ye, L.L. Rolf, Jr., and N. Zuhdi. 1991. The pig as a potential organ donor for man. In Cooper, D.C.K., Kemp, E., Reemtsma, K., and White, D.J.G. (eds), Xenotransplantation: The Transplantation of Organs and Tissues Between Species. Berlin: Springer, 481–500.

Cramer, D.V., and L. Makowka. 1994. The use of xenografts in experimental transplantation, In Cramer, D.V., Podesta, L.G., and Makowka, L. (eds), Handbook of Animal Models in Transplantation Research. Boca Raton, FL: CRC Press, 299–310.

Institute of Medicine. 1996. Xenotransplantation: Swine, Ethics and Public Policy. Washington, DC: National Academy Press.

Kalter, S.S., and R.L. Heberling. 1995. Xenotransplantation and infectious diseases. ILAR J. 5(37) 31–37.

Kaufmann, C.L., B.A. Gaines, and S.T. Ildstad. 1995. Xenotransplantation. Annu. Rev. Immunol. 13(3): 339–367.

Lin, S.S., and J.L. Platt. 1996. Immunologic advances towards clinical xenotransplantation. In Tumbleson, M.E., and Schook, L.B. (eds), Advances in Swine in Biomedical Research, Vol. 1. New York: Plenum Press, pp. 147–162.

Matthews, P.J., and G.W. Beran. 1996. Assessment of public health aspects of porcine xenotransplantation. In Tumbleson, M.E., and Schook, L.B. (eds), Advances in Swine in Biomedical Research, Vol. 1. New York: Plenum Press, pp. 163–170.

Michaels, M.G., and R.L. Simmons. 1994. Xenotransplant-associated zoonoses. Strategies for prevention. Transplantation 57(1): 1–7.

Pinkert, C.A. 1994. Transgenic Animal Technology. New York: Academic Press.

Prentice, E.D., I.J. Fox, R.S. Dixon, D.L. Antonson, and T.A. Lawson. 1994. History, donor considerations and ethics of xenotransplantation. In Smith, A.C., and Swindle, M.M. (eds), Research Animal Anesthesia, Analgesia and Surgery. Greenbelt, MD: Scientists Center for Animal Welfare, pp. 25–36.

Public Health Service. 1996. Draft Public Health Service Guideline on Infectious Disease Issues in Xenotransplantation. Fed. Reg. 61(185): 49920–49932.

Pursel, V.G., M.B. Solomon, and R.J. Wall. 1996. Genetic engineering of swine. In Tumbleson, M.E., and Schook, L.B. (eds), Advances in Swine in Biomedical Research, Vol. 1. New York: Plenum Press, pp. 189–206.

Smith, T.P.L., and C.W. Beattie. 1996. Identifying tumor initiator/suppressor and penetrance associated genes by gene mapping. In Tumbleson, M.E., and Schook, L.B. (eds), Advances in Swine in Biomedical Research, Vol. 1. New York: Plenum Press, pp. 239–249.

Swindle, M.M. 1996. Considerations of specific pathogen free swine (SPF) in xenotransplantation. J. Invest. Surg. 9(3): 267–271.

Swindle, M.M. In press. Defining appropriate health status and management programs for specific pathogen free (SPF) swine for xenotransplantation. Ann. NY Acad. Sci.

World Health Organization (WHO). 1996. Draft WHO recommendations on xenotransplantation and infectious disease prevention. Geneva: WHO.

World Health Organization (WHO). 1998a. Report of WHO Consultation on Xenotransplantation. Geneva, Switzerland: WHO.

World Health Organization (WHO). 1998b. Xenotransplantation: Guidance on Infectious Disease Prevention and Management. Geneva, Switzerland: WHO.

Ye, Y., S. Niekrasz, R. Kosanke, R. Welsh, H.E. Jordan, J.C. Fox, W.C. Edwards, C. Maxwell, and D.K.C. Cooper. 1994. The pig as a potential organ donor for man. Transplantation 57(6): 694–703.

15 MAGNETIC RESONANCE ANGIOGRAPHY: Imaging of Thoracic, Neck, Brain, and Abdominal Vessels in the Normal Large White Pig

M. Rahbek Schmidt, S. B. Kristiansen, E. Lundorf, E. V. Stenbøg , and J. C. Djurhuus

Magnetic resonance (MR) angiography was used for imaging of blood vessels of the brain, neck, thorax, and abdomen in healthy adult pigs. This noninvasive method is suitable for anatomic labeling of vessels. When placing standard saturation pulse inferior or superior to the scanned volume, arteries and veins are separated on the angiographies. To ensure correct and stable positioning of pigs in the scanner, a specially designed nonmagnetic restraint box has been developed at this institution; this is advantageous if routine animal MR studies are performed. Complete relaxation and, hence, endotracheal intubation is preferable for optimal scanning results.

Materials and Methods

Animals and Anesthesia

MR angiography was performed in two female pigs, mixed Danish Landrace and Yorkshire, age 3 months, weighing 40 kg. The animals were preanesthetized with ketamine 15 mg/kg and midazolam 0.75 mg/kg. After endotracheal intubation anesthesia was maintained with ketamine 7.5 mg/kg/h and midazolam 0.35 mg/kg/h, using a Servo ventilator (NO_2: 4 l/min and O_2: 2 l/min). To ensure complete relaxation, pancuronium, 0.2 mg/kg/h, was given.

Measuring Procedure

MR angiography was performed on a GE Signa 1.5 Tesla whole body scanner (General Electrics, WI, USA). The animals were examined in the supine position, and body coil was used. The scanning protocol included an initial series of scout images to determine localization and direction of the vessels to be examined. Slice spacing was set contiguous and the matrix used was 256 × 192.

General Parameters Used

Volume spoiled GRASS (SPGR), 2D time of flight, 16 kHz receiver bandwidth (variable bandwidth), and flow compensation.

Thoracic, Neck, and Brain Vessels

Parameters

Field of view was 32 × 32 cm, yielding a pixel size of 0.125 × 0.166 cm. Slice thickness was 2 mm. A 60-degree flip angle was used, repetition time (TR) was 16 milliseconds, echo time (TE) 4.4 milliseconds. No phase wrap, extended dynamic range, or swap phase frequency was used. Standard saturation pulse was not used. A total of 140 slices were acquired sequentially with two signal averages in a scan time of 15 minutes.

Abdominal Vessels

Parameters

Field of view was 40 × 30 cm, yielding a pixel size of 0.156 × 0.156 cm. Slice thickness was 2.9 mm. A 45-degree flip angle was used, TR was 22 milliseconds, TE 3.9 milliseconds. Standard saturation pulse was placed inferior (arteries) and superior (veins) to the scanned volume. A total of 89 slices were acquired sequentially with one signal average in a scan time of 7 minutes.

After acquisitions three-dimensional angiographies were reconstructed using the independent console (Figs. 15.1–15.7).

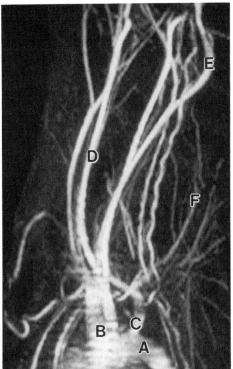

FIGURE 15.1   Sagittal view. *A*-Aortic arch, *B*-Origin of the brachiocephalic trunck, *C*-Left subclavian artery, *D*-Common carotid artery, *E*-External jugular vein, *F*-Vertebral arteries.

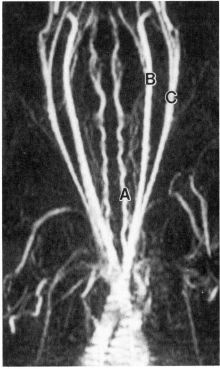

FIGURE 15.2   Coronal view angiography. *A*-Vertebral artery, *B*-Carotid artery, *C*-External jugular vein and their systems.

294

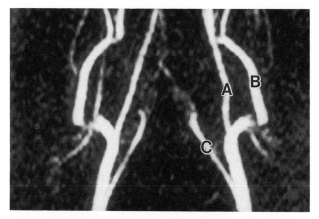

FIGURE 15.3   Coronal view of the brain and angiography of the carotid arterial system. *A*-Internal carotid artery, *B*-External carotid artery, *C*-Branches for anastomoses with the vertebral arteries.

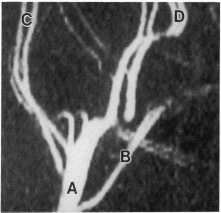

FIGURE 15.4   Sagittal view of the brain and angiography of the carotid arterial system. *A*-Common carotid artery, *B*-External carotid artery, *C*-Internal carotid artery, *D*-Branches for anastomoses with the vertebral arteries.

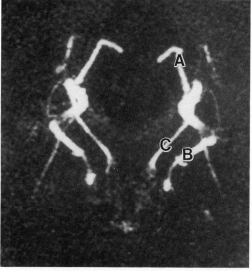

FIGURE 15.5   Rostral view of the brain and angiography of cerebral arteries disclosing part of the circulus arteriosus cerebri of Willis. *A*-Rostral cerebral artery, *B*-Caudal communicating cerebral artery, *C*-Internal carotid artery.

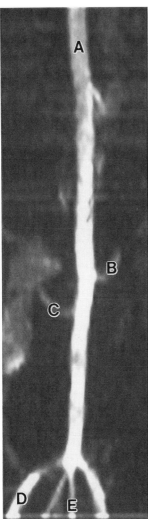

FIGURE 15.6   Coronal view and angiography of the lower abdominal aorta. *A*-Origin of
both renal arteries, *B*-Left renal artery, *C*-Right renal artery, *D*-External iliac artery, *E*-Internal iliac artery.

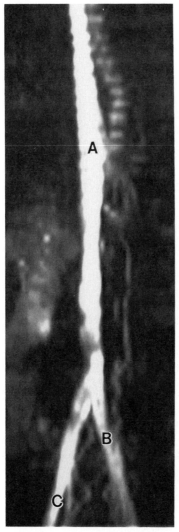

FIGURE 15.7   Coronal view and angiography. *A*-Lower inferior caval vein, *B*-Origin of common iliac veins, *C*-Branching in external veins.

APPENDIX

Table A1. Age/weight correlations

Minipig—Hanford		Minipig—Yucatan		Micropig—Yucatan	
Age (mo)	Weight (kg)	Age (mo)	Weight (kg)	Age (mo)	Weight (kg)
1	4–7	1	3–6	1	3– 5
2	8–11	2	7–9	2	6– 8
3	12–19	3	10–15	3	9–12
4	20–27	4	15–20	4	12–14
5	25–33	5	20–25	5	14–16
6	34–42	6	25–30	6	16–20
8	40–50	8	35–45	8	25–35
10	45–55	10	45–55	10	30–40
12	55–70 male 50–65 female	12	55–65 male 45–50 female	12	55–65 male 35–45 female

SOURCE: Reprinted with permission of Charles River Laboratories, Inc.

Table A2. Physiology

	Microswine	Miniswine
Breed	Yucatan	Hanford, Yucatan
Growth		
Birth weight	600–700 g	600–1000 g
Weight at sexual maturity	15–20 kg	Hanford 28–42 kg; Yucatan 20–30kg
Adult weight	40–60 kg (at 12–14 mo)	
Life span	10–15 y	68–80 kg (at 2 y) 10–15 y
Reproduction		
Gestation period	111–114 days	111–114 days
Average litter size	5–6	Hanford 6–8; Yucatan 5–6
Weaning age	28–35 days	28–35 days
Sexual maturity	5–6 mo	5–6 mo
Breeding age	6–8 mo	6–8 mo

SOURCE: Reprinted with permission of Charles River Laboratories, Inc.

Table A3.   Recommended diets

Age	Model	Recommended diet
Pigs 1–2 mo old	Micro and mini	0.25–0.75 lb/day (0.11–0.34 kg/day) of a 50/50 mix of starter and maintenance/breeder diet
Pigs 2–3 mo old	Micro and mini	0.75–1.25 lb/day (0.34–0.57 kg/day) maintenance/breeder diet
Pigs over 3 mo old	Micro	1.25–1.75 lb/day (0.57–0.79 kg/day) maintenance/breeder
	Mini	1.75–2.2 lb/day (0.79–1.00 kg/day) maintenance/breeder

NOTE: Individual animals and conditions vary, so new users of swine should be observant, especially at first, to get a feel for optimum feed levels; weight loss and weight gain are the best indicators.

SOURCE: Reprinted with permission of Charles River Laboratories, Inc.

Table A4.   Serum biochemical values of 30 healthy, mature Yucatan miniature swine

	Reference range		
	Mean	mean ± 2 SD	Range observed
Glucose (mg/dl)	79.8	36.4–123.2	56.0–153.0
SUN (mg/dl)	19.2	9.2–29.2	10.0–29.0
Creatinine (mg/dl)	1.6	1.2–2.0	1.2–2.0
Total protein (gm/dl)	7.5	6.1–8.9	6.3–9.4
Albumin (gm/dl)	4.7	3.9–5.5	4.1–5.6
Globulin (gm/dl)	2.8	1.6–4.0	1.4–3.6
A/G	1.8	0.8–2.8	1.11–3.49
Sodium (mEq/1)	147.0	144–152.6	142.0–153.0
Potassium (mEq/1)	4.6	4.0–5.2	3.9–5.2
Chloride (mEq/1)	104.2	94.4–114.0	95.0–114.0
Calcium (mg/dl)	10.6	9.6–11.6	9.3–11.6
Phosphorus (mg/dl)	6.9	5.1–8.1	5.0–8.3
Total bilirubin (mg/dl)	0.1	0.0–0.3	0.0–0.3
AST (IU/I)	28.2	10.4–56.0	15.0–53.0
ALT(IU/I)	33.6	20.4–46.8	20.0–48.0
CPK (IU/I)	168.0	48.0–288.0	37.0–270.0
Cholesterol (mg/dl)	101.8	38.4–165.2	47.3–173.0

NOTE: SUN, serum urea nitrogen; A/G, albumin globulin ratio; AST, aspartate aminotransferase; ALT, alanine aminotransferase; CPK, creatine phosphokinase.
SOURCE: Reprinted with permission from Radin et al., 1986, Hematologic and serum biochemical values for Yucatan miniature swine, Lab. Anim. Sci. 36(4): 425–427.

Table A5.   Clinical chemistry reference values for fasted Yucatan miniature pigs

	Mean		Pooled SD	Median	Observed range
	Male	Female			
Glucose (mmol/l)	3.65	3.85	64.	3.66	2.28–5.11
Urea (mmol/l)	7.00	8.68	2.64	7.14	5.00–16.1
Creatinine (µmol/l)	106.1	123.8[a]	15.9	114.9	88.4–150.3
Uric acid (µmol/l)	3.6	7.1	7.1	5.9	0.0–29.7
Total protein (g/l)	77.0	71.0	9.0	76.0	44.0–83.0
Albumin (g/l)	53.0	46.0[a]	6.0	51.0	26.0–57.0
Globulin (g/l)	24.0	25.0	4.0	24.0	18.0–36.0
Albumin/Globulin	2.2	1.9[a]	.3	2.1	1.3–2.7
Bilirubin total (µmol/l)	3.42	3.42	1.37	3.42	1.7–6.84
Triglyceride (mg/l)	192.	341[a].	134	235	100–530
Total cholesterol (mmol/l)	1.81	1.89	.38	1.85	1.03–2.67
Alkaline phosphatase (U/l)	90.1	87.7	21.5	84.5	39.0–128.0
Gamma glutamyl transferase (U/l)	61.1	62.1	11.2	61.5	41.0–86.0
Alanine aminotransferase (U/l)	71.9	73.0	13.6	71.0	49.0–106.0
Lactate dehydrogenase (U/l)	450.8	556.7[a]	88.0	492.0	389.0–727.0
Aspartate aminotransferase (U/l)	38.7	41.8	5.9	39.0	32.0–55.0
Sodium (mmol/l)	139.3	141.7	4.2	141.0	132.0–149.0
Potassium (mmol/l)	4.0	4.2	.3	4.0	3.5–4.8
Chloride (mmol/l)	101.2	105.0	4.3	102.0	96.0–111.0
Iron (µmol/l)	22.7	23.6	3.5	23.1	11.8–37.6
Calcium (mmol/l)	2.72	2.52	.18	2.65	2.08–2.92
Phosphorus (mmol/l)	2.42	2.39	.26	2.33	1.97–2.91

NOTE: SD, standard deviation.
[a]Significant difference ($p < .05$) between genders, $N = 24$.
SOURCE: Reprinted with permission from Parsons, A. H., and R. E. Wells, 1986, Serum biochemistry of healthy Yucatan miniature pigs. Lab. Anim. Sci., 36(4):428–430.

Table A6.   Hematologic values of 30 healthy, mature Yucatan miniature swine

	Mean	Reference range mean ± 2 SD	Range observed
RBC (10^6/μl)	7.0	5.4–8.6	5.6–8.8
Hemoglobulin (g/dl)	14.9	12.5–17.3	13.1–17.0
Hematocrit (%)	44.6	36.4–52.8	36.3–53.7
MCV (fl)	64.4	57.0–71.8	58.2–72.5
MCH (pg)	21.4	18.8–24.0	18.9–24.3
MCHC (g/dl)	33.2	31.6–34.8	31.1–34.5
RDW	19.4	16.2–22.6	15.7–23.8
Platelets (10^3/μl)	440.6	201.4–679.8	217.0–770.0
WBC (10^3/μl)	12.6	6.6–18.6	6.9–21.2
100 cell manual differential			
% segmented neutrophils	41.9	17.5–66.3	18.0–64.0
% bands	0.2	0.0–1.2	0.0–2.0
% lymphocytes	45.6	19.2–72.0	21.0–71.0
% monocytes	7.5	1.1–13.9	2.0–15.0
% eosinophils	4.1	0.0–10.0	0.0–13.0
% basophils	0.5	0.0–2.5	0.0–5.0

NOTE: RBC, red blood cells; MCV, mean corpuscular volume; MCH, mean corpuscular hemoglobin; MCHC, mean corpuscular hemoglobin concentration; RDW, red cell distribution width; WBC, white blood cells.
SOURCE: Reprinted with permission from Radin et al., 1986, Hematologic and serum biochemical values for Yucatan miniature swine, Lab. Anim. Sci., 36(4):425–427.

Table A7.   Population data for fetal values that follow

	Pigs (N = 54)			
	Early gestation (n = 11)	Late gestation (n = 43)	Sows (n = 12)	
No. of females	8	25	No. of early gestation	3
No. of males	3	18	No. of late gestation	9
Body weight (g)	366 ± 26	653 ± 200	Body weight (kg)	61 ± 15
Gestation			Age (months)	17 ± 9
Days	82 ± 6	104 ± 6		
Range	(76–88)	(98–110)		

SOURCE: Reprinted with permission from Schantz et al., 1995, Normal hematology, serology and serum protein electrophoresis values in fetal Yucatan miniature swine, Lab. Anim. Sci. 45(3): 285–289.

Table A8. Erythrocytic data for fetal pigs

	Pigs (N = 54)		
	Early gestation (n = 11)	Late gestation (n = 43)	Sows (n = 12)
Erythrocytes			
($\times 10^6$/µl)	4.30 ± 0.49	4.74 ± 0.55	4.22 ± 0.39
Hemoglobin (g/dl)	9.3 ± 0.7	10.3 ± 1.1	9.0 ± 1.3
Hematocrit (%)	32.7 ± 2.4	34.6 ± 3.9	27.3 ± 3.4
MCV (fl)	77 ± 7	65 ± 2	
	73 ± 4		
MCH (pg)	22.0 ± 2.8	21.8 ± 0.9	21.2 ± 1.0
MCHC (%)	28.6 ± 1.2	29.8 ± 1.5	32.9 ± 0.5
Nucleated erythrocytes			
(/100 leukocytes)[a]	148 ± 26	11 ± 18	0

NOTE: MCV, mean corpuscular volume (femtoliters); MCH, mean corpuscular hemoglobin (picograms); MCHC, mean corpuscular hemoglobin concentration.

[a] Age differences were significant ($p < 0.05$).

SOURCE: Reprinted with permission from Schantz et al, 1995, Normal hematology, serology and serum protein electrophoresis values in fetal Yucatan miniature swine, Lab. Anim. Sci. 45(3): 285–289.

Table A9. Leukocytic data for fetal pigs

	Pigs (N = 54)		
	Early gestation (n = 11)	Late gestation (n = 43)	Sows (n = 12)
Leukocytes[a]			
($\times 10^3$/µl)	21 ± 0.3	4.1 ± 2.1	9.7 ± 0.6
Neutrophils[a] (%)	281 ± 1.0	35 ± 17	66 ± 4
Bands (%)	01 ± 1.0	0	1 ± 1
Lymphocytes[a] (%)	701 ± 2	63 ± 18	31 ± 4
Monocytes (%)	11 ± 1	1 ± 1	2 ± 0
Eosinophils (%)	0	0	0
Basophils (%)	0	0	0
Metamyelocytes (%)	0	0	0

[a] Age differences were significant between sow and fetal values ($p < 0.05$).

SOURCE: Reprinted with permission from Schantz et al., 1995, Normal hematology, serology and serum protein electrophoresis values in fetal Yucatan miniature swine, Lab. Anim. Sci. 45(3): 285–289.

Table A10. Serum electrolyte data for fetal pigs

	Pigs (N = 54)		Sows (n = 12)
	Early gestation (n = 11)	Late gestation (n = 43)	
Ca[a] (mg/dl)	10.8 ± 0.7	11.4 ± 0.9	9.7 ± 0.1
P (mg/dl)	8 ± 0.8	8.7 ± 0.9	7.4 ± 0.2
Na[b] (mEq/l)	130 ± 1.0	141 ± 5.0	139 ± 1.0
K[a] (mEq/l)	8.1 ± 2.3	6.5 ± 1.0	4.7 ± 0
Cl (mEq/l)	95 ± 3.0	100 ± 4.0	103 ± 2.0

[a] Age differences were significant ($p < 0.05$).
[b] Age differences were significant between sow and fetal values ($p < 0.05$).
SOURCE: Reprinted with permission from Schantz et al., 1995, Normal hematology, serology and serum protein electrophoresis values in fetal Yucatan miniature swine, Lab. Anim. Sci. 45(3): 285–289.

Table A11. Serum enzyme data for fetal pigs

	Pigs (N = 54)		Sows (n = 12)
	Early gestation (n = 11)	Late gestation (n = 43)	
ALP (IU/l)	333 ± 145	531 ± 230	66 ± 31
LD (IU/l)	1207 ± 545	491 ± 174	497 ± 26
AST (IU/l)	178 ± 129	47 ± 40	46 ± 10
ALT (IU/l)	15 ± 11	6 ± 3	29 ± 9
GGT (IU/l)	94 ± 23	65 ± 15	42 ± 1
Amylase[a] (U/l)	641 ± 171	1044 ± 281	1711 ± 39

NOTE: ALP, alkaline phosphatase: age difference was significant between sow and fetal values ($p < 0.01$); LD, lactate dehydrogenase; AST, aspartate transaminase; ALT, alanine transaminase: age difference was significant between sow and fetal values ($p < 0.05$); GGT, glutamyltransferase.
[a] Age differences were significant ($p < 0.05$).
SOURCE: Reprinted with permission from Schantz et al., 1995, Normal hematology, serology and serum protein electrophoresis values in fetal Yucatan miniature swine, Lab. Anim. Sci. 45(3): 285–289.

Table A12.   Serum metabolite data for fetal pigs

	Pigs (N = 54)		
	Early gestation (*n* = 11)	Late gestation (*n* = 43)	Sows (*n* = 12)
Glucose[a] (mg/dl)	32 ± 5.0	65 ± 42	79 ± 1.0
BUN (mg/dl)	20 ± 2.0	15 ± 5.0	19 ± 4.0
Uric acid (mg/dl)	0	0.3 ± 0.3	0
Cholesterol[a] (mg/dl)	44 ± 7.0	59 ± 11	60 ± 3.0
Bili[c] (mg/dl)	0.4 ± 0.1	0.2 ± 0.1	0.3 ± 0.1
Creatinine[a,b] (mg/dl)	0.7 ± 0.0	1.4 ± 0.4	1.3 ± 0.3
Triglyceride[a,c] (mg/dl)	18 ± 3.0	20 ± 4.0	42 ± 1.0
BUN/creatinine[d] ratio	28 ± 1.0	13 ± 8.0	12 ± 4.0

NOTE: BUN, blood urea nitrogen; Bili, total bilirubin.
[a] Age difference was significant between early fetal group and sow ($p < 0.05$).
[b] Age difference was significant between early and late fetal groups ($p < 0.05$).
[c] Age difference was significant between late fetal group and sow ($p < 0.05$).
[d] Age differences were significant ($p < 0.05$).
SOURCE: Reprinted with permission from Schantz et al., 1995, Normal hematology, serology and serum protein electrophoresis values in fetal Yucatan miniature swine, Lab. Anim. Sci. 45(3): 285–289.

Table A13.   Population data for protein electrophoresis for fetal pigs

	Pigs (N = 54)			
	Early gestation (*n* = 9)	Late gestation (*n* = 35)	Sows (*n* = 8)	
No. of females	7	19	No. of early gestation	2
No. of males	2	16	No. of late gestation	6
Body weight (g)	380 ± 15	641 ± 220	Body weight (kg)	59 ± 14
			Age (months)	59 ± 6
Gestation, days				
Mean ± SD	86 ± 1	03 ± 7		
(Range)	(85–87)	(96–110)		

SOURCE: Reprinted with permission from Schantz et al., 1995, Normal hematology, serology and serum protein electrophoresis values in fetal Yucatan miniature swine, Lab. Anim. Sci. 45(3): 285–289.

Table A14.   Serum protein electrophoresis data for fetal pigs

	Pigs ($N = 44$)		Sows	
	Early gestation	Late gestation	Early gestation	Late gestation
Tp (g/dl)	1.75 ± 0.04	2.22 ± 0.39	5.44 ± 0.08	6.32 ± 0.67
ALB (g/dl)	0.24 ± 0	0.50 ± 0.25	2.64 ± 0.09	2.93 ± 0.37
GLOB (g/dl)	1.52 ± 0.05	1.73 ± 0.30	2.81 ± 0.01	3.39 ± 0.53
α_1[a,b] (g/dl)	0.42 ± 0.02	0.24 ± 0.11	0.14 ± 0.06	0.04 ± 0.03
α_2[a,b] (g/dl)	0.66 ± 0.13	0.94 ± 0.25	1.01 ± 0.13	1.27 ± 0.24
β[a,c] (g/dl)	0.30 ± 0.02	0.41 ± 0.14	0.85 ± 0.07	1.04 ± 0.35
γ[a,c] (g/dl)	0.15 ± 0.17	0.14 ± 0.13	0.81 ± 0.01	1.15 ± 0.54
ALB/GLOB[c]	0.16 ± 0.01	0.31 ± 0.18	0.94 ± 0.04	0.89 ± 0.20

NOTE: Tp, total protein concentration: difference between sow groups was significant ($p < 0.05$) and age difference was significant between early and late fetal groups; ALB, albumin: age difference was significant between sow and fetal values ($p < 0.05$); GLOB, total globulin concentration: difference between sow groups was significant ($p < 0.05$) and age difference was significant between sow and fetal values ($p < 0.05$).

[a] Globulin fraction.

[b] Age difference was significant between early fetal group and sows ($p < 0.05$).

[c] Age difference was significant between sow and fetal values ($p < 0.05$).

SOURCE: Reprinted with permission from Schantz et al., 1995, Normal hematology, serology and serum protein electrophoresis values in fetal Yucatan miniature swine, Lab. Anim. Sci. 45(3): 285–289.

Table A15.   Age-related whole-body composition and body weight of the female Sinclair miniature swine

Age	N	Bone mineral content (kg)	Lean mass (kg)	Total fat (kg)	Body weight (kg)
1.0	6	0.806[a]	25.000[a]	9.014[a]	34.819[a]
1.5	6	1.216[b]	33.812[b]	16.702[a,b]	51.730[b]
2.0	6	1.556[c]	43.853[c]	24.396[b,c]	69.806[c]
2.5	6	1.745[c,d]	44.710[c]	30.384[c,d]	76.839[c,d]
3.0	6	1.849[d,e]	49.552[d]	37.071[d,e]	88.472[d,e]
3.5	6	1.804[d,e]	49.319[d]	28.140[b,c,d]	79.262[c,d,e]
4.0	6	1.991[e]	52.427[d]	37.665[d,e]	92.083[e,f]
>6.0	6	2.021[e]	52.115[d]	47.892[e]	102.029[f]

NOTE: Whole-body composition measured using a Dual Energy X-ray Absorptiometer (QDR 2000-Plus, Hologic, Waltham, MA); body weights of miniature swine older than 2.5 years of age are exaggerated due to obesity.

[a,b,c,d,e,f] Means with different superscripts within the same column are different at $p < 0.05$.

SOURCE: Reprinted with permission from Bouchard, et al., 1995, Retrospective evaluation of production characteristics in Sinclair miniature swine—44 years later, Lab. Anim. Sci. 45(4):408–414.

Table A16.   Effect of parity on reproductive parameters of Sinclair miniature swine

Parity	N	Litter size	Stillborn	Weaned piglets	N	Litter weight (kg)
1	150	6.5 ± 2^a	$0.64 \pm 0.09^{a,b}$	5.0 ± 0.2^a	124	3.5 ± 0.1^a
2	100	$7.6 \pm 0.2^{b,c}$	$0.47 \pm 0.11^{a,b}$	$6.4 \pm 0.2^{b,c}$	85	$4.4 \pm 0.2^{b,c}$
3	60	$7.9 \pm 0.3^{b,c}$	$0.52 \pm 0.14^{a,b}$	6.7 ± 0.3^c	55	4.5 ± 0.2^c
4	35	$7.2 \pm 0.4^{a,b}$	0.91 ± 0.18^b	5.4 ± 0.4^a	34	$3.9 \pm 0.2^{a,b}$
5	16	$7.5 \pm 0.5^{a,b,c}$	$0.63 \pm 0.27^{a,b}$	$5.5 \pm 0.6^{a,b}$	13	$4.0 \pm 0.4^{a,b,c}$
>6	10	8.9 ± 0.7^c	1.90 ± 0.34^c	$5.8 \pm 0.7^{a,b,c}$	9	$4.3 \pm 0.5^{a,b,c}$

NOTE: Data collected between 1985 and 1993, mean + SEM; N, number of litters applies to the columns on the right; under certain circumstances some litters were not weighed.
[a,b,c]Means with different superscripts within column are different at $p < 0.05$.
SOURCE: Reprinted with permission from Bouchard et al., 1995, Retrospective evaluation of production characteristics in Sinclair miniature swine—44 years later, Lab. Anim. Sci. 45(4): 408–414.

Table A17.   Effect of the sow age on reproductive parameters of Sinclair miniature swine

Sow age (years)	N	Litter size	Stillborn	Weaned Piglets	N	Litter weight (kg)
1	72	6.4 ± 3^a	0.39 ± 0.13^a	5.2 ± 0.3^a	69	3.4 ± 2^a
2	164	$7.4 \pm 0.2^{b,c}$	$0.54 \pm 0.8^{a,b}$	6.2 ± 0.2^b	142	4.2 ± 0.1^b
3	88	$7.2 \pm 0.2^{b,c}$	$0.72 \pm 0.12^{b,c}$	$5.7 \pm 0.2^{a,b}$	68	4.1 ± 0.2^b
4	34	$7.7 \pm 0.4^{b,c}$	1.09 ± 0.19^c	$5.6 \pm 0.4^{a,b}$	30	4.1 ± 0.3^b
5	6	$6.0 \pm 0.9^{a,b}$	$0.67 \pm 0.44^{a,b,c}$	$4.5 \pm 0.9^{a,b}$	5	$3.8 \pm 0.6^{a,b}$
>6	7	8.6 ± 0.8^c	2.00 ± 0.41^d	4.4 ± 0.9^a	6	$3.3 \pm 0.6^{a,b}$

NOTE: Data collected between 1985 and 1993, mean + SEM; N, number of litters applies to the columns on the right; under certain circumstances some litters were not weighed.
[a,b,c,d]Means with different superscripts within a column are different at p <0.05.
SOURCE: Reprinted with permission from Bouchard et al., 1995, Retrospective evaluation of production characteristics in Sinclair miniature swine—44 years later, Lab. Anim. Sci. 45(4): 408–414.

Table A18. Range[a] of observed hematologic reference values[b] for Sinclair pigs

Analyte[c]	Reference value range
WBC	4700–15,300/µl
RBC	$4.97–8.69 \times 106/µl$
High	9.8–17.3 g/dl
PCV (calculated)	27–49 vol%
PCV (centrifuged)	28–50 vol%
MCV	52–61 fl
MCH	18.6–21.4 pg
MCHC	34.0–35.7 g/dl
Neutrophils (S)	46.2–5661/µl
Neutrophils (B)	0–153/µl
Lymphocytes	3102–8840/µl
Monocytes	0–1572/µl
Eosinophils	0–544/µl
Basophils	0–162/µl
Platelets ($N = 19$)	$311–585 \times 10^3/µl$
Plasma T. protein	6.7–7.8 g/dl

NOTE: $N = 20$ for all analytes except platelets, 10 males and 10 females (all were 1.5 years old); reference intervals were established by determining the nonparametric central 0.95 interfractile interval as recommended by the International Federation of Clinical Chemistry; WBC, white blood cells; RBC, red blood cells; PCV, packed cell volume; MCV, mean corpuscular volume; MCH, mean corpuscular hemoglobin; MCHC, mean corpuscular hemoglobin concentration; S, segmented; B, bands.

[a] Too few reference values to establish reference interval by either parametric or nonparametric methods.

[b] WBC, RBC, Hgb, MCV, and platelets measured with Coulter 6 Plus 4; PCV (centrefuged) via microhematocrit method; 100 cell WBC differential counts; plasma total protein by refractometry; rest of values calculated.

[c] Analytes measured using Kodak clinical chemistry systems except for serum osmolality, which was measured by a freezing point osmometer; some reference values were calculated from measured value.

SOURCE: Courtesy of Guy Bouchard, DVM, Sinclair Research Center; values from the Clinical Pathology Laboratory, Department of Veterinary Pathology. Columbia, MO, USA.

Table A19.   Reference intervals for clinical chemistry values of Sinclair pigs

Analyte	Reference intervals	Analyte	Reference intervals
A/G ratio	0.9–1.7	CO_2 (total)	26–35 amol/L
Albumin	3.3–4.8 g/dl	Creatinine	0.8–1.9 mg/dl
ALP	42–89 U/L	GGT	19–86 U/L
ALT	23–62 U/L	Glucose	48–290 mg/dl
AMS	365–1871 U/L	LDH	883–1450 U/L
Anion gap[a]	13.2–24.0 mmol/L	LPS	14–343 U/L
AST	16–43 U/L	Magnesium	1.7–2.3 mg/dl
Bilirubin (total)	0.1–0.3 mg/dl	Osmolality (meas)	285–324 mosm/kg
Bilirubin (dir)	0.1–0.3 mg/dl	Osmolality (calc)[b]	276–307 mosm/kg
Bilirubin (conj)	0.0–0.0 mg/dl	Osmolal gap[c]	3–20 mosm/kg
Bilirubin (delta)	0.1–0.3 mg/dl	Phosphorus	5.8–7.8 g/dl
Calcium	10.0–11.3 mg/dl	Potassium (K)	3.9–5.6 mmol/L
Chloride	98–106 mmol/L	Protein, total	6.7–7.8 g/dl
Cholesterol	47–124 mg/dl	Urea nitrogen (UN)	7–13 mg/dl
CK	219–1411 U/L		

NOTE: N = 40 for all analytes, 20 males and 20 females (all were 1.5 years old); A/G, albumin/globulin; ALP, alkaline phosphatase; ALT, alanine aminotransferase; AMS, amylase; AST, aspartate aminotransferase; CK, creatinine kinase; conj, conjugated; dir, direct; GGT, glutamyltransferase; LDH, lactate dehydrogenase; LPS, lipopolysaccharides.

[a] Anion gap = (Na + K) – (Cl + CO_2).
[b] Calculated Osmolatity = 1.86 (Na + K) + UN/2.8 + Glucose/18.
[c] Osmolal gap = measured osmolality – calculated osmolality.

SOURCE: Courtesy of Guy Bouchard, DVM, Sinclair Research Center. Values from the Clinical Pathology Laboratory, Department of Veterinary Pathology. Columbia, MO, USA.

Table A20.   Weight development (kg) of the Göttingen minipig at the full-barrier breeding facility in Dalmose

Period	Body weight (kg) 1995
Birth	0.45
1 month	2.7
2 months	5.3
3 months	7.2
6 months	13.7
9 months	17.7
12 months	23.9
18 months	32.4
24 months	34.9

SOURCE: Courtesy of Peter Bollen, Ellegaard Göttingen Minipigs; reprinted with permission from Bollen, P.J.A., and L. Ellegaard, 1996. Developments in breeding Göttingen minipigs. In Tumbleson, M.E., and Snook, L. (eds.), Advances in Swine Biomedical Research, Vol. 1, New York: Plenum Press, pp. 59–66.

Table A21. Hematology of the Göttingen minipig

Parameter	Abbre-viation	Unit		Male (3 mo)	Female (3 mo)	Male (6 mo)	Female (6 mo)
Hemoglobin	Hb	mmol/L	mean	7.45	7.40	7.89	7.66
			SD	0.35	0.54	0.51	0.50
Red blood cell count	RBC	10^{12}/L	mean	8.01	8.06	7.92	8.03
			SD	0.44	0.68	0.56	0.58
Hematocrit	PCV	ml/100 ml	mean	36.80	36.67	38.20	37.60
			SD	1.52	2.29	1.82	2.41
Reticulocyte count	RETIC	%	mean	1.31	1.71	1.65	1.09
			SD	0.50	0.75	0.85	0.54
Reticuloycte count	RETIC	10^{12}/L	mean	0.10	0.13	0.13	0.09
			SD	0.04	0.06	0.07	0.04
Mean cell volume	MCV	10^{-15}/L	mean	46.03	45.75	48.39	46.88
			SD	2.59	4.25	3.07	2.29
Mean cell hemoglobin	MCH	mmol	mean	0.94	0.93	1.00	0.97
			SD	0.06	0.10	0.09	0.06
Mean cell hemoglobin conc.	MCHC	mmol/L	mean	20.25	20.18	20.66	20.37
			SD	0.51	0.52	0.67	0.31
White blood cell count	WBC	10^6/L	mean	11.95	11.36	8.68	8.60
			SD	2.45	1.37	1.50	2.18
Segmented neutrophils	NEUTRO SEG	%	mean	27.20	27.87	32.53	29.07
			SD	9.6	13.17	6.77	8.46
Segmented neutrophils	NEUTRO SEG	10^9/L	mean	3.27	2.93	2.85	2.52
			SD	1.41	1.31	0.85	1.02
Band neutrophils	NEUTRO BAND	%	mean	1.33	1.53	1.60	0.93
			SD	0.98	1.19	1.12	0.96
Lymphocytes	LYMPHO	%	mean	68.80	67.60	61.80	66.07
			SD	10.28	13.88	7.84	8.78
Lymphocytes	LYMPHO	10^9/L	mean	8.19	6.98	5.34	5.65
			SD	2.02	1.38	0.99	1.44
Eosinophils	EOS	%	mean	0.87	0.93	1.33	2.13
			SD	1.25	1.53	1.18	2.26
Eosinophils	EOS	10^9/L	mean	0.10	0.10	0.12	0.19
			SD	0.15	0.17	0.11	0.23
Basophils	BASO	%	mean	0.67	0.53	0.73	0.33
			SD	0.90	0.74	0.88	0.62
Basophils	BASO	10^9/L	mean	0.08	0.07	0.06	0.02
			SD	0.12	0.10	0.07	0.04
Monocytes	MONO	%	mean	1.13	1.53	2.00	1.47
			SD	1.25	1.51	1.07	1.19
Monocytes	MONO	10^9/L	mean	0.14	0.20	0.17	0.14
			SD	0.15	0.21	0.09	0.13
Platelet count	THROMB	10^9/L	mean	513.1	490.30	348.30	364.50
			SD	88.34	115.2	79.47	51.72
Activated partial throm-boplastin time	APTT	sec.	mean	45.86	44.08	42.65	43.22
			SD	5.77	9.99	8.17	9.83

Table A21. (*continued*)

Parameter	Abbre-viation	Unit		Male (3 mo)	Female (3 mo)	Male (6 mo)	Female (6 mo)
Thrombin time	TT	sec	mean	25.80	28.36	23.91	23.69
			SD	4.16	5.00	3.59	4.55
Prothrombin time	PTT	sec	mean	11.71	11.54	11.94	11.65
			SD	0.34	0.46	0.62	0.41
Fibrinogen	FIBR	g/l	mean	6.50	5.37	6.85	4.80
			SD	1.39	0.66	1.24	0.59

SOURCE: Courtesy of Peter Bollen, Ellegaard Göttingen Minipigs; reprinted with permission from Bollen, P.J.A., and L. Ellegaard. 1996. Developments in breeding Göttingen minipigs. In Tumbleson, M.E., and Snook, L. (eds.), Advances in Swine Biomedical Research, Vol. 1, New York: Plenum Press, pp. 59–66.

Table A22.   Clinical chemistry of the Göttingen minipig

Parameter	Abbre-viation	Unit		Male (3 mo)	Female (3 mo)	Male (6 mo)	Female (6 mo)
Alanine	ALAT	pkat/L	mean	1.12	1.00	0.92	0.96
			SD	0.16	0.17	0.07	0.27
Ornithine carbamyl transferase	OCT	10/L	mean	4.49	4.13	4.43	4.79
			SD	0.28	0.53	0.44	0.74
Sorbitol dehydrogenase	SDH	pkat/L	mean	0.01	0.01	0.01	0.01
			SD	0.01	0.01	0.01	0.01
Aspartate aminotransferase	ASAT	pkat/L	mean	0.38	0.34	0.36	0.34
			SD	0.13	0.09	0.10	0.07
Alkaline phosphatase	ALKPH	pkat/L	mean	4.29	3.88	3.49	2.71
			SD	0.92	1.11	0.75	0.98
Bilirubin	BILI	pmol/L	mean	2.69	2.27	2.32	1.87
			SD	0.49	0.74	0.48	0.56
γ-glutamyl transferase	GGT	pkat/L	mean	0.80	0.79	0.89	0.77
			SD	0.10	0.12	0.12	0.18
Cholesterol	CHOL	mmol/L	mean	1.72	2.40	1.33	0.96
			SD	0.33	0.49	0.20	0.43
Creatine kinase	CK	pkat/L	mean	5.99	1.17	7.89	9.38
			SD	2.25	2.20	4.85	3.88
Lactate dehydrogenase	LDH	pkat/L	mean	16.68	17.45	13.59	15.27
			SD	2.34	2.32	2.03	5.39
Amylase	AmYL	IU/L	mean	49.04	50.08	49.33	52.17
			SD	11.59	13.97	10.53	15.23
Protein (total)	PROT	g/L	mean	58.43	57.58	61.02	61.66
			SD	3.97	3.63	3.33	3.60
Triglicerides	TRIG	mmol/L	mean	0.40	0.59	0.36	0.47
			SD	0.07	0.12	0.07	0.12
Carbamid	UREA	mmol/L	mean	2.49	2.37	2.12	2.35
			SD	0.56	0.59	0.50	0.59
Creatinine	CREAT	pmol/L	mean	103.10	97.60	109.70	95.73
			SD	2.02	1.38	10.21	10.22
Glucose	GLUC	mmol/L	mean	3.47	3.71	3.17	3.16
			SD	0.43	0.42	0.38	0.35
Sodium	Na	mmol/L	mean	143.80	143.90	143.20	144.10
			SD	2.48	2.62	1.18	1.76
Potassium	K	mmol/L	mean	4.89	5.00	4.58	4.72
			SD	0.48	0.60	0.42	0.58
Calcium	Ca	mmol/L	mean	2.78	2.76	2.66	2.71
			SD	0.09	0.13	0.11	0.12
Inorganic phosphorus	P	mmol/L	mean	2.73	2.78	2.85	2.73
			SD	0.23	0.17	0.16	0.14
Chloride	Cl	mmol/L	mean	100.90	101.50	101.50	102.60
			SD	1.99	1.15	2.18	1.98
Albumin	ALB	%	mean	57.27	56.69	55.75	54.04
			SD	3.01	2.43	1.76	3.40
Albumin	ALB	g/L	mean	33.44	32.64	34.01	33.26
			SD	2.66	2.58	1.94	1.98

Table A22. (*continued*)

Parameter	Abbre-viation	Unit		Male (3 mo)	Female (3 mo)	Male (6 mo)	Female (6 mo)
α1-globulin	ALPHA 1	%	mean	3.83	3.39	3.73	3.39
			SD	1.27	0.78	0.76	0.51
α1-globulin	ALPHA 1	g/L	mean	2.23	1.95	2.27	2.07
			SD	0.72	0.48	0.45	0.33
α2-globulin	ALPHA 2	%	mean	18.00	18.55	16.63	17.6
			SD	2.23	2.41	2.32	3.05
α2-globulin	ALPHA 2	g/L	mean	10.49	10.64	10.16	10.84
			SD	1.23	1.20	1.56	1.94
β-globulin	BETA	%	mean	12.30	12.71	13.66	13.53
			SD	1.49	1.38	1.45	1.20
β-globulin	BETA	g/L	mean	7.19	7.33	8.33	8.35
			SD	1.02	0.99	0.97	0.94
γ-globulin	GAMMA	%	mean	8.60	8.76	10.21	11.12
			SD	2.00	1.56	1.32	2.86
γ-globulin	GAMMA	g/L	mean	5.07	5.02	6.24	6.91
			SD	1.41	1.11	0.98	2.04
Albumin/ globulin ratio	A/G ratio		mean	1.35	1.32	1.26	1.19
			SD	0.17	0.13	0.09	0.17

SOURCE: Courtesy of Peter Bollen, Ellegaard Göttingen Minipigs; reprinted with permission from Bollen, P.J.A., and L. Ellegaard. 1996. Developments in breeding Göttingen minipigs. In Tumbleson, M.E., and Snook, L. (eds.), Advances in Swine Biomedical Research, Vol. 1. New York: Plenum Press, pp. 59–66.

Table A23. Percentage of body weight of various tissues and organs in the 12-week-old pig (mean weight, 22.74 ± 3.45 kg)

Organ	Percentage of body weight
Body weight	100
Cerebrum	0.31 ± 0.06
Cerebellum	0.06 ± 0.02
Spinal cord	0.14 ± 0.08
Thyroid gland	0.02 ± 0.004
Larynx–trachea	0.21 ± 0.03
Lungs	1.09 ± 0.18
Heart	0.49 ± 0.06
Aorta	0.11 ± 0.05
Esophagus	0.13 ± 0.05
Stomach	1.22 ± 0.16
Small intestine	4.46 ± 0.38
Large intestine	2.74 ± 0.59
Liver	3.16 ± 0.41
Spleen	0.19 ± 0.05
Pancreas	0.29 ± 0.18
Kidneys	0.55 ± 0.01
Adrenal glands	0.0104 ± 0.0018
Skeletal muscle	35.97 ± 2.3
Fat	12.52 ± 1.04
Skeleton	16.73 ± 0.89
Rind ±	6.32 ± 0.54
Blood	5.53 ± 0.42
GI tract content	5.61 ± 2.22
Various connective tissues	3.33 ± 0.62

NOTES: Data are expressed as mean ± 1 Standard Deviation; GI, stomach, small, and large intestine.

SOURCE: Reprinted with permission from Elowsson et al., 1997, Body composition of the 12 week old pig studied by dissection, Lab. Anim. Sci. 47(2): 200–202.

Table A24. Percentage of body weight of specified muscles (left and right sides) of the 12-week-old pig (mean weight, 22.74 ± 3.45 kg)

Muscle	Percentage of body weight
Longissimus dorsi	3.17 ± 0.27
Biceps femoris	2.14 ± 0.12
Quadriceps femoris	1.91 ± 0.17
Semitendinosus	0.66 ± 0.06
Semimembranosus	2.58 ± 0.21

SOURCE: Reprinted with permission from Elowsson et al., 1997, Body composition of the 12 week old pig studied by dissection, Lab. Anim. Sci. 47(2): 200–202.

Table A25. Commonly used therapeutic agents (see Chapter 2 for anesthetic, analgesic, and emergency drugs)

Antibiotics	
Amoxicillin	10 mg/kg b.i.d. po
Ampicillin	2–5 mg/kg b.i.d. im
Ceftiofur	3–5 mg/kg s.i.d. im
Ceftriaxone	50–75 mg/kg t.i.d. im or iv
Cephaloridine	10 mg/kg b.i.d. im or sc
Cephradine	25–50 mg/kg b.i.d. po
Enrofloxacin	5 mg/kg b.i.d. im or po
Erythromycin	2–5 mg/kg b.i.d. im or iv
Gentamicin	2 mg/kg b.i.d. im
Griseofulvin	20 mg/kg s.i.d. po
Kanamycin	6 mg/kg b.i.d. im
Lincomycin	5–10 mg/kg b.i.d. po
	2–5 mg/kg im
Penicillin, procaine/benzathine	10,000–40,000 units im every 3 days
Tetracycline/oxytetracycline	10–25 mg/kg po b.i.d.; 2–5 mg/kg s.i.d. im
Trimethoprim/sulfadiazine	5 mg/kg s.i.d. im
	25–50 mg/kg s.i.d. po
Metronidazole	66 mg/kg s.i.d. po
Tylosin	8.8 mg/kg po b.i.d.
	2–4 mg/kg b.i.d. im
Anthelmintics	
Amprolium	10 mg/kg po
Fenbendazole	5 mg/kg po
Ivermectin	200 µg/kg im
Levamazole	8 mg/kg po
Thiabendazole	75–100 mg/kg po

SOURCES: Brooks et al., 1984, Ungulates as laboratory animals, In Fox et al. (eds.), Laboratory Animal Medicine, New York: Academic Press, pp. 274-295.

Flecknell, 1996, Laboratory Animal Anesthesia, 2nd ed., New York: Academic Press.

Hawk and Leary, 1995, Formulary for Laboratory Animals, Ames: Iowa State University Press.

GENERAL REFERENCES

Cramer, D.V., L.G. Podesta, and L. Makowka. 1994. Handbook of Animal Models in Transplantation Research. Boca Raton, FL: CRC Press.

Flecknell, P.A. 1996. Laboratory Animal Anaesthesia, 2nd ed. New York: Academic Press.

Getty, R. (ed). 1975. Sisson and Grossman's The Anatomy of the Domestic Animals—Porcine, Vol. 2. Philadelphia: W.B. Saunders, pp. 1215–1422.

Gilbert, S.G. 1966. Pictoral Anatomy of the Fetal Pig, 2nd ed. Seattle: University of Washington Press.

Hawk, C.T., and S.L. Leary. 1995. Formulary for Laboratory Animals. Ames: Iowa State University Press.

Kohn, D.H., S.K. Wixson, W.J. White, and G.J. Benson (eds). 1997. Anesthesia and Analgesia in Laboratory Animals. New York: Academic Press.

Pond, W.G., and K. Houpt. 1978. Biology of the Pig. Ithaca, NY: Comstock Publishing Associates.

Popesko, P. 1977. Atlas of Topographical Anatomy of the Domestic Animals, Vol. 1, 2nd ed. Philadelphia: WB Saunders.

Riebold, T.W., D.O. Goble, and D.R. Geiser. 1995. Large Animal Anesthesia: Principles and Techniques, 2nd ed. Ames: Iowa State University Press.

Sack, W.O. 1982. Essentials of Pig Anatomy and Harowitz/Kramer Atlas of Musculoskeletal Anatomy of the Pig. Ithaca, NY: Veterinary Textbooks.

Stanton, H.C., and H.J. Mersmann (eds). 1986. Swine in Cardiovascular Research, Vol. 1. Boca Raton, FL: CRC Press.

Stanton, H.C., and H.J. Mersmann (eds). 1986. Swine in Cardiovascular Research, Vol. 2. Boca Raton, FL: CRC Press.

Swindle, M.M. 1983. Basic Surgical Exercises Using Swine. Philadelphia: Praeger Press.

Swindle, M.M. (ed). 1992. Swine as Models in Biomedical Research, Ames: Iowa State University Press.

Swindle, M.M., and R.J. Adams (eds). 1988. Experimental Surgery and Physiology: Induced Animal Models of Human Disease, Baltimore: Williams and Wilkins.

Thurmon, J.C., and G.J. Benson (eds). 1996. Lumb and Jones Veterinary Anesthesia, 3rd ed. Baltimore: Williams and Wilkins.

Tumbleson, M.E. (ed). 1986. Swine in Biomedical Research, Vol. 1. New York: Plenum Press.

Tumbleson, M.E. (ed). 1986. Swine in Biomedical Research, Vol. 2. New York: Plenum Press.

Tumbleson, M.E. (ed). 1986. Swine in Biomedical Research, Vol. 3. New York: Plenum Press.

Tumbleson, M.E., and L.B. Schook (eds). 1996. Advances in Swine in Biomedical Research, Vol. 1. New York: Plenum Press.

Tumbleson, M.E., and L.B. Schook (eds). 1996. Advances in Swine in Biomedical Research, Vol. 2. New York: Plenum Press.

INDEX

317

ISBN 0-8138-1829-X

9 780813 818290

90000